A clinical guide to implants in dentistry

2nd edition

A clinical guide to implants in dentistry

2nd edition

Richard M. Palmer
Professor of Implant Dentistry and Periodontology

Paul J. Palmer
Head of Conservative Dentistry

Leslie C. Howe
Consultant in Periodontology

Thanks to Peter Floyd and Vincent Barrett who contributed to the first edition
and Claire Morgan for the new chapter on Implant Overdentures

2008

Published by the British Dental Association
64 Wimpole Street, London, W1G 8YS, UK

ISBN 978 0904588 927

Printed and bound by
Dennis Barber Limited. Lowestoft, Suffolk

Foreword

The prime aim of this book is to present an overview of the application of osseointegrated implants in dental practice. It is not based upon a single implant system, but upon our experience of a few well known and tested systems which have all produced highly sucessful and predictable results. It is not intended to be a step-by-step instruction manual of 'how to do it', but to give the clinician a wide appreciation of treatment planning, the various stages of treatment and how implant dentistry relates to and compares with other treatment options. There is a trend to present implant dentistry as a simple, straightforward procedure requiring minimal training. We trust that this book also demonstrates some of the complexities and pitfalls of this treatment modality, and the need for comprehensive education and training in this demanding field of dentistry.

This second edition has been extensively revised in light of developments in the last 10 years.

Richard M. Palmer
Paul J. Palmer
Leslie C. Howe
Kings College London Dental Institute
at Guy's King's College and St Thomas' Hospitals
Guy's Campus
London SE1 9RT

Contents

Introduction to dental implants

Implants have been used to support dental prostheses for many decades, but they have not always enjoyed a favourable reputation. This situation changed dramatically with the development of endosseous osseointegrated dental implants. They are the nearest equivalent replacement to the natural tooth, and are therefore a useful addition in the management of patients who have missing teeth because of disease, trauma or developmental anomalies. There are a number of dental implant systems which offer predictable long-term results backed by good scientific research and clinical trials. In the first place it may be helpful to clarify some of the commonly used terms in implant dentistry (*Table 1*).

Sucess criteria

It is important to establish success criteria for implant systems, and for implants to be tested in well controlled clinical trials. The minimum success criteria proposed by Albrektsson *et al* (IJOMI 1986;1;11) is set out in *Table 2*.

The most obvious sign of implant failure is mobility. However, some criteria in *Table 2* apply to the overall requirements of an implant system, and are not as useful when judging the success of individual implants. This is well illustrated by considering the radiographic criteria. Bone remodelling occurs in the first year of function in response to occlusal forces and establishment of the normal dimensions of the peri-implant soft tissues (See Chapter 2). The 'ideal' bone level is usually judged against a specific landmark on the implant (such as the implant head or implant/abutment junction) and it may differ therefore between implant systems (*Fig.6*). Subsequently the bone levels are usually more or less stable, and small changes such as 0.2mm per annum are impossible to measure with conventional radiographs. These bone level measures therefore do not apply to individual implants but to mean (average) changes measured across a large number of implants. For example, a detectable change of 1mm or more may occur at very few implants in contrast to the majority which remain unchanged or in a steady state. It is also difficult to stipulate what level of change in an individual implant over a given period of time would constitute failure. A rapid change in bone level may be followed by a long period of stability. On the other hand, progressive or continuous bone loss is a worrying sign of impending failure. An implant with marked loss of bone may therefore be judged as 'surviving' rather than 'successful'. (Most published clinical studies report mean (standard deviation) changes in bone levels, but it is usually more helpful to describe the frequency distributions of bone level change (e.g. number/proportion of implants losing 1mm or more over a given time period).

The original osseointegrated implants such

Table 1 Basic terminology in implant dentistry	
Osseointegration	A direct structural and functional connection between ordered, living bone and the surface of a load-carrying implant (Albrektsson *et al*. Acta Orthopaedica Scand 1981; **52**: 155 (*Fig. 1*).
Endosseous dental implant	A device inserted into the jaw bone (endosseous) to support a dental prosthesis. It is the 'tooth root' analogue and is often referred to as a 'fixture' (*Fig. 2*).
Implant abutment	The component which attaches to the dental implant and supports the prosthesis. A transmucosal abutment (TMA) is one which passes through the mucosa overlying the implant. A temporary or healing abutment may be used during the healing of the peri-implant soft tissue before the definitive abutment is chosen (*Fig. 3*).
Abutment screw	A screw used to connect a dental abutment.
Single stage implant surgery	Surgical placement of a dental implant which is left exposed to the oral cavity following insertion. This is the protocol used in non-submerged implant systems (*Fig. 4*).
Two stage implant surgery	Initial surgical placement of a dental implant which is buried beneath the mucosa and then subsequently exposed with a second surgical procedure some months later. This is used in submerged implant systems (*Fig. 5*).

Figure 1- Histological section of an implant with bone growing in intimate contact with the surface. The dense bone which contains a small medullary space fills the area between two thread profiles which are 0.6mm apart.

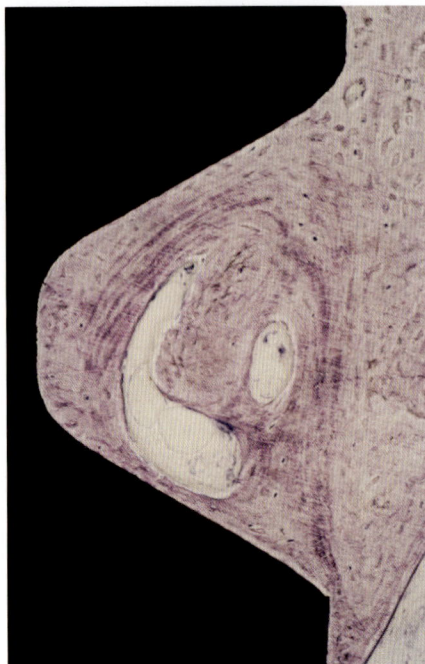

Figure 2- Three different designs of endosseous implants being inserted into prepared sites within the jaw bone. Figure 2a is a machined threaded implant of the Branemark design (Nobel Biocare). Figure 2b is an Astra ST implant which has a microthreaded coronal portion, a macro-threaded apical portion and a surface treatment which makes it appear dull grey. Figure 2c is a Straumann implant which has a smooth transmucosal collar, a macro-threaded body and a surface treatment which gives it a light grey appearance.

as the Branemark system showed that implants placed in the mandible (particularly anterior to the mental foramina) enjoyed a higher success rate than the maxilla (approximately 95% success for implants in the mandible compared with 85 to 90% for the maxilla). An example of the lowest recorded success rates were for short implants (7mm) used in the maxilla to support overdentures, especially when the implants were not joined together. Further studies showed that the overall mean failure rate in smokers was about twice that in non-smokers. Development of implant systems over the last decade, particularly with refinement of implant surfaces (see below), have led to significantly lower rates of failure to achieve initial osseointegration and better long-term success. Some studies have suggested that these improvements apply equally to smokers, with near equivalent success rates to non-smokers. However, it is recommended that smoking should still be considered a significant risk factor and patients warned of this association. The overall lifetime exposure of the patient to smoking (e.g. pack years – number of packs per day x number of years smoking) is important with regard to the chronic detrimental effects on the healing potential and inflammatory and immune responses. It should also be noted that reported failure rates are not evenly distributed throughout the patient population. Rather, implant failures are more likely to cluster in certain individuals. Implant studies sometimes do not provide this information and provide substantial data based on analysis of individual implants assuming that they are independent of the subject. This is inappropriate and more sophisticated analysis taking account of subjects and implants should be used.

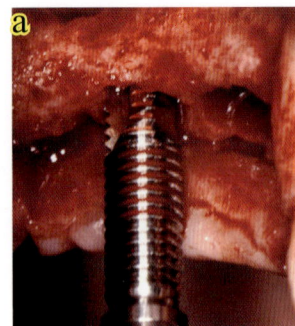

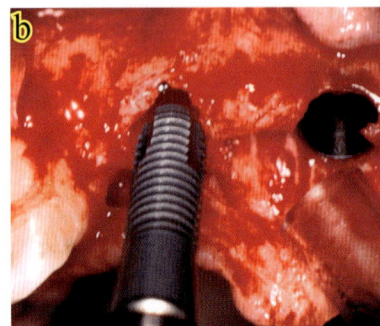

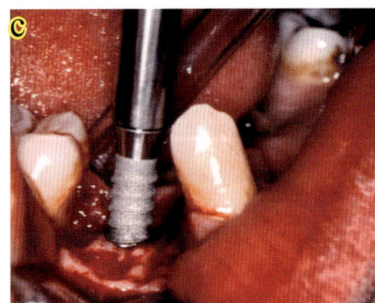

Basic guide to osseointegration

Figure 1 shows an histological section of a titanium screw threaded implant which has been in function in bone for 1 year. There is very close apposition of bone over most of the implant surface at this level of magnification using a light microscope. At the ultrastructural level there is an unmineralised zone at the surface and the precise nature of the biological attachment is not well defined. The micromechanical interlocking of unmineralised bone and the microsurface of the implant provides a relatively strong union. Various definitions of

Table 2 Suggested minimum success criteria for dental implants *
1. An individual, unattached implant is immobile when tested clinically
2. Radiographic examination does not reveal any peri-implant radiolucency
3. After the first year in function, radiographic vertical bone loss is less than 0.2mm per annum.
4. The individul implant performance is characterised by an absence of signs and symptoms such as pain, infections, neuropathies, paraesthesia or violation of the inferior dental canal
5. As a minimum the implant should fulfil the above criteria with a success rate of 85% at the end of a 5 year observation period and 80% at the end of a 10 year period.
* after Albrektsson *et al.* IJOMI 1986; 1:11

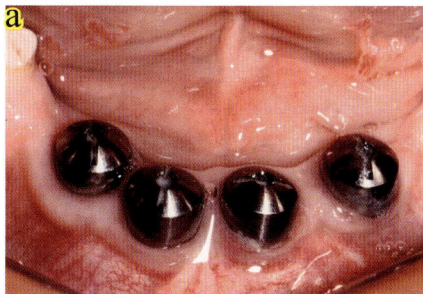

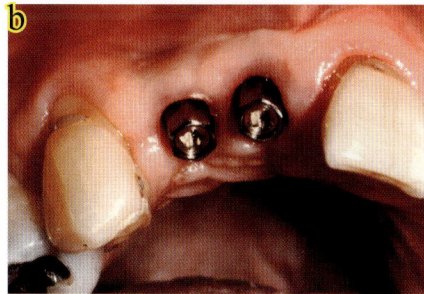

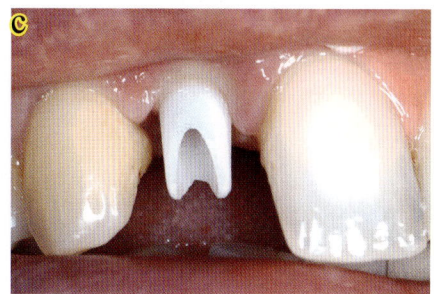

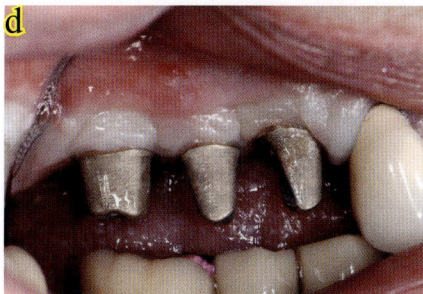

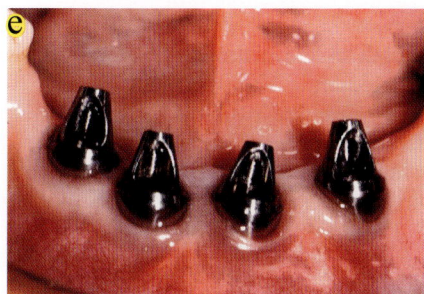

Figure 3 – Various forms of implant abutment are illustrated.

Figure 3a shows some simple cylindrical healing abutments which are used during the healing stage of the mucosa before definitive abutments are selected.

Figure 3b shows abutments which are used to support individual crowns in single tooth restorations. The crowns are cemented on the parallel sided hexagon.

Figure 3c shows a prepared alumina abutment that will support an all porcelain crown.

Figure 3d shows cast gold customised abutments used to support a cemented bridge.

Figure 3e shows angled abutments that have been selected to provide a screw retained bridge with access holes on the lingual aspects of the reconstruction.

osseointegration have been proposed, but perhaps the most useful is that given in *Table 1*. It has been proposed that the biological process leading to and maintaining osseointegration is dependent upon a number of factors which include:

Biocompatibility and implant design

Implants made of commercially pure titanium have established a benchmark in osseointegration, against which few other materials compare. Related materials such as niobium are able to produce a high degree of osseointegration and in addition, successful clinical results are reported for titanium alloys (Ti/Al/V) and hydroxyapatite coated implants. More recently resorbable coatings have been developed which aim to improve the initial rate of bone healing against the implant surface and then resorb within a short time frame to allow establishment of a bone to metal contact. In addition, there is interest in incorporating growth

factors that could improve bone healing.

The implant design has a great influence on initial stability and subsequent function. The main design parameters are:

- Implant length – implants are generally available in lengths from about 6mm to as much as 20mm. The most common lengths employed are between 8 and 15mm which correspond quite closely to normal root lengths.

- Implant diameter – most implants are approximately 4mm in diameter. At least 3mm in diameter is required to ensure adequate implant strength of commercially pure titanium. Narrower implants may be designed as one piece components that simply support a crown. This avoids the difficulty of producing abutment connections that are strong enough, but has the disadvantage of reduced

Figures 4a and 4b - An implant of the Straumann type has been inserted and left protruding through the mucosa in a one stage surgical procedure. A wide screw has been placed on the top to protect the inner aspect of the implant until a definitive abutment is connected. Sutures adapt the soft tissue around the smooth collar.

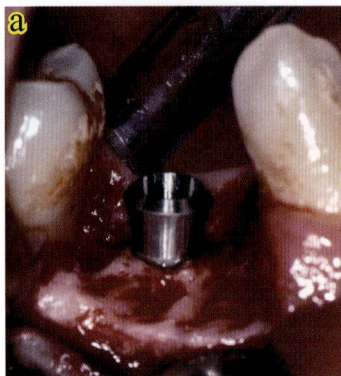

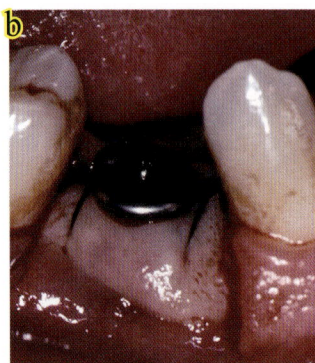

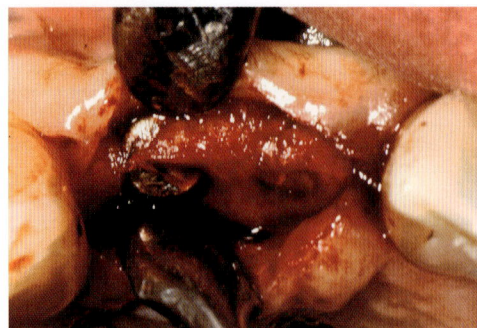

Figure 5- Exposure of two implants that have been buried beneath the mucosa for a period of 6 months. Bone has grown over the top of them and this needs to be removed before a healing abutment is connected.

prosthodontic options/flexibility. Implant diameter may be more important than implant length in the distribution of loads to the surrounding bone. Implant diameters of 5 - 6mm are available, which are considerably stronger, but they are not so widely used because sufficient bone width is not so commonly encountered.

- Implant shape – hollow-cylinders, solid-cylinders, hollow screws or solid screws have all been employed. They are designed to maximise the potential area for osseointegration. The majority of implants currently available are solid screws, which provide good initial stability and offer good load distribution characteristics in function (*Fig. 2*).

- Surface characteristics – the degree of surface roughness and topography varies between different systems. Surfaces which are machined, grit-blasted, etched, plasma sprayed, electrolytically roughened and coated are available. *Figs. 7 to 10* show the characteristics of these surfaces viewed with the scanning electron microscope, showing considerable increases in potential surface area. The optimum surface morphology has yet to be defined, and some may perform better in certain circumstances. By increasing surface roughness there is the potential to increase the surface contact with bone. It has been determined that a surface roughness of about $2\mu m$ (Ra value) enhances cellular responses and results in a more rapid bone to implant contact, thereby shorten-

ing the healing period. Very rough/porous surfaces such as titanium plasma sprayed are not commonly employed because of concerns about ionic exchange, surface corrosion and bacterial contamination if they become exposed within the mouth.

Bone factors

The stability of the implant at the time of placement is very important and is dependent upon bone quantity and quality as well as implant design and site preparation. The edentulous ridge can be classified in terms of shape and bone quality (*Fig.11*). Following loss of a tooth the alveolar bone resorbs in width and height. In extreme cases bone resorption proceeds to a level which is beyond the normal extent of the alveolar process and well within the basal bone of the jaws. Radiographic determination of bone quantity and quality is considered in Chapter 5 and procedures which can be used to augment bone in Chapter 8. The most favourable quality of jaw bone for implant treatment is that which has a well formed cortex and densely trabeculated medullary spaces with a good blood supply. Bone which is predominantly cortical may offer good initial stability at implant placement but is more easily damaged by overheating during the drilling process, especially with sites more than 10mm in depth. At the other extreme, bone with a thin or absent cortical layer and sparse trabeculation offers very poor initial implant stability and fewer cells with a good osteogenic potential to promote osseointegration. Success is highly dependent upon a surgical technique which avoids heat-

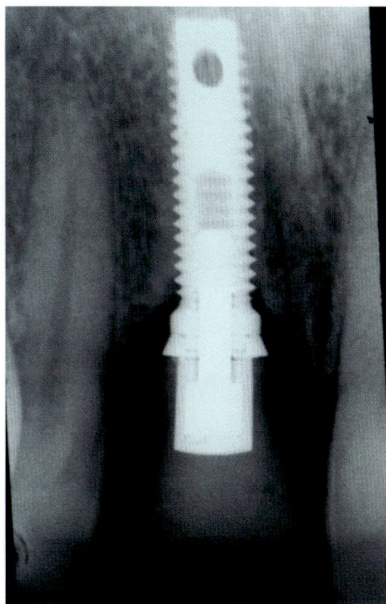

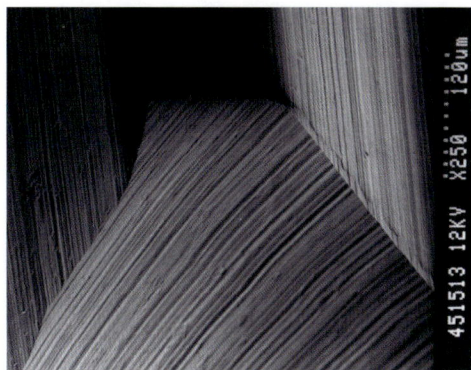

Figure 7- A scanning electron micrograph of a Branemark/Nobel Biocare implant illustrating tiny grooves produced during the machine process.

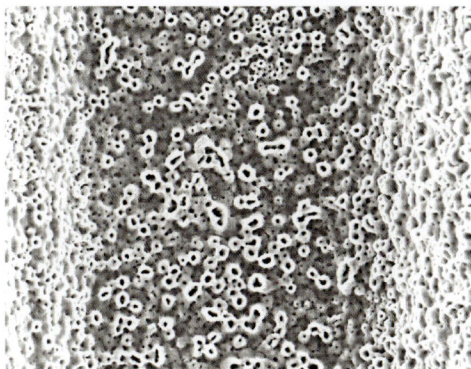

Figure 8- A scanning electron micrograph of the Nobel Biocare Ti-unite surface produced with an electrolytic process.

Figure 6- A periapical radiograph of a single tooth implant. The bone contacts the implant up to the most coronal thread. An abutment screw which is more radio-opaque can be seen connecting the abutment to the implant. The crown is all porcelain and is cemented to the abutment. In this system (Branemark) the landmark for measuring the bone level is from the junction between the implant and the abutment.

ing the bone. Slow drilling speeds, the use of successive incrementally larger sharp drills and copious saline irrigation aim to keep the temperature below that at which bone tissue damage occurs (around 47°C for 1 minute). Methods by which these factors are controlled are considered in more detail in Chapter 6 (Basic Implant Surgery). Factors which compromise bone quality are infection, irradiation and heavy smoking. The effects of the latter two are a result of a diminution of the vascular supply to the bone which compromises the healing response, a feature which has been well described in healing fractures. There have also been reports of bone necrosis of the jaws in patients treated with bisphosphonates, but this is more of a problem in those who have received intravenous bisphosphonates (*Fig. 12*) rather than those on oral medication.

Loading conditions

Following installation of an implant it is important that it is not overloaded during the early healing phase. Micromovement of less than 100μm may allow osseointegration, but there is no precise way of controlling this. Movement of the implant above this level during healing results in fibrous tissue encapsulation rather than osseointegration. This has been

compared to the healing of a fracture where stabilisation of the bone fragments is very important to prevent non-union. In partially dentate subjects it is helpful to provide temporary/ provisional prostheses which are tooth supported or are well relieved in the area where the implants have been installed. However, in patients who wear mucosa supported complete dentures it may be necessary to avoid denture wear for at least one week. This also helps to prevent breakdown of the soft tissue wound. The original Branemark system advised leaving implants unloaded beneath the mucosa for around 6 months in the maxilla and 3 months in the mandible, mainly because of differences in bone quality. Most systems recommend a healing period of 6-12 weeks for routine protocols. However, these are largely empirical guidelines, and bone quality and implant stability will vary greatly between individuals, jaws and sites within jaws. Currently there is no accurate measure which precisely determines the optimum period of healing before loading can commence. Bone quality can be assessed by measuring the cutting torque during preparation of the implant site. The stability of an implant and increasing bone-to-implant contact over time has been quantified using resonance frequency analysis. This non-invasive tool measures the stiffness of the implant at the bone interface. In defined

Figure 9- A scanning electron micrograph of an Astra Tech implant surface produced by blasting with titanium dioxide. Latest versions of this surface also incorporate fluoride.

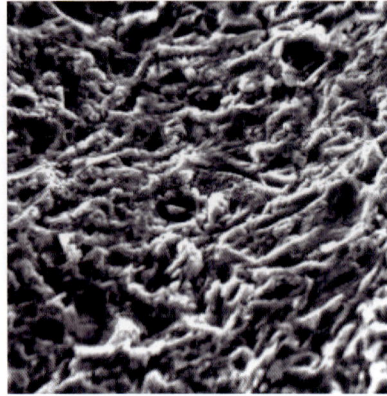

Figure 12- Bone necrosis in a patient who has received intravenous bisphosphonates.

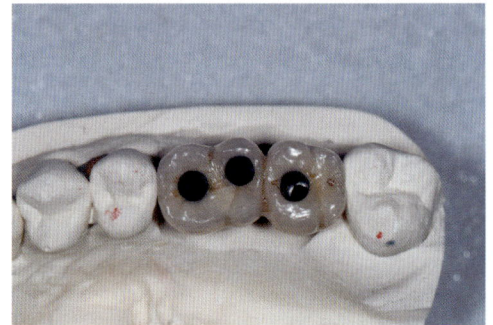

Figure 10- A scanning electron micrograph of a Straumann surface produced by blasting with small and large particles and acid etching.

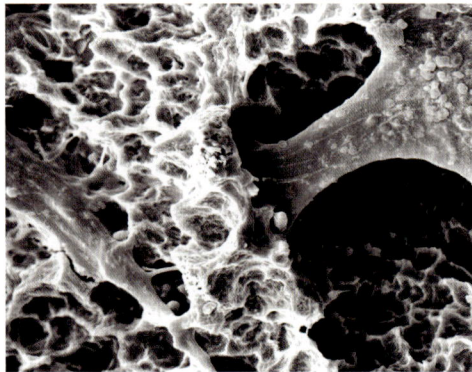

Figure 13- The so-called 'tripod' arrangement of three implants is recommended in situations of high load.

circumstances it has been shown that immediate loading is compatible with subsequent successful osseointegration, providing the bone quality is good and the functional forces can be adequately controlled. The latter may involve placing an adequate number of implants and connecting them together as soon as possible with a rigid framework. However, these latter protocols should only be used by experienced clinicians, and there is much data to support the more cautious approach advocated by Branemark in ensuring a high level of predictable implant success. The loading of the implant supported prosthesis is a further important consideration which will be dealt with in the following section.

Prosthetic considerations

Carefully planned functional occlusal loading will result in maintenance of osseointegration and possibly increased bone to implant contact. In contrast, excessive loading may lead to bone loss and/or component failure. Clinical loading conditions are largely dependent upon:

Figure 11- Shows examples of dental panoramic tomograms of edentulous jaws. Both show extensive resorption of the maxillary ridge. There is far less resorption of the mandible in figure 11a than figure 11b. In the latter case there is reasonable bone volume in the anterior mandible but resorption close to the level of the inferior dental canal in the posterior part.

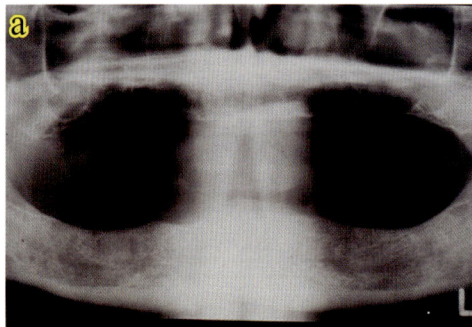

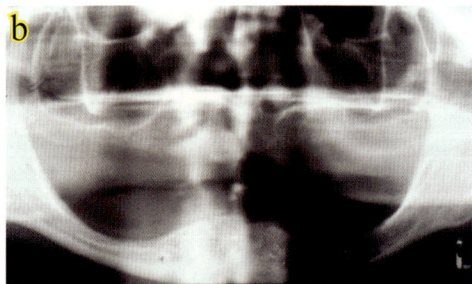

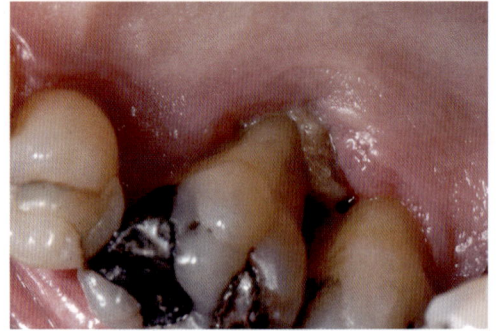

The type of prosthetic reconstruction

This can vary from a single tooth replacement in the partially dentate case to a full arch reconstruction in the edentulous individual. Implants which support overdentures may present particular problems with control of loading as they may be largely mucosal supported, entirely implant supported or a combination of the two.

The occlusal scheme

The lack of mobility in implant supported fixed prostheses requires provision of shallow cuspal inclines and careful distribution of loads in lateral excursions. With single tooth implant restorations it is important to develop initial tooth contacts on the natural dentition and to carefully control guidance in lateral excursions on the implant restoration. Loading will also depend upon the opposing dentition which could be natural teeth, another implant supported prosthesis or a conventional removable prosthesis. Surprisingly high forces can be generated through removable prostheses.

The number, distribution, orientation, and design of implants

The distribution of load to the supporting bone can be spread by increasing the number and dimensions (diameter, surface topography, length) of the implants. The spacing and 3-dimensional arrangement of the individual implants will also be very important. The so-called 'tripod' arrangement of three implants is recommended in situations of high load, such as replacement of molar teeth in the partially dentate individual (*Fig 13*). Evidence for this is derived more from biomechanical theory than comparative clinical trials.

The design and properties of implant connectors

Multiple implants are joined by a cast or milled framework. A rigid connector provides good splinting and distribution of loads between implants. It is equally important that the connector has a passive fit on the implant abutments so that loads are not set up within the prosthetic construction.

Dimensions and location of cantilever extensions

Some implant reconstructions are designed with cantilever extensions to provide function (and appearance) in areas where provision of additional implants is difficult due to lack of bone. Cantilever extensions have the potential to create high loads, particularly on the implant adjacent to the cantilever. The extent of the leverage of any cantilever should be considered in relation to the anteroposterior distance between implants supporting the reconstruction. The cantilever extension should not exceed this length and the cross sectional design of the framework should be adequate to prevent flexing.

Patient parafunctional activities

Great caution should be exercised in treating patients with known parafunctional activities. Excessive loads may lead to loss of marginal bone or component fracture.

Conclusion

There are a great many factors to take into account to ensure predictable successful implant treatment. There is no substitute for meticulous attention to detail in all of these areas. Failure to do so will result in higher failure rates and unnecessary complications.

Teeth and implants

An osseointegrated implant restoration may closely resemble a natural tooth. However, the absence of a periodontal ligament and connective tissue attachment via cementum, results in fundamental differences in the adaptation of the implant to occlusal forces, and the structure of the gingival cuff.

Clinicians who use dental implants in the treatment of their patients require an understanding of the nature of osseointegration and the important fundamental differences between dental implants and natural teeth. The main comparisons are summarised in *Table 1* and illustrated in *Figure 1* which shows a single tooth implant and the adjacent natural teeth. The tooth originally formed within the jaws and erupted through the overlying mucosa in a complex series of biological events that are by no means fully understood. The implant on the other hand was surgically placed within the jaw bone, and is one of the few prosthetic devices that has been shown to successfully and permanently breach the surface epithelium with minimal or no complications.

Gingiva versus periimplant soft tissues

In healthy teeth the gingival margin is located on enamel. The gingival margin is scalloped and forms a shallow sulcus at the tooth surface. The gingiva rises between the teeth to form the interdental papillae, which are complex structures. Between the anterior teeth the papillae are pyramidal structures with the attachment of the gingivae following the contour of the cement enamel junction (*Fig.2*). In the molar regions, the buccal and lingual papillae at natural tooth embrasures are separated by the 'col', an area of gingivae which forms a slight dip beneath the contact point. A complex array of gingival connective tissue fibres form well defined bundle groups:

- Interdental fibres
- Dento-gingival fibres
- Circular fibres
- Alveolar crest fibres

Many of these fibres are inserted into the root cementum between the alveolar crest and cement enamel junction, and are therefore dependent upon the presence of natural teeth.

In the case of an implant, a transmucosal element (an abutment, neck of the implant or the restoration) protrudes through the overlying mucosa which heals and adapts around it without a cementum attachment. The collagen fibres within the periimplant mucosa run parallel to the abutment with no insertion into the abutment surface. There have been descriptions of more ordered fibre arrangements in relation

Table 1 Healthy teeth versus healthy implants		
	Healthy teeth	**Healthy implant**
Gingival sulcus depth	Shallow in health	Dependent upon abutment length and restoration margin
Junctional epithelium	On enamel	On titanium or other prosthetic material
Gingival fibres	Complex array inserted into cementum above crestal bone	No organised collagen fibre attachment – parallel fibres
Crest of bone	1 to 2mm apical to CEJ	According to implant design eg at or about first thread in threaded implants or at the level of change in surface morphology
Connective tissue attachment	Well organised collagen fibre bundles inserted as Sharpey's fibres into alveolar bone and cementum	Bone growing into close contact with implant surface: oxide layer/bone proteoglycan and collagen
Physical characteristics	Physiologic mobility caused by viscoelastic properties of the ligament	Rigid connection to bone – as if ankylosed
Adaptive characteristics	Width of ligament can alter to allow more mobility with increased occlusal forces	No adaptive capacity to allow mobility. Orthodontic movement impossible
Proprioception	Highly sensitive receptors present within the periodontal ligament	No ligament receptors

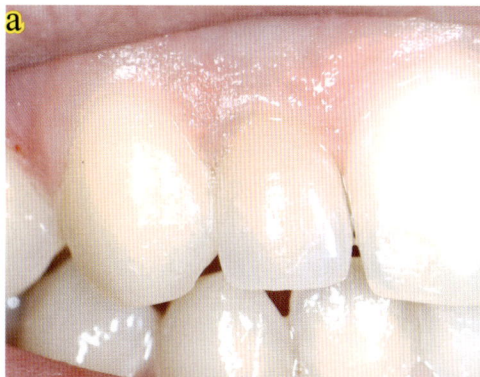

Figure 1a – Clinical photograph of a single tooth implant replacing the upper right lateral incisor. The porcelain fused to metal crown emerges from the gingiva with interdental tissue which appears very similar to normal papillae.

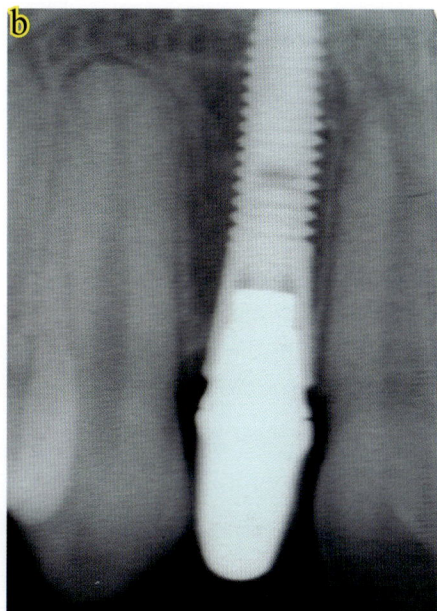

Figure 1b – Radiograph of the single tooth implant and adjacent teeth. The bone contacts the implant surface with no intervening radiolucent space which would be observed if there were fibrous tissue encapsulation. The bone margin is coincident with the implant/abutment junction. The adjacent teeth have a normal periodontal ligament space.

tacts and a basal lamina-like structure formed by the epithelial cells. The biological attachment mechanism is now thought to be mediated through particular adhesins or integrins, which are fundamental in cell to cell adhesion as well as cell to matrix adhesion. It is well established that a junctional epithelium will also form on root surface cementum, dentine and various dental materials including implant components (*Fig.5*). A normal junctional epithelium can be regenerated from adjacent oral mucosa/gingival following excision, and the new junctional epithelium is indistinguishable from that which previously existed. It is thought that the properties of the junctional epithelium are dictated by the influence of the underlying connective tissue, the presence of an inflammatory infiltrate and the presence of a tooth/implant surface to which it adheres (rather than the inherent properties of the epithelial cells). The junctional epithelium has a particularly high turnover and is permeable to both the ingress of substances and to the passage of components of the immune and inflammatory system. It is therefore well equipped to deal with the problems of a breach in the epithelial integrity caused by an emerging tooth or implant. The junctional epithelium may be found on the implant itself or on the abutment. This will be because of differences in the designs of implants, the biological requirements of the attachment of the soft tissue cuff and the level of the junction between abutment and implants.

Biological width

In teeth, the concept of the biological width is well established, in that a zone of attached connective tissue separates the underlying alveolar bone from the apical termination of the junctional epithelium (*Fig.6a*). The connective tissue zone is about 1.5 - 2mm wide and the length of the junctional epithelium about 1.5mm. Figures 6b and c show two different designs of implants and the corresponding biological width. In the first case the implant design is typical of a traditional submerged (two stage) system with a flat-top connection between implant and abutment, such as the Branemark. After 1 year of function the bone margin is usually located at the first thread. The junctional epithelium (1.5mm to 2 mm apicocoronal width) is located on the abutment, and a zone of connective tissue of about 1mm to 2mm in width intervenes. The join between abutment and implant head is located within this zone. In contrast the non submerged (single stage) implant (typical of the ITI Straumann type) is placed so that its roughened surface is placed within bone, but the smooth neck which is an integral part of the implant performs the function of the transmucosal element. The junctional epithelium is therefore routinely located on the implant, and the implant/abutment join is located coronal to this level. It has been postulated that the

to transmucosal implant surfaces which have a rougher surface (such as plasma spraying). In this situation some fibres appear to run at right angles to the implant surface, but there is no good evidence of an attachment mechanism. However a rough abutment surface does have potential negative properties, such as increased corrosion potential and microbial contamination if it becomes exposed within the oral cavity.

The papillae which forms around a single tooth implant may be supported by collagen fibres attached to the adjacent natural teeth. However, in cases where there are adjacent implants rather than teeth, the formation of soft tissue papillae is less predictable and their form is dependent upon the presence of an adequate thickness of soft tissue, bone height, implant spacing and careful contouring of the crown profiles to encourage the appearance and maintenance of a papillary form (*Fig.3*). The soft tissue between multiple posterior unit implants is more likely to have a flat contour but again may be influenced by soft tissue thickness and crown morphology.

Junctional epithelium

In healthy teeth the junctional epithelium (*Fig.4*) is attached to enamel by hemidesmosomal conjoin within the flat-top design may influence the level of soft tissue attachment and biological width. This may be caused by micromovement between the two components or by allowing microbial penetration of the microgap between implant and abutment. Other systems which have an internal conical connection between the implant and abutment such as Astra Tech or Ankylos can maintain the bone level close to this junction. At present the theoretical differences between the types do not reveal any major differences in their clinical performance.

Probing depth examination

Periodontal probing of natural teeth is an important part of any dental examinations. It is well established that the probe penetrates the junctional epithelium to some degree in health, and that this penetration increases in the presence of inflammation. Under these latter circumstances the probe is stopped by the most coronal intact gingival connective tissue fibres, about 2mm from the bone. The situation around the dental implant is different and the sulcus depth is more dependent upon the thickness of the soft tissue cuff. Probing depths around implants are generally deeper than around teeth, bleeding on probing may be more common, but penetration of the soft tissue at the base of the sulcus occurs to a similar degree with the probe tip finishing short of the bone margin by about 2mm. Some clinicians advocate routine recording of probing depths (and attachment levels from the abutment restoration margin) around implants. Others prefer to record visible signs of inflammation or the use of digital pressure on the external surface of the periimplant soft tissue to elicit signs of inflammation such as bleeding or suppuration. Others rely on radiographic assessment of bone levels to monitor stability.

Periodontal ligament versus osseointegration

Periodontal ligament

The periodontal ligament is a complex structure, about 0.1 to 0.2mm in width, providing support to the teeth in a viscoelastic manner (*Fig.7*). The ligament comprises collagen fibres which are embedded as Sharpey's fibres in the root cementum and the alveolar bone, together with the blood supply and connective tissue ground substance, which provide the other key elements to the supporting mechanism. The periodontal ligament has a sensitive proprioceptive mechanism which can detect minute changes in forces applied to the teeth. These forces are dissipated through compression and redistribution of the fluid elements as well as through the fibre system. Forces transmitted through the periodontal ligament can result in remodelling and tooth movement as seen in orthodontics or in the widening of the ligament and an increase in tooth mobility in response to excessive forces

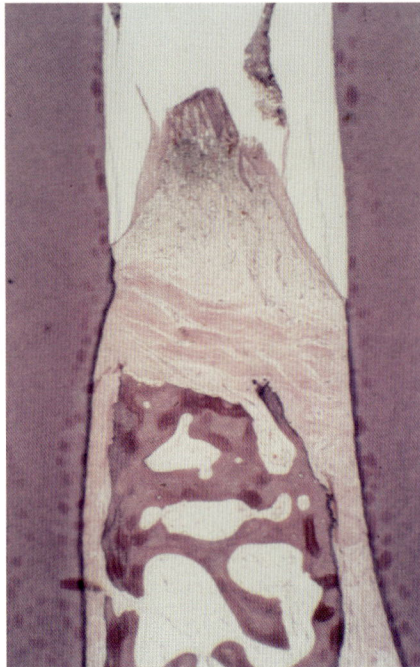

Figure 2 – A histological section of an interdental space between two teeth. The enamel has been removed by the demineralisation process. The junctional epithelium outlines the enamel space and terminates at the level of the root cementum. The interdental bone septum is situated just below the cement enamel junction (in health 1-2 mm) and there is a well developed transeptal fibre arrangement. There is a small inflammatory infiltrate in the gingival connective tissue at the top of the papilla.

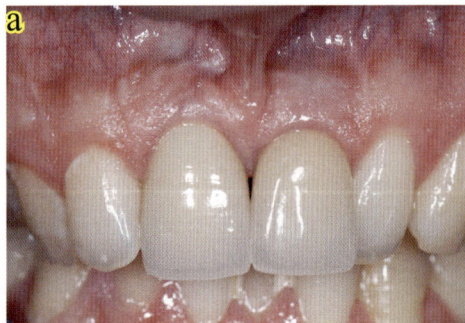

Figure 3a- The maxillary central incisors in this patient have been replaced with single tooth implants. The gingival morphology is good but there is a slight discrepancy in the level of the gingival margin and the interdental tissue is more complete between natural tooth and implant compared with the mid line space between the two implant restorations. The mid line interdental tissue is not supported by a normal gingival fibre arrangement seen at tooth surfaces.

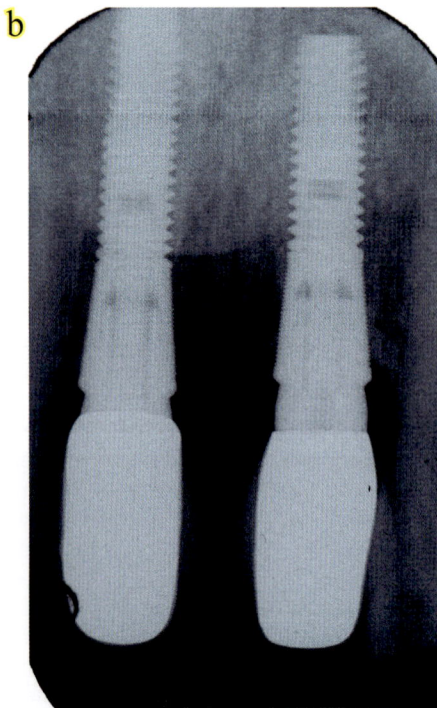

Figure 3b- A radiograph of the clinical case shown in figure 3. The implants are slightly different lengths and at slightly different levels. The titanium abutment on the right implant is shorter than that on the left implant. Bone levels are close to the heads of the implant and there is a slightly higher crestal bone height between the two implants.

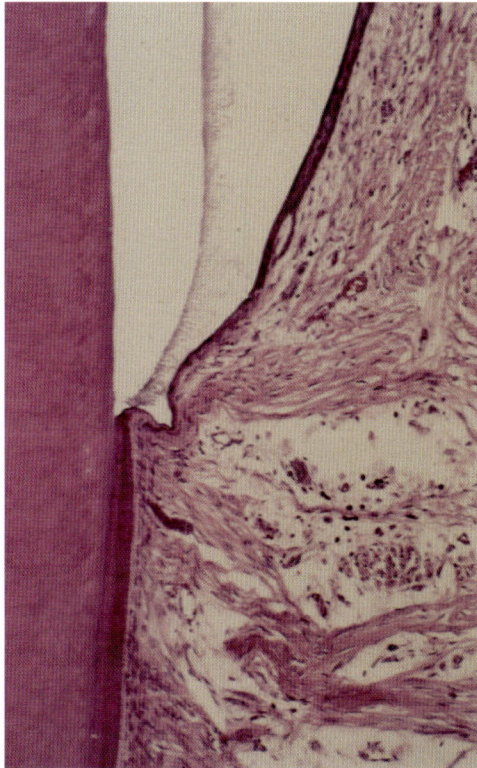

Figure 4- A histological section of junctional epithelium at a natural tooth. It terminates at the cement enamel junction and was attached to the enamel by hemidesmosomes and a basal lamina-like structure. Collagen fibres are inserted into the cementum and radiate into the gingival connective tissue.

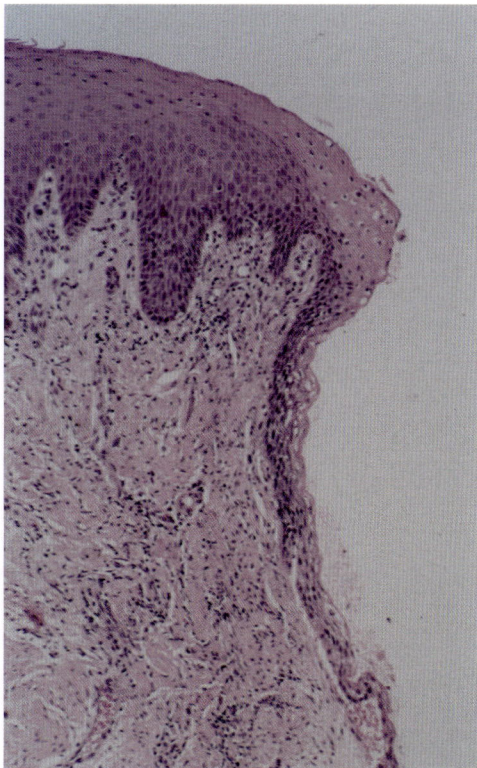

Figure 5- A histological section of the soft tissue cuff excised from around an implant. A non-keratinised sulcular and junctional epithelium is present and is very similar to that which exists around teeth. The collagen fibre bundles are not so well organised as there is no attachment to the abutment/implant surface.

(eg occlusal trauma). The periodontal ligament is therefore capable of detecting and responding to a wide range of forces.

Osseointegration

The precise nature of osseointegration at a molecular level is not fully understood. At the light microscopical level there is a very close adaptation of the bone to the implant surface (*Fig.8*). At the higher magnifications possible with electron microscopy, there is a gap (about 100 NM in width) between the implant surface and bone. This is occupied by an intervening collagen rich zone adjacent to the bone and a more amorphous zone adjacent to the implant surface. Bone protecoglycans may be important in the initial attachment of the tissues to the implant surface, which in titanium implants consists of a titanium oxide layer (this has the properties of a ceramic). Osseointegration is not an absolute phenomenon and can be measured as the proportion of the total implant surface that is in contact with bone. Greater levels of bone contact occur in cortical bone than in cancellous bone, where marrow spaces are often adjacent to the implant surface. The degree of bone contact may increase with time and function. When an implant is first placed in the bone there should be a close fit to ensure stability. The space between implant and bone is initially filled with blood clot and serum/ bone proteins. Although great care is taken to avoid damaging the bone, the initial response to the surgical trauma is resorption, which is then followed by bone deposition. There is a critical period in the healing process at around 2 weeks post implant insertion when bone resorption will result in a lower degree of implant stability than that achieved initially. Subsequent bone formation will result in an increase in the level of bone contact and stability. This has been demonstrated in unloaded implants in the early healing period and over longer time periods following loading of implants. Thus osseointegration should be viewed as a dynamic process in which bone turnover occurs, but not as the same adaptive process that occurs within the ligament of natural teeth. Osseointegration is more akin to an ankylosis, where the absence of mobility and no intervening fibrous tissue capsule is the sign of successful integration. Under these circumstances there is no viscoelastic damping system although proprioceptive mechanisms may operate within bone and associated oral structures. Forces are distributed to the bone and may be concentrated in certain areas, particularly around the neck of the implant. Some designs, particularly those with threads, may dissipate the forces more effectively. Excessive forces applied to the implant may result in remodelling of the marginal bone i.e. apical movement of the bone margin with loss of osseointegration. The exact mechanism of how this occurs is not entirely clear but it has been suggested that microfractures may propagate within the adjacent bone. This type

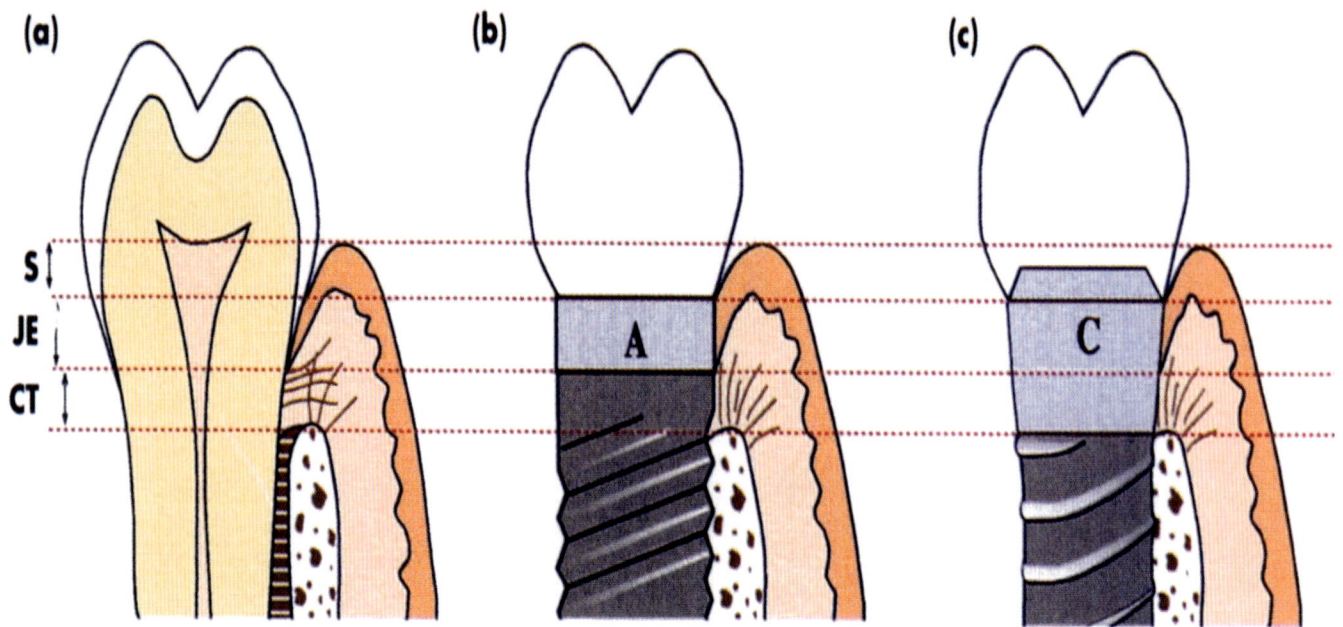

Figure 6 a,b,c - The biological width of the dentogingival junction in (a) teeth and (b) around implants typical of the Branemark system, and (c) the non-submerged ITI implant system. S= sulcus which is approximately 0.5 to 1 mm deep; JE= junctional epithelium which is about 1.5 to 2 mm in apicocoronal width; CT= connective tissue zone (1 to 2 mm in width) in which the fibres are attached to root cementum in teeth but run parallel to the implant surface; A=abutment – The abutment to implant junction is situated beneath the soft tissue in the Branemark system; C= smooth transmucosal collar of the ITI system.

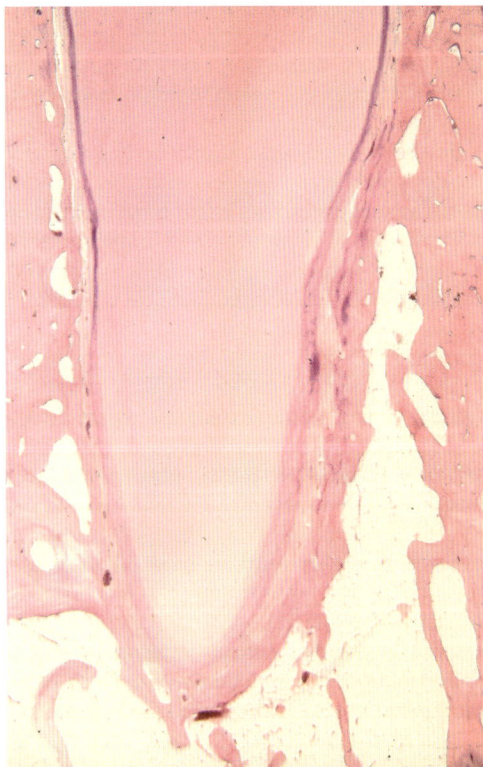

Figure 7- A histological section of a tooth root, periodontal ligament and alveolar bone. The periodontal ligament is inserted into the cementum and the lamina dura as Sharpey's fibres. The viscoelastic properties of the ligament give the tooth a degree of mobility and the ligament is able to respond to increased forces by remodelling processes.

of bone loss caused by excessive loading may be slowly progressive to a point where there is catastrophic failure of the remaining osseointegration or fracture of the implant. Fortunately, either event is rare. Excessive forces are usually suspected prior to this stage through radiographic marginal bone loss or mechanical failure of the superstructure and/or abutments (See Chapter 11).

It has been shown that well controlled forces may result in an increase in the degree of bone to implant contact. Adaptation is therefore possible, though osseointegration does not permit movement of the implant in the way that a tooth may be orthodontically repositioned. Therefore the osseointegrated implant has proved itself to be a very effective anchorage system for difficult orthodontic cases, and may be used as an alternative anchorage system to head gear. The fact that the implant behaves as an ankylosed unit also restricts its use to individuals who have completed their jaw growth (*Fig.9*). Placement of an osseointegrated implant in a child will result in relative submergence with growth of the surrounding alveolar process during normal development. It is therefore advisable to delay implant placement until after growth is complete. This can be 16 years of age for females and 18 years of age for males, although small amounts of alveolar bone development can continue into their early 20s.

Periodontitis and peri-implantitis
It is quite possible that bacteria that are implicated in periodontitis, such as Porphryromonas gingivalis, are also the major pathogens in destructive

Figure 8a- A histological section through an osseointegrated screw shaped implant which has been in place for 6 months. Bone is in close apposition over a large proportion at the surface.

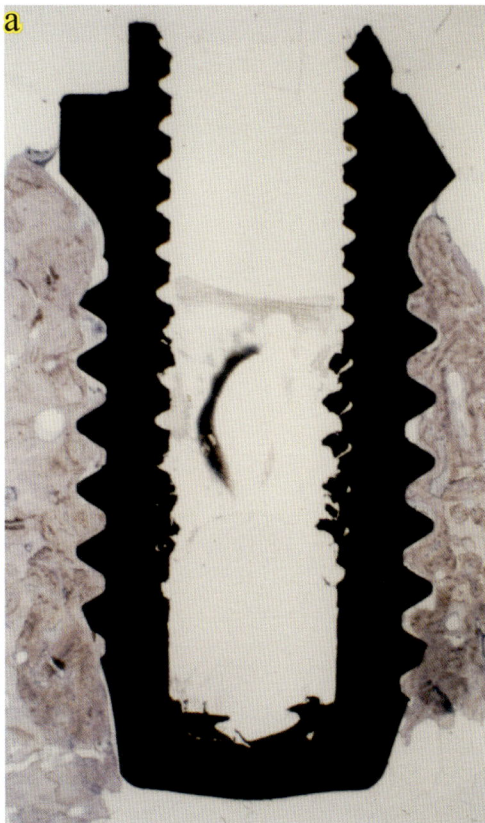

Figure 8b- A higher power view of an area of figure 8a showing bone filling the thread profiles and contacting the implant surface without a visible gap (at this magnification), except for a small area of narrow space.

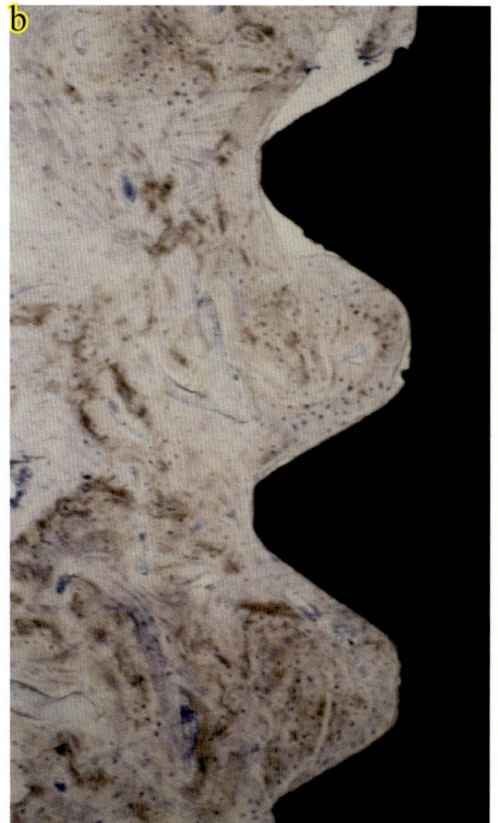

Figure 9- An ankylosed upper left central incisor tooth following trauma. Damage to the periodontal ligament has led to a bony ankylosis and resorption which can be seen in figure 9b. The tooth has no detectable mobility and has not developed into a normal vertical position with the adjacent teeth. In this respect it is behaving like an osseointegrated implant. An osseointegrated implant should not be placed in a child until growth is complete.

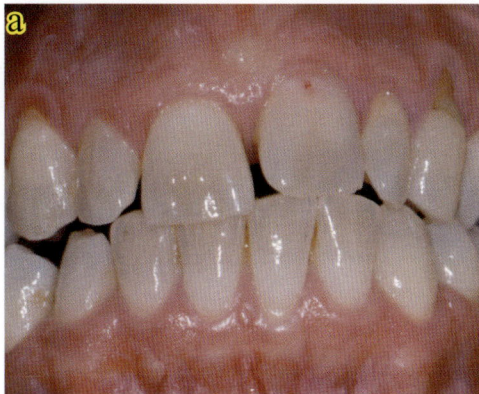

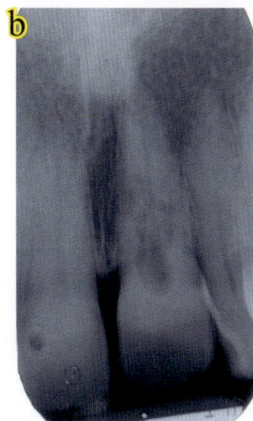

inflammatory lesions around implants (peri-implantitis). There is therefore a possibility of colonisation or infection of the implant surfaces from periodontopathic bacteria. The destruction of the supporting tissues of teeth and implants have many similarities but there are important differences caused by the nature of the supporting tissues (see earlier). This is particularly noticeable with the different patterns of tissue destruction observed. Peri-implantitis affects the entire circumference of the implant resulting in a 'gutter' of bone loss filled with inflammatory tissue extending to the bone surface (*Fig.10*). In contrast, periodontitis-affected teeth commonly have irregular loss of supporting tissues, often confined to proximal surfaces and resulting in complex infrabony defects. In addition, for the most part the periodontal tissues are capable of 'walling off' the inflammatory lesion from the alveolar bone and periodontal ligament with a zone of fibrous tissue. It would seem probable that destructive inflammatory lesions affecting both teeth and implants have stages in which the disease process is more rapid (burst phenomenon) followed by periods of relative quiescence. The incidence of peri-implantitis would appear to be low, but can result in rapid destruction of the marginal bone and is difficult to differentiate from bone loss because of excessive forces. This problem is dealt with in Chapter 11.

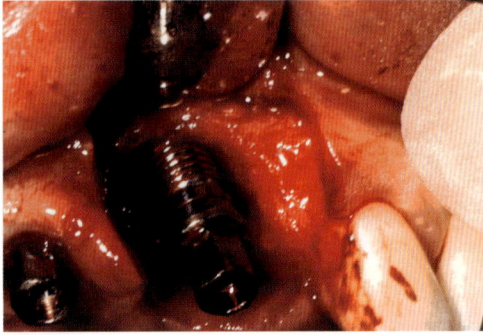

Figure 10- An exposed implant following destruction of the most coronal bone by an inflammatory infiltrate. There was a plaque induced inflammation caused by retention of cement at the crown abutment junction which was situated subgingivally.

Conclusion

Modern osseointegrated implants are a useful alternative to natural teeth. There are fundamental differences between them, and an understanding of the attachment mechanisms of hard and soft tissues and their responses to the harsh environment of the oral cavity is essential to the dental surgeon who is involved in providing this form of treatment.

Assessment of the dentition and treatment options for the replacement of missing teeth

In most cases the patient and dentist have a number of choices for the replacement of missing teeth. The advantages and disadvantages of these options can be presented to the patient following careful clinical and radiographic examinations.

The restorative dentist has a wide range of options for replacement of teeth lost through dental disease, trauma or other causes such as developmental abnormalities.

The most common causes of tooth loss are dental caries (and its sequelae) and periodontal disease. Both diseases have an impact on the condition and prognosis of the remaining teeth which will therefore require very careful assessment to determine whether they require remedial treatment and furthermore whether they would provide suitable abutments for fixed or removable prostheses. It is essential that all caries, endodontic lesions and periodontal diseases have been treated before embarking on definitive replacement of missing teeth by whatever method is finally chosen.

Initial examination and considerations

The minimal clinical examination should assess the restorative status of the teeth, a periodontal screening, mucous membranes, TMJs, jaw relationship and occlusion. Vitality testing should also be carried out where appropriate and a complete periodontal examination for all those whose screening indicates significant periodontitis (BPE score 4 in any sextant) (*Fig.1*).

The most convenient overall radiographic examination is the dental panoramic tomogram (*Fig.2*). This may need to be supplemented with intra-oral radiographs where the image quality does not permit proper assessment. Bitewing radiographs are adequate for dentitions minimally affected by caries or early periodontitis (*Fig.3*). Periapical radiographs using a paralleling technique should be considered advisable for all potential abutment teeth, heavily restored teeth, teeth with known or suspected endodontic problems and teeth with moderate to advanced periodontitis (*Fig.4*).

Following a full clinical and radiographic examination, it may be helpful to assign a prognosis to individual teeth, taking into account all factors; restorative, endodontic, periodontal. The prognosis may be simply categorised eg excellent/good, fair, questionable/poor, hopeless. In addition, the individual tooth prognosis may be affected by the type of planned restoration. For example, a tooth with a post crown may have a fair prognosis if it is to be kept as a free standing unit, but would be severely compromised if used to support a denture or fixed bridge. Features that adversely affect the prognosis are described in *Table 1* and illustrated in *Figure 5*.

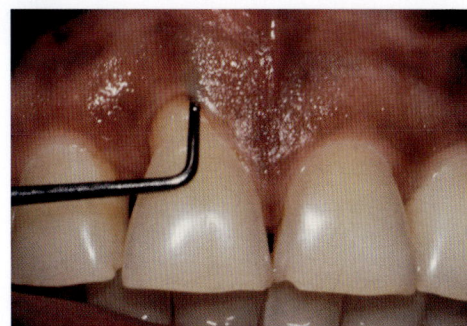

Figure 1 – Probing to assess the periodontal status of the patient. In this case a relatively healthy looking gingival margin has a probing depth of nearly 10mm.

Figure 2- (Left) The dental panoramic tomogram is a very useful screening tool. This individual has a heavily restored dentition and moderate to advanced periodontitis. The image in the mid-line is not quite so clear but it does indicate advanced bone loss on the incisor teeth.

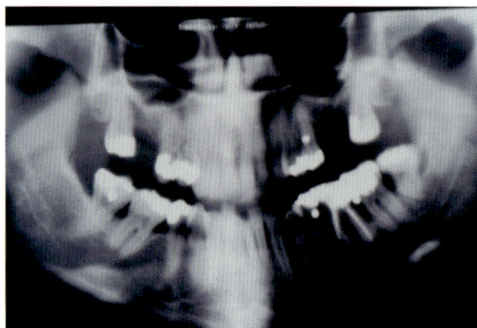

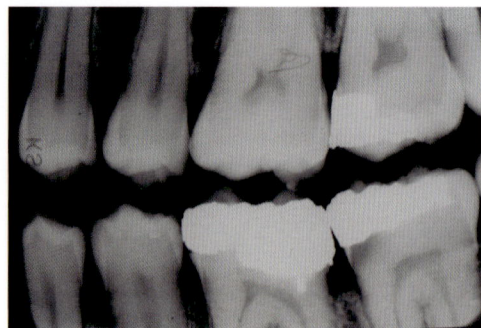

Figure 3- (Right) Bitewing radiographs are useful for diagnosis of caries and early periodontal disease. Recurrent caries is visible on the mesial aspect of the lower second molar but the interdental bone crests are at a normal level.

Figure 4a- This periapical radiograph shows an upper right central incisor with an inadequate root filling, an apical radiolucency and a very short post. This tooth would not be considered to be a suitable bridge abutment.

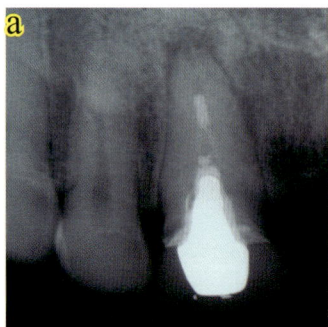

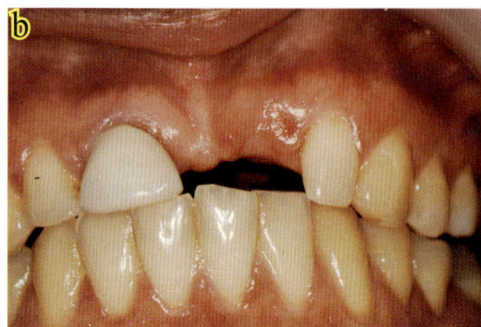

Figure 4b- The clinical status of the patient illustrated in figure 4a. The missing upper left central incisor space is large. The patient had a mid-line diastema prior to tooth loss.

Figure 5a- The upper anterior teeth in this patient are very broken down. They were bridge abutments which have suffered from caries and fracture. Restoration of these teeth would be very difficult. If individual restorations were possible it is unlikely that they would be considered to be adequate bridge abutments.

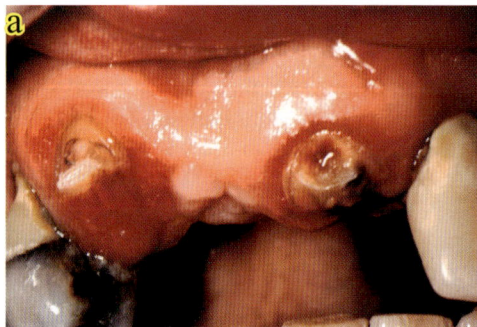

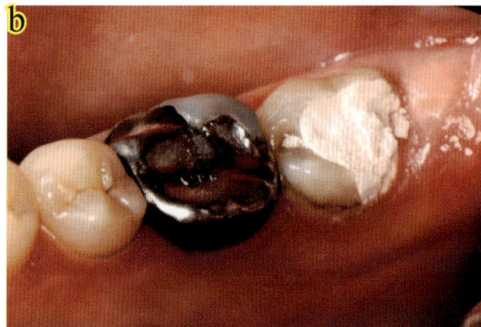

Figure 5b- The first and second molars are heavily restored. The second molar requires a replacement restoration but this extends subgingivally to a considerable extent. This retromolar area is difficult to perform periodontal surgery to expose restoration margins.

Figure 5c- These heavily worn teeth have been crown lengthened but restoration is still difficult. The lower right central incisor is non-vital and has a labial sinus. This tooth was considered to be untreatable.

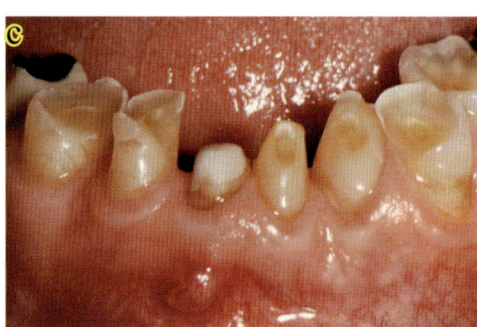

Figure 5d- This shows surgical exposure of a complex bone defect affecting the upper right first pre-molar. A deep periodontal pocket was detected on the mesial aspect in relation to the groove and the bifurcation of this tooth. Recurrent abscesses have destroyed most of the buccal and mesial bone. This tooth has a very poor prognosis.

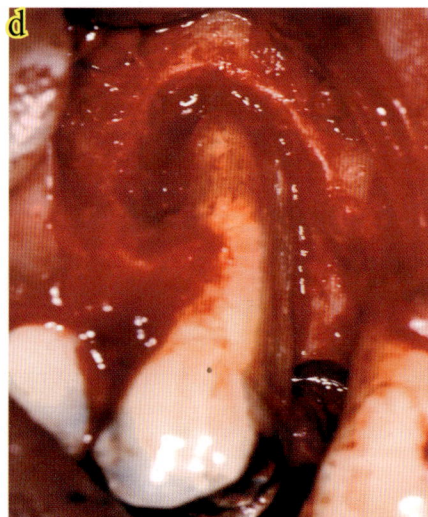

Table 1 Important factors which adversely affect individual tooth prognosis	
Restorations and caries	Extensions subgingivally or onto root surfaces
	Extension within the pulp chamber or root canal
	Minimal remaining coronal tooth substance
	Inadequate or overextended posts in root filled teeth
Endodontic factors	Periapical symptoms/signs
	Inability to control the coronal seal
	Inadequate previous RCT including broken instruments in root canal
	Sclerosed canals
	Fractures / splits
Periodontal factors	Probing depths over 6mm
	Attachment loss over 6mm
	Bone loss more than 50%
	Poor root morphology – especially short roots
	Involvement of furcations – especially grade II/III
	Mobility – especially grade III
Occlusal factors	Signs of parafunction or severe attrition
	History of repeated tooth restoration / fractures

The basic questions to be asked about individual teeth are:

1. Can the tooth be restored successfully?

2. Can the tooth be endodontically treated successfully?

3. Can the tooth be treated periodontally?

4. Following treatment will the tooth be a suitable abutment?

5. How important is the tooth strategically?

6. What impact will the loss of the tooth have on the overall plan?

The individual tooth assessment and prognosis then needs to be put into the context of the treatment requirements of the entire dentition. In addition to the above considerations, many subjects are seen with missing teeth due to trauma or developmental absence of teeth in whom the remaining dentition is very healthy. The potential abutment teeth, the size and location of the edentulous space and the occlusal relationships will have a great effect on the possible restorative solutions.

Potential abutment teeth

The size and shape of the natural crown and root form are important considerations. Teeth with short and/or conical crown forms offer poor retention and support. Procedures such as periodontal surgical crown lengthening or adhesive restorations may overcome many of the difficulties (*Figs 6 and 7*). Certain teeth, particularly canines, are very difficult to re-place with routine restorations because of the lack of suitable adjacent abutments (*Fig.8*). For example, loss of the canine in a distal free end saddle situation leaves only the lateral incisor as a distal abutment for a removable prosthesis. This is a most unsatisfactory situation and often leads to progressive loss of the incisors.

Healthy unrestored teeth make the best abutments for fixed bridges but the damage that occurs to teeth following preparation must be considered. Conversely heavily restored teeth may be unsuitable abutments - further tooth preparation may remove the only remaining tooth substance and restorations retained by pins or posts are prone to failure.

The edentulous area

The requirements for restoring an edentulous area depend upon its location and size. Many subjects will accept or prefer non-replacement of missing molars. The concept of the shortened arch is well established and most patients will accept a dentition extending from first molar to first molar or from second premolar to second premolar (*Fig 9*). Patients with fewer teeth than this often have an aesthetic problem and/or a functional disadvantage. The point at which replacement of missing posterior teeth in the free end saddle situation is carried out is very much dependent upon patient wishes. The alternative to an implant supported prosthesis is a removable prosthesis or a limited extension distal cantilever bridge. Replacement of molar teeth to prevent over-eruption of teeth in the opposing arch, which may compromise future restorative options, is important in some subjects (*Fig.10*).

Figure 6a- (left) - The upper left lateral incisor has a short clinical crown due to delayed apical migration of the gingival margin.

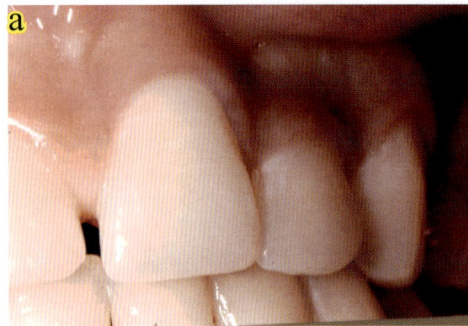

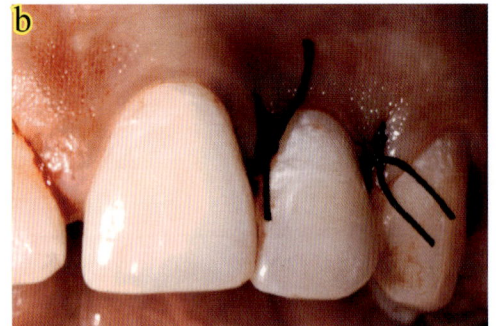

Figure 6b- (right) - Minor crown lengthening surgery has been performed on the upper lateral incisor to improve the aesthetics.

Figure 7a – (left) Shows replacement of an upper left canine with a resin bonded bridge and acceptable aesthetics from the buccal aspect. The pontic has been ridge lapped.

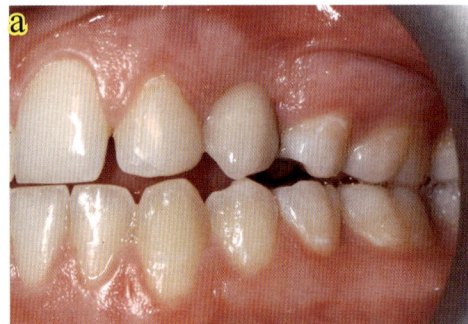

Figure 7b- (right) Shows the cantilever design and very good coverage of the palatal aspect of the premolar abutment.

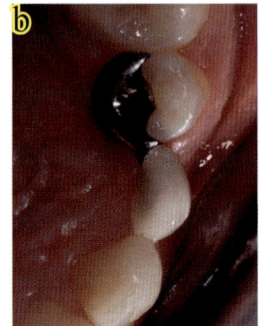

Figure 7c- (left) The periapical radiograph illustrates a very wide space between adjacent roots which would permit implant replacement should the bridge fail. The space has been partially closed with an adhesive restoration on the lateral incisor tooth.

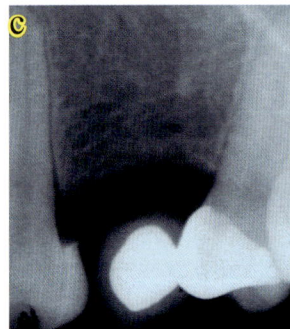

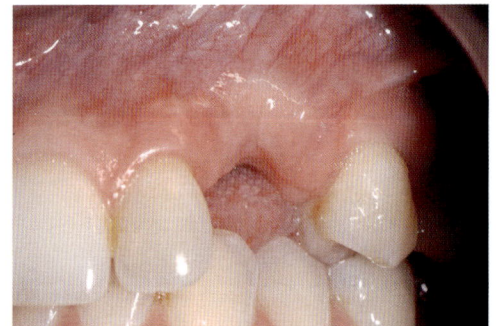

Figure 8- (right) Progressive resorption of a transplanted canine has led to loss of this tooth. In most of these cases a single tooth implant would be considered a good option.

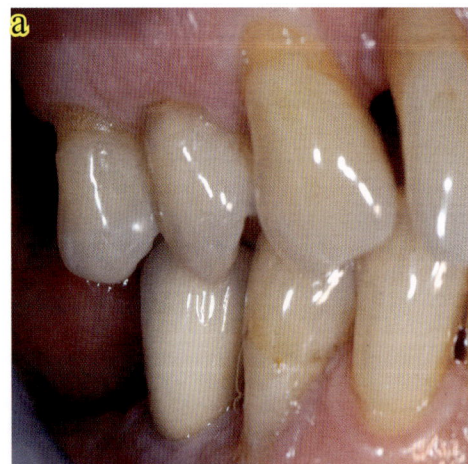

Figure 9a- (left) A patient with a shortened dental arch. The lower right second premolar has been replaced with a single tooth implant.

Figure 9b- (right) Radiograph of the premolar implant.

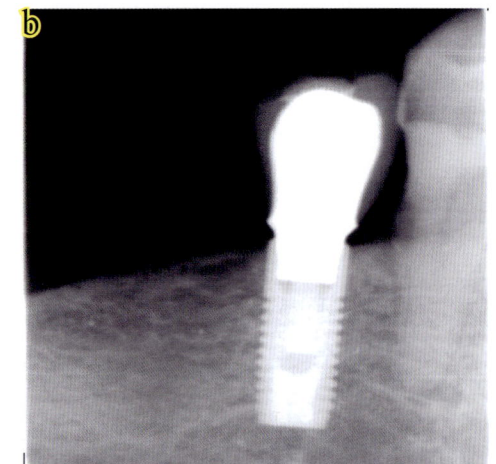

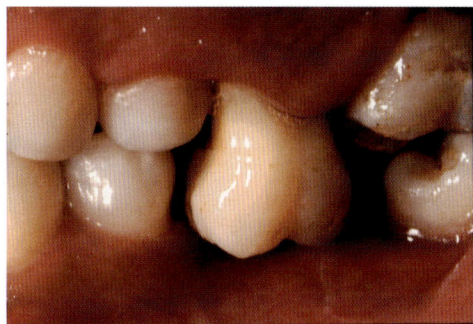

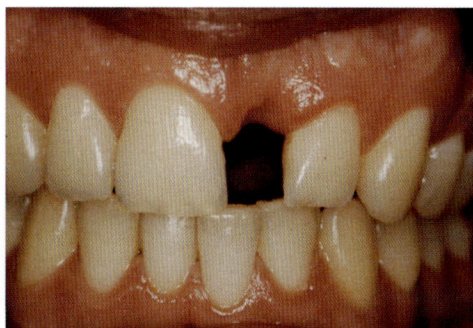

Figures 10 –(left) Severe overeruption of an upper first molar into the opposing edentulous space.

Figure 11- (right) Following loss of the upper left central incisor there has been considerable space closure and simple provision of a replacement tooth with normal dimensions is not possible..

Few patients will accept non-replacement of missing incisors/canines. The full range of prosthetic options can be considered and an explanation of their advantages and disadvantages given to the patient. There are, however, a few general considerations.

Single missing teeth

The size of the edentulous space of single missing units varies enormously. At one extreme there is barely enough space for the missing unit (*Fig.11*). Orthodontic realignment may need to be considered to either eliminate the space or provide enough to accommodate the missing unit (*Fig.12*). This decision can be particularly difficult in the orthodontic management of missing maxillary canines. In other cases the single tooth space may be larger than the natural tooth. In spaced dentitions the prosthetic options for replacement of the single missing tooth are more limited (*Fig.13*).

Multiple missing teeth

In many cases patients will present with an existing prosthesis that gives information about the aesthetic requirements, including the number and size of teeth, which can be accommodated. In other cases it will be necessary to carry out a diagnostic wax-up or provision of a temporary denture to establish this. The height and shape of the edentulous ridge is another important consideration. It should be remembered that following tooth loss, alveolar resorption may occur in both a horizontal and vertical plane (*Fig.14*). Factors which influence the degree of resorption include previous periodontal and endodontic infections, surgical trauma during extraction, postoperative infection, and the type and quality of the previous prosthesis. Loss of ridge height and width may necessitate prosthetic replacement of the missing soft and hard tissues to provide adequate aesthetics at the gingival margin and lip support. In removable prostheses this can be achieved with a labial flange but if a fixed restoration is to be chosen, then some form of ridge augmentation may be necessary. The provision of a diagnostic temporary denture is extremely useful, particularly to determine whether a labial flange is needed (*Fig.15*).

Occlusal relationships

Examination of the occlusion should encompass basic jaw relationships and determination of the intercuspal position. The patient's mandible should be manipulated into its most retruded position and the presence of any contacts in this retruded arc should be sought. Movement of the mandible laterally and anteriorly should demonstrate the existing occlusal relationships and presence of any significant interferences. For individuals with more extensive edentulous spans it is advisable to take accurate study casts and mount these in a semi-adjustable articulator using a facebow. This will allow a clear assessment of the occlusal scheme and any implications of the treatment alternatives to be more accurately assessed.

Some cases, such as Class 2 division 2 incisor relationships, can pose particularly difficult problems with any type of prosthesis due to space and angulation limitation (*Fig 16*). Tilted and overerupted teeth may need to be corrected before a satisfactory restoration can be provided. Restoration of individuals with parafunctional activities or severe occlusal wear demand special care (*Fig 17*).

Figure 12- Shows a young patient who has undergone orthodontic treatment and replacement of the maxillary lateral incisors with the resin bonded bridges.

Figure 12a- (left) Labial view showing good aesthetics.

Figure 12b- (right) Palatal view showing retainers on the central incisors and canines. This design has been chosen to ensure orthodontic stability. Measurement with the periodontal probe suggests that there would be adequate space for an implant restoration if the resin bonded bridge should fail.

Figures 12c – 12d – Demonstrate good radiographic root alignment following orthodontic treatment.

Figures 12e – 12f – These radiographs show an earlier stage in orthodontic treatment where marked root conversion would not allow implant placement even though clinically there may appear to be adequate space at the crown level.

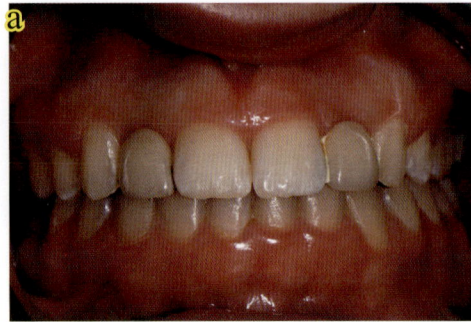

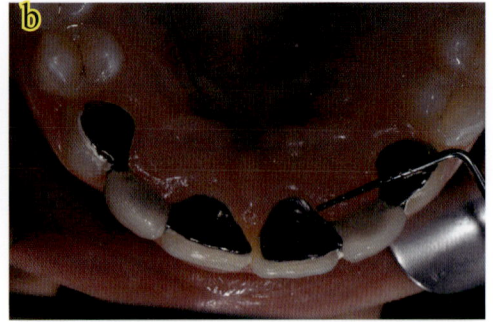

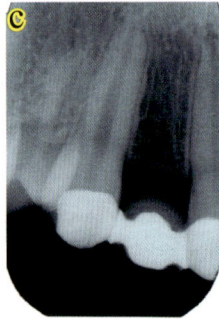

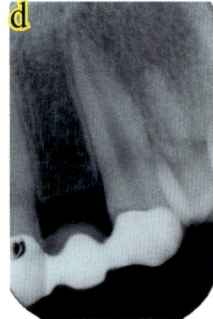

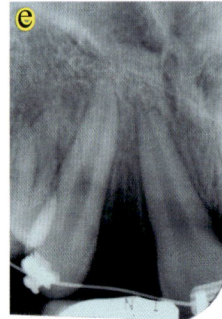

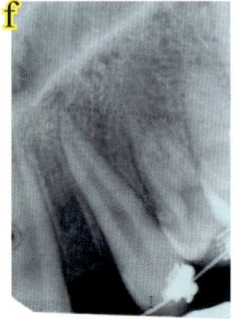

Figure 13a- Replacement of the upper left central incisor with a removable denture.

Figure 13b- Palatal view of the same individual showing extensive coverage of the palatal tissue by the chrome cobalt framework. Replacement of an incisor in a spaced dentition may be achieved using a removable denture, a spring cantilevered bridge or a single tooth implant.

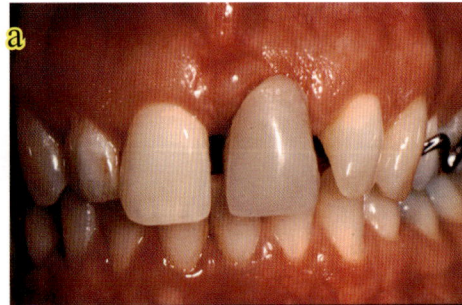

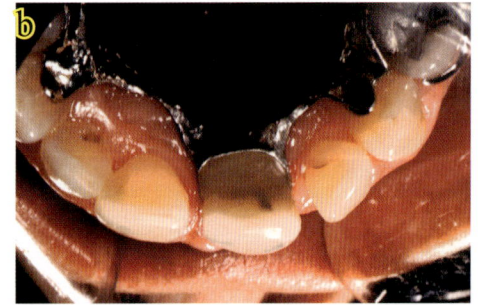

Figure 14a- An anterior edentulous space with loss of ridge height in the mid-line. Replacement of the missing tissue would be necessary to achieve a satisfactory aesthetic result. This may be achieved using surgical reconstruction or as part of the prosthesis.

Figure 14b – The same ridge seen from the occlusal aspect showing a concavity on the patient's left side following loss of the buccal plate when the tooth was avulsed.

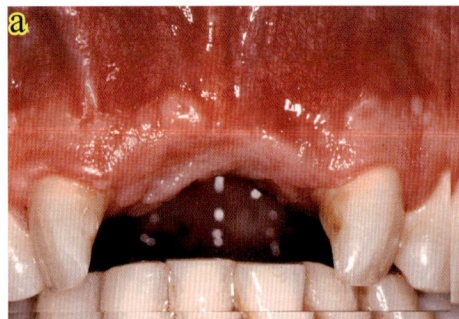

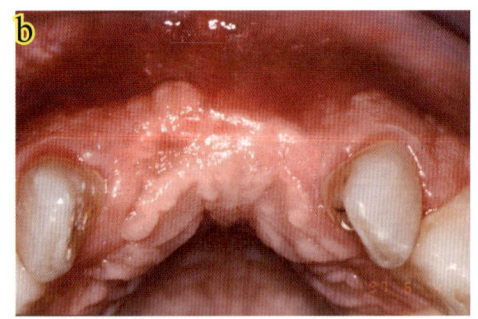

Figure 15a- Loss of the central incisors and left lateral incisor with minor ridge resorption.

Figure 15b- A removable acrylic partial denture with ridge lap teeth and good aesthetics.

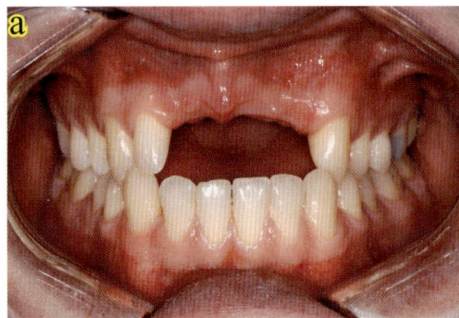

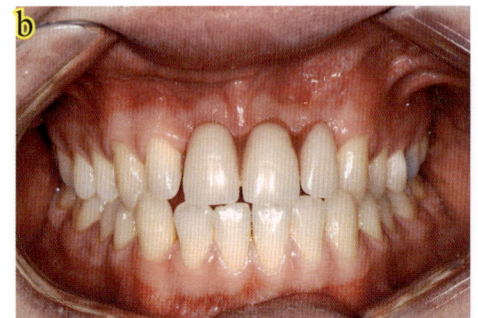

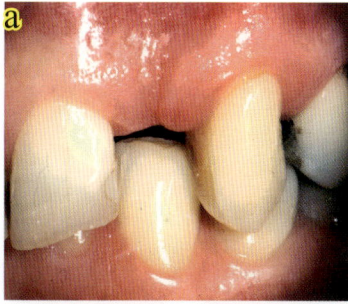

Figure 16a – A severe class II division II incisor relationship with little space between the mandibular tooth and the maxillary ridge.

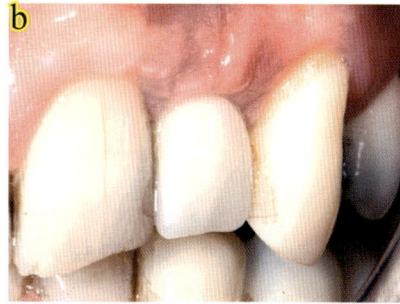

Figure 16b- Satisfactory replacement of the missing lateral incisor with a single tooth implant.

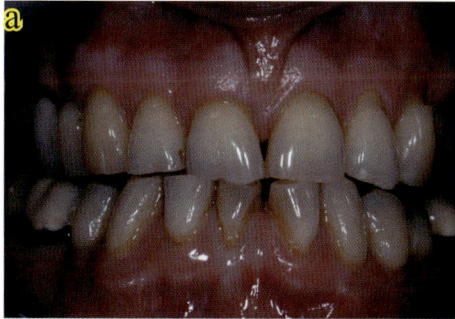

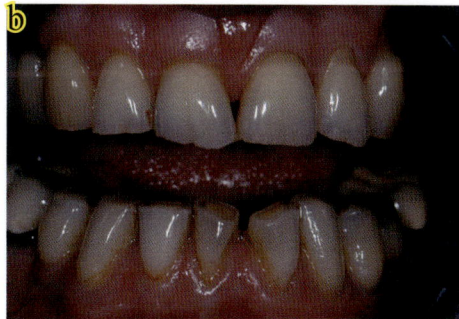

Figure 17 a and b- A patient with moderate wear of the anterior teeth suggesting a parafunctional activity. This patient requested replacement of some molar units with implant restorations. The cause of the tooth wear needs to be identified and managed.

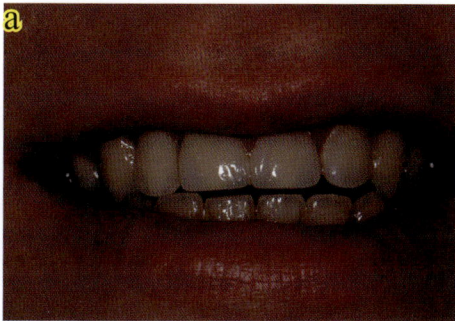

Figure 18a- A removable partial denture showing acceptable aesthetics.

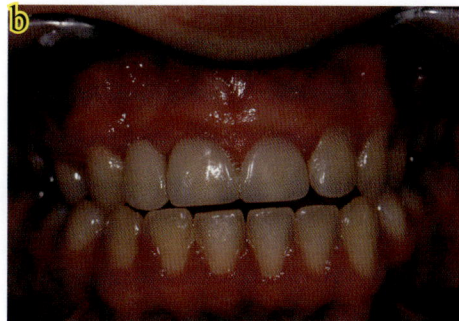

Figure 18b – The intraoral appearance of the partial denture. The ridge lap teeth give a natural appearance. Gingivitis affects the lower teeth and some inflammation is present under the denture pontics.

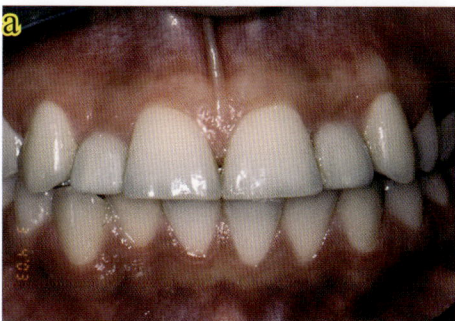

Figure 19a- Resin bonded bridges used to replace missing lateral incisors. The labial view shows short unaesthetic pontics.

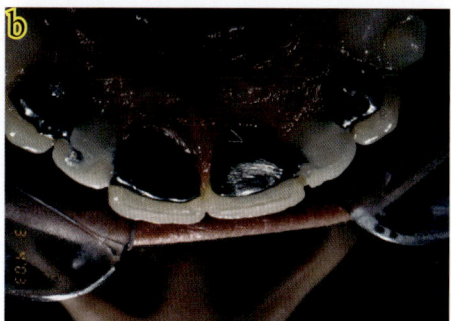

Figure 19b – The palatal view shows narrow spaces where the lateral incisors are missing. Unless orthodontic retention is required a cantilever bridge is normally recommended.

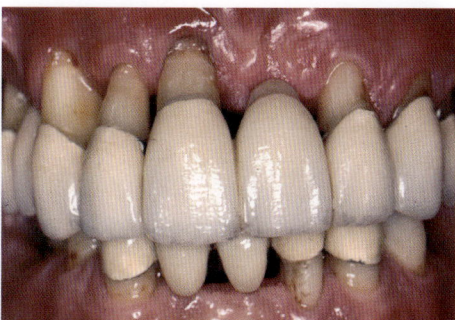

Figure 20- A full arch fixed bridge in a patient who has lost many of the upper teeth through periodontitis. The design of the bridge is an effective splint for the remaining teeth which have very much reduced periodontal support.

Figure 21a- A patient treated with an implant supported maxillary anterior bridge. The upper right central incisor is a pontic and implant are located in the sites of the other four missing teeth.

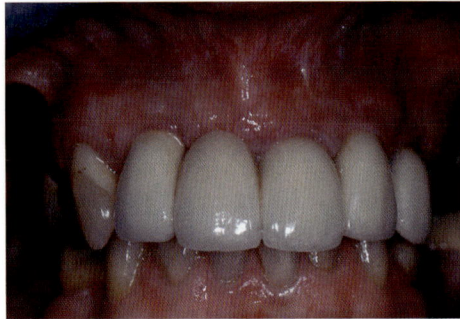

Figure 21b- Radiographs of the four supporting implants.

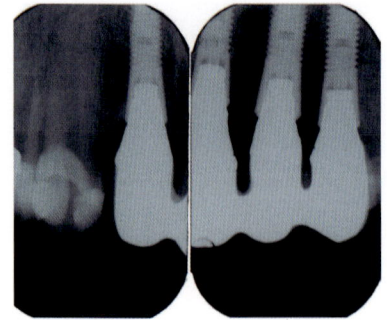

Advantages and disadvantages of treatment options

Removable prostheses

These are a commonly prescribed treatment option and may be used as a long-term restoration or provisional restoration prior to a fixed prosthesis (*Fig.18*).

Advantages
• Replace multiple teeth in multiple sites.
• Support obtained from mucosa and/or teeth.
• Generally do not require extensive preparation of abutment teeth.
• May be designed to accommodate future tooth loss.
• Can be used to replace missing soft tissue.
• Can provide good lip support by incorporating labial flanges.
• Aesthetics may be very good.
• The least expensive of restorations.

Disadvantages
• Removable prostheses may not be liked by patient and may reduce self-confidence.
• Connectors cover soft tissue such as the palate and gingiva.
• In subjects with less than ideal oral hygiene they may compromise the health of the periodontal tissues and promote caries around abutment teeth.
• Retentive elements such as clasps may spoil aesthetics.
• Moderate maintenance requirements and durability.

Fixed prostheses

Fixed prostheses fall into two main categories
1. Resin bonded bridgework (*Fig.19*).
2. Conventional partial or full coverage bridgework (*Fig.20*).

Resin bonded bridgework

Advantages
• Minimal or no preparation required.
• Fixed restoration.
• Good aesthetics if ideal spacing exists and abutment teeth are satisfactory.
• Less expensive than conventional bridges.
• Consequence of failure are relatively small –caries is readily diagnosed in most

instances. Cantilever designs for single tooth replacements minimise potential problems.

Disadvantages
• Lack of predictability: decementation leading to loss of retention or caries under one of the retainers – average life span 5 to 7 years.
• Dependent upon meticulous technique and available enamel/surface area for bonding.
• Change in colour/translucency of abutment teeth due to presence of retainer
• May interfere with occlusion, particularly incisal guidance.
• Patients may feel sense of insecurity with restoration, especially if their bridge has debonded previously.

Conventional partial or full coverage bridgework

Advantages
• Fixed.
• Good appearance, including that of abutment teeth if they need to be improved/harmonised.
• Medium term predictability is good for short span bridges.
• Good control of occlusion possible.
• Minimally compromise oral hygiene.

Disadvantages
• Involve considerable tooth preparation which sometimes result in pulpal sequelae.
• Failure due to decementation and caries of abutment teeth may lead to further tooth loss.
• Moderately expensive.
• Highly operator dependent requiring exacting techniques both clinically and technically.
• Requires lengthy clinical time and temporary restorations.
• Irreversible.

Implant retained prostheses

An implant retained fixed bridge prosthesis is shown in *Fig. 21*.

Advantages
• Fixed or removable.
• Independent of natural teeth – can provide fixed restoration where no abutment teeth exist.

- Immune to dental caries.
- High level of predictability.
- Good maintenance of supporting bone.

Disadvantages
- Dependent upon presence of adequate bone quantity and quality.
- Involves surgical procedure(s).
- Highly operator/technique dependent.
- High initial expense and lengthy treatment time.
- Moderate maintenance requirements especially for removable or extensive fixed prostheses.

Treatment choices

In situations where all types of prosthesis are possible the final choice may rest with the patient, and is largely dependent upon their expectations/desires, financial budget and willingness to undergo treatment. It is important that the patient's expectations are realistic and achievable. However, some factors may dictate that a certain type of restoration is not feasible or is undesirable. This can best be illustrated by considering a number of case studies (see Case A to Case C).

Conclusion
The patient should be presented with the treatment alternatives and an indication of their respective advantages and disadvantages in their particular case. The treatment plans should be outlined in writing and an estimate of the relative costs given. Complex treatment plans require more detailed descriptions and a projected timetable for completion and costings. It is important to ensure that the patient understands the proposals and is given the opportunity to clarify any matters. A written consent to the agreed treatment plan is advisable.

Case A – Figure 22a and 22b

Figure 22 shows a young female (aged 27 years) who had a developmentally missing lateral incisor replaced with a 3 unit fixed bridge. The preparation of the adjacent teeth is destructive but does allow changing the size, shape and colour of all the involved teeth. The available space for the lateral incisor crown was small and a simple cantilever resin bonded bridge should have been a better alternative. The radiograph in figure 22b shows that the roots of the incisor and canine are divergent providing good space apically to accommodate an implant but limited space at the crestal region. Emergence of an implant crown through a site with little space can compromise the soft tissue health. If a single tooth implant had been considered then prior orthodontic treatment could have improved this situation.

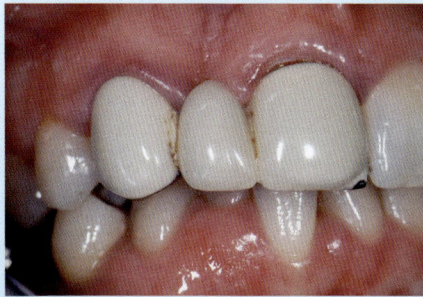

Figure 22a- A young patient with a conventional three unit fixed bridge replacing the upper right lateral incisor.

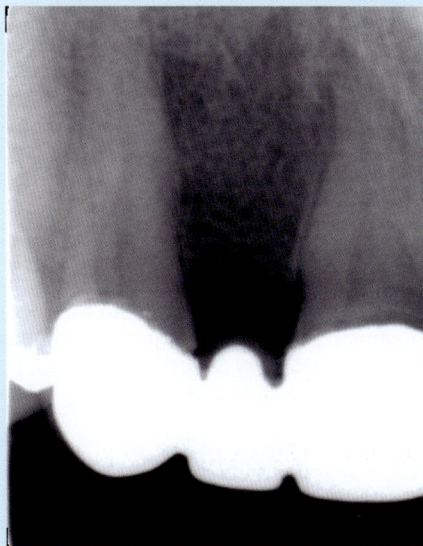

Figure 22b- Radiograph of the supporting teeth demonstrating divergent roots and a narrow space at crown level.

Figure 23a- A large anterior edentulous space following traumatic loss of teeth.

Figure 23b- The patient wearing a removable partial denture bearing 4 teeth with spaces between them.

Figure 23c- The same patient with a diagnostic set up placing five teeth in the gap and no spaces.

Case B – Figure 23

Figure 23 illustrates a young female (aged 35 years) who lost four anterior teeth in an accident (figure 23a). The edentulous span is wide and the abutment teeth not ideal. The edentulous ridge form is good and a labial flange is not required for aesthetics or lip support. The present removable prosthesis (figure 23b) provides good aesthetics with a natural looking spaced dentition. She requests a fixed prosthesis. A diagnostic set up which eliminates the diastemas by increasing the number of prosthetic teeth is shown in figure 23c. This setup would be required for a conventional fixed bridge but was unacceptable to the patient as she wanted to maintain the appearance of a spaced dentition. She therefore has two choices – a removeable prosthesis or four individual single tooth implants.

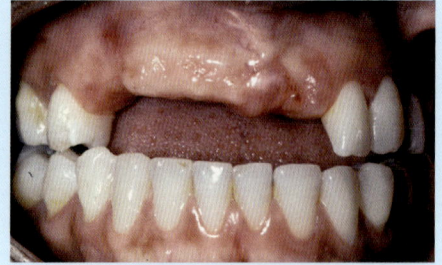

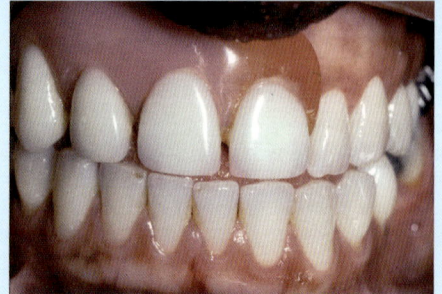

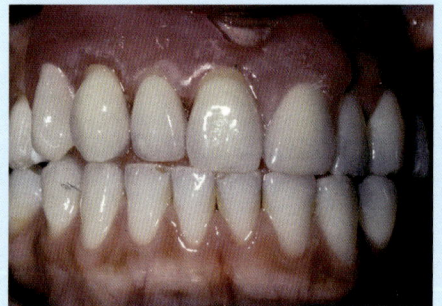

Figure 24a- A three unit posterior maxillary bridge replacing the first molar.

Figure 24b- A radiograph of the bridge and associated structures showing a large maxillary air sinus and a large post in the premolar root.

Case C – Figure 24

Figure 24 shows a patient with a failing posterior maxillary bridge with decementation of the posterior abutment (second molar). Replacement of this bridge is difficult. The bridge could be sectioned to allow removal of the crowns and assessment of the condition of the individual abutments. Restoration of the individual teeth with single crowns and replacement of the missing first molar with an implant is a possibility. But there is a large air sinus that would need extensive bone grafting prior to implant placement and the second premolar has an unfavourable prognosis as it has been root treated and a large post crown provided. The second premolar tooth could also be replaced with an implant. If the second molar has a good prognosis a new fixed bridge extending to the first premolar could be considered, replacing both the second premolar and first molar, but this is a long span and the long term prognosis would be uncertain.

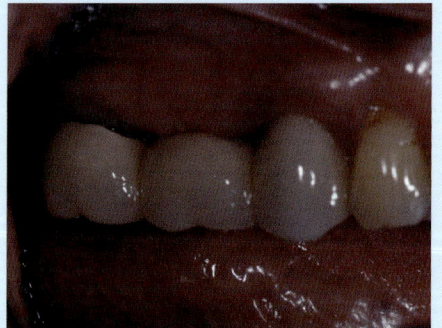

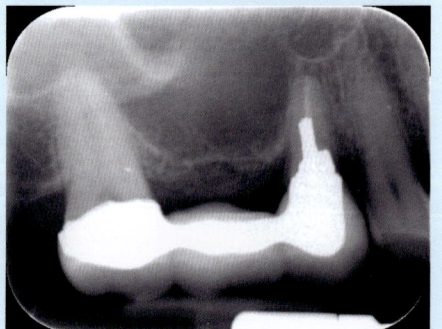

Treatment planning for implant restorations

Treatment planning may be facilitated by determining the desired result that meets the need of the patient, and then planning in reverse order to achieve this goal.

Treatment planning for the provision of an implant retained restoration is essentially the same as that for a conventional prosthesis, except it also has to consider the provision of an adequate number, type, position and distribution of implants. It therefore involves a surgical phase of treatment (Chapter 6) and usually a time delay for the process of osseointegration to take place. The treatment plan should begin with a clear idea of the end result, which should fulfil the functional and aesthetic needs of the patient. It is important that these goals are realistic, predictable and readily maintainable.

Types of implant restoration

Before considering the more detailed aspects of planning the following types of implant retained restorations are described:
- Fixed bridges
- Overdentures
- Single tooth restorations

Fixed bridges

Implant retained fixed bridges range from limited span bridges to complete arch restorations for the edentulous jaw. There are two basic bridge designs, the original type as described by Branemark which has a cast metal bar with acrylic teeth and 'gumwork' attached to a number of implants and resembles a "denture on stilts" (*Fig.1*), and the more aesthetic approach where it resembles conventional bridgework with implants placed so that the prosthetic teeth appear to emerge from the natural soft tissues (*Fig.2*). These two designs will be considered in more detail.

The original Branemark 'bone anchored bridge' is the design on which many of the long-term success reports are based. It was largely used in the mandible and required the placement of four to six implants between the mental foramina. A cast metal framework is cantilevered distally, generally to a distance

of no more than 12mm but determined by the size of the bar and the maximum antero-posterior distance between implant centres.

In the mandibular arch, prosthetic stability has been reported for 99% of fixed prostheses over a 15-year period. However, lack of facial support and cheek biting can lead to poor appearance and functional limitations, especially in patients with more advanced bone resorption. Fixed prostheses in the mandible opposing a complete denture may also cause more bone loss in the opposing jaw than a mandibular overdenture. More frequent maxillary denture relines and increased retention problems have been noted.

Although maxillary prosthetic survival rates of 92% have been reported over a 15-year period, more complications are encountered. Phonetic problems are the most frequent complaint. Spaces between the bridge and the underlying soft tissues result in breaks in the palatal contour and speech disruption. Oral hygiene may be compromised if acrylic flanges are extended over abutments and soft tissue hyperplasia may occur. Although the situation can be improved by placing a removable gingival veneer, they are complex and technically demanding restorations. The appearance can be very good but in patients with less ridge resorption or a high smile line, there is a likelihood of aesthetic problems.

The alternative bridge design is similar to a conventional fixed bridge prosthesis constructed on natural teeth and can be cemented or screw retained. In favourable circumstances, with minimal bone resorption, it is possible to achieve optimal aesthetics. Conversely when there has been substantial loss of bone, or when soft tissue replacement is required, it may be impossible to achieve the desired aesthetic result with this type of prosthesis. Where there is considerable resorption, the prosthetic teeth become progressively long, with large spaces apparent interproximally [so called "black tri-

Figure 1- The upper crowned natural teeth oppose a full arch implant-supported bridge in the lower jaw. The bridge is similar in design and concept to that described by Branemark. Titanium abutments protrude a few millimetres through the mucosa and a space separates the bridge superstructure from the underlying mucosa. The prosthetic teeth are acrylic and have 'gumwork' in much the same fashion as a complete denture. This bridge is very rigid and is not removable by the patient.

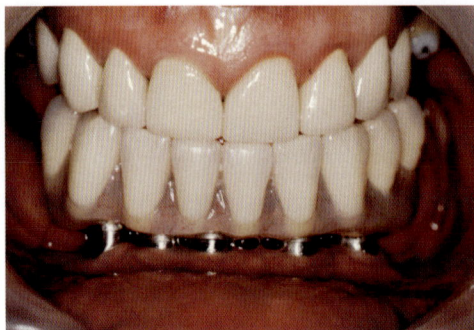

Figure 2- An implant supported maxillary bridge opposing a crowned natural dentition. Maxillary bridges usually require a more aesthetic approach and the design of bridge gives the impression that the teeth are emerging from the gum. The bridge design in figure 1 would not be suitable in this case.

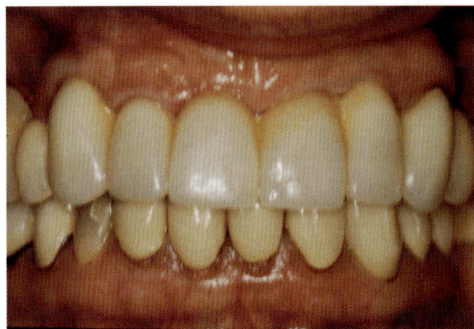

Figure 3a- The upper right central incisor has been replaced with a single tooth implant in this patient with a spaced dentition. The soft tissue contours are very good even though the diastemas are quite large.

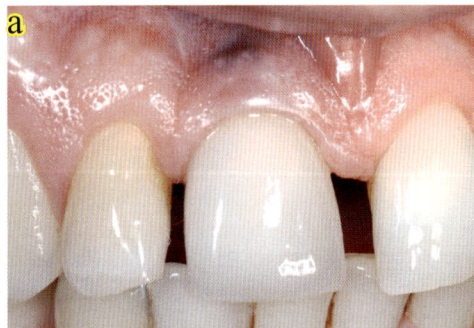

Figure 3b- A Periapical radiograph of the case shown in figure 3a. The bone levels are at an ideal location at the top of the implant.

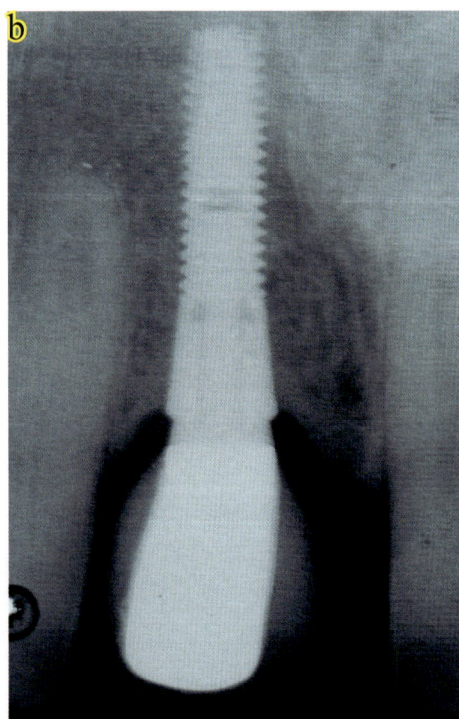

angles"]. In patients with a high lip line, the result may be aesthetically unacceptable and the large spaces also compromise speech.

Bone grafting may be necessary to avoid this problem (Chapter 7) or an alternative restoration chosen, such as an overdenture or patient detachable bridgework. In the latter design a cast metal bar is attached to an equivalent number of implants used for fixed bridgework. A superstructure bearing the prosthetic teeth and a labial flange can be removed by the patient for daily oral hygiene. The restoration is implant supported and although the teeth and labial flange are detachable there is a high level of 'security'. The restoration is difficult to manufacture, requiring a high level of precision with retention of the removable section of the prosthesis dependent on the accuracy of fit onto the milled bar.

Overdentures

These are patient removable complete dentures retained usually by implants joined with a bar or with 'ball' attachments. This subject is dealt with in more detail in Chapter 10.

Single tooth restorations

Single tooth restorations are individual free-standing units not connected to other teeth or implants (*Fig.3*). They are similar to conventional single crowns and are normally cemented to prefabricated or customised abutments. Cantilever units are not normally recommended, and if two adjacent teeth are missing the requirement is usually for placement of two implants. If more than two adjacent teeth are missing, for example four incisor teeth, the decision has to be made whether to restore the space with four single units or a fixed bridge using fewer implants. The latter option is the one most often used because space is not normally available to provide an implant per tooth (see later section on implant spacing).

High success rates have been reported for single tooth restorations, particularly those replacing anterior teeth. Replacement of single molars is more problematic because of the size discrepancy between implant and tooth and the high occlusal loads. Therefore, wider diameter (5-6mm) or two standard diameter implants may be used if space and finances allow.

Planning considerations

- Functional and aesthetic considerations
- Evaluation of the edentulous ridge
- Study casts and diagnostic set-ups
- Implant numbers and spacing

For simplicity, it will be assumed that treatment options other than implant retained restorations have been considered (Chapter 3) and there are no contra-indications. Planning begins with an assessment of the aesthetic and functional requirements, and proceeds to more detailed planning with intra-oral examination, diagnostic set-ups, appropriate radiographic examination (Chapter 5), and construction of provisional restorations and surgical guides.

Functional and aesthetic considerations

Reduced or insufficient function is a common complaint for patients who have removable dentures or who have lost many molar teeth. Function of an otherwise adequate denture may be improved by providing implants to aid stability and retention. The alternative treatment is to replace the denture with a fixed bridge. The overdenture may be the treatment of choice where:

- The patient does not have a psychological problem with dentures and is quite happy to wear a removable restoration.
- There is considerable resorption of the jaws allowing too few implants to be placed for a fixed bridge.
- The opposing jaw is restored with a satisfactory denture or the opposing teeth may be compromised by the occlusal forces generated by a fixed implant supported restoration.

The fixed bridge may be the treatment of choice where:

1. There is a good dentition in the opposing jaw which may de-stabilise the denture. This is a particular problem where a natural dentition in the maxilla opposes an edentulous mandible (*Fig.1*).
2. Patients have such a strong gag reflex that they cannot tolerate a removable prosthesis.
3. Resorption of the jaws is not too advanced thereby allowing placement of an adequate number of implants, and the prosthetic replacement of large amounts of soft and hard tissue is not required.

A shortened dental arch extending to the first molar or second premolar should be considered. Providing there are sufficient well distributed implants in the anterior part of the jaw, a distal cantilever extension can be used thereby avoiding placement of implants in more difficult anatomical locations. Patients who request replacement of missing molar teeth need sufficient bone above the inferior dental canal or below the maxillary sinus floor to allow implants of sufficient size to withstand high occlusal forces. For example, replacement of the first and second molars would normally require three standard 4mm diameter implants joined together with a fixed bridge. The occlusion should be carefully assessed, particularly in all excursive movements. It may be helpful to examine the occlusion with the existing prosthesis or the provisional prosthesis to assess the type of loading to which the implant restoration will be subjected. It is also important to determine the available vertical space for the prosthesis (*Fig. 4*).

Aesthetic considerations can be of great importance in many patients. The coverage of the anterior teeth (and gingivae) by the lips during normal function and smiling should be carefully assessed (*Figs. 5 and 6*). An anterior restoration should also provide adequate lip support. The appearance of the planned restoration can be judged by providing a diagnostic set up or a provisional prosthesis. They may also serve extremely well as a model for the surgical stent or guide to assist in the optimal placement of the implants (see chapter 6), and as a transitional restoration during the treatment programme. Ideally, the patient should be examined with and without their current or provisional prosthesis to assess facial contours, lip support, tooth position and how much of the prosthesis is revealed during function (*Fig.7*).

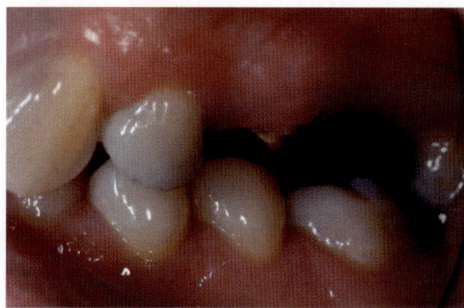

Figure 4- A patient with missing maxillary posterior teeth.

Figure 4a- The clinical view showing relatively little vertical space between the maxillary ridge and the opposing teeth. There may have been some overeruption of the unopposed mandibular premolar.

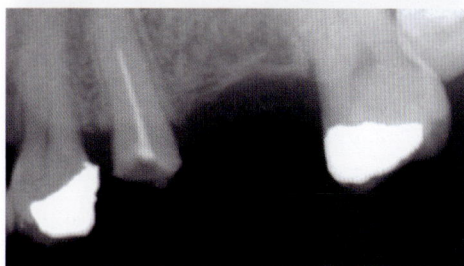

Figure 4b- The radiograph of the same case showing a retained root at the upper left second premolar and good bone height in the first molar space.

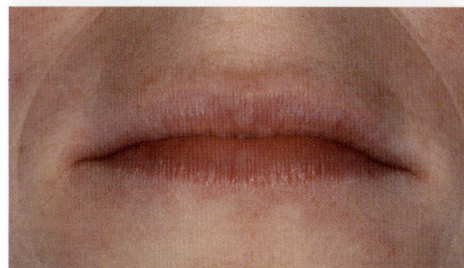

Figure 5a- The lips at rest in a patient with missing central incisor teeth who wishes to have a fixed prosthesis.

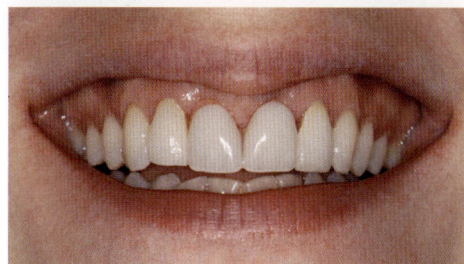

Figure 5b- The patient smiling revealing several millimetres of gingivae and a good appearance with his existing partial denture.

Figure 5c- A intra-oral view showing a nice dentition and ridge lap pontics on the partial denture.

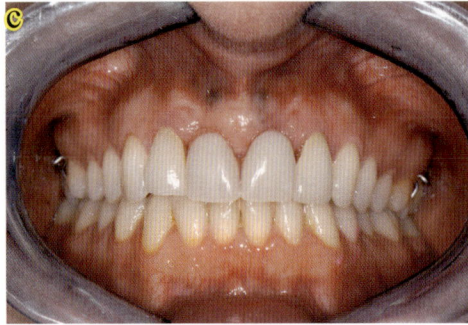

Figure 5d- The ridge height in the central incisor region is good.

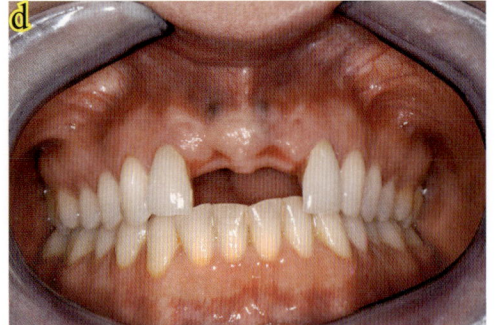

Figure 5e- An occlusal view indicating that there is probably good ridge width.

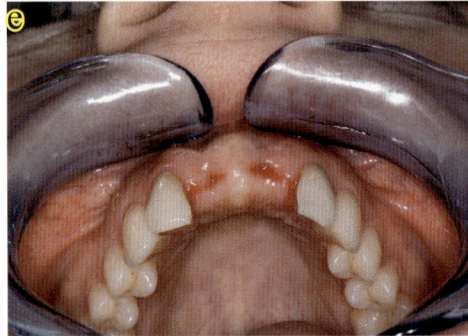

Figure 5f- An intra-oral periapical radiograph showing good bone height.

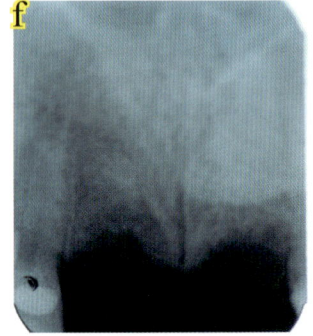

Figure 6a- This smile line does not have great aesthetic demands and it is difficult to determine which tooth has been replaced with a prosthesis.

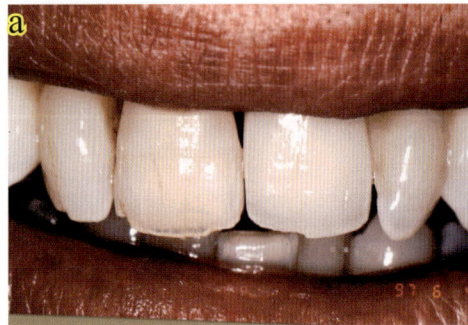

Figure 6b- An intra-oral view of the same individual revealing the implant retained crown at the upper left central incisor. The patient was happy to have a restoration which did not have a gingival margin at a level more consistent with the other teeth.

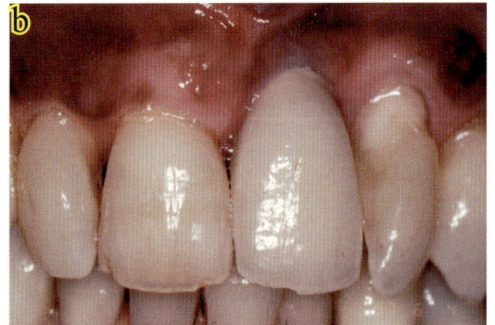

Figure 6c- Another patient who has had the left incisor tooth replaced with a single tooth implant showing acceptable aesthetics when smiling.

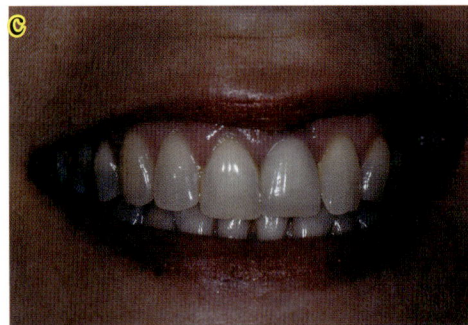

Figure 6d- The intra-oral radiograph of the case shown in Figure 6c.

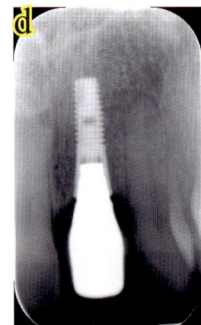

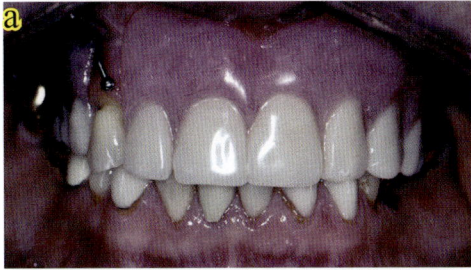

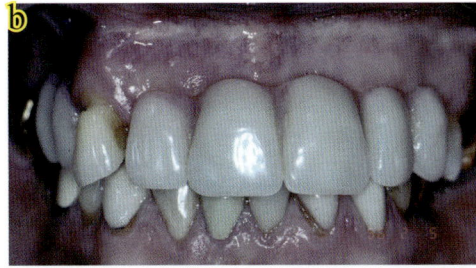

Figure 7a- A female patient with the maxillary anterior teeth replaced with an acrylic removable partial denture which has a labial flange. The patient requested an implant supported bridge and did not want a denture.

Figure 7b- The diagnostic set-up. Denture teeth have been set up in a ridge lap fashion without a labial flange.

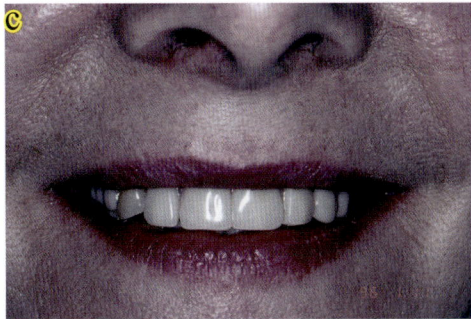

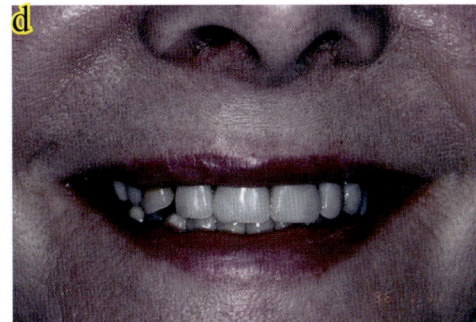

Figure 7c- The patient smiling with the original denture complete with labial flange.

Figure 7d- The patient smiling with the diagnostic set up. There is less lip support without the labial flange.

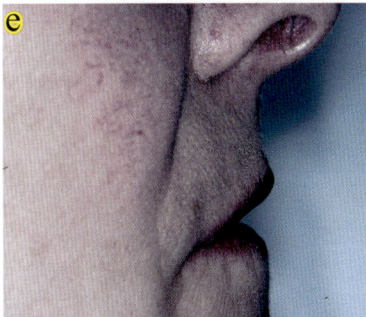

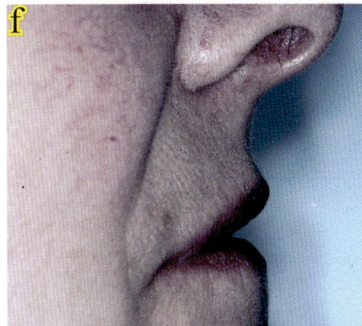

Figure 7e- Lip support in profile with the original denture.

Figure 7f- Lip support in profile with the diagnostic set up. Although there is less lip support the patient is satisfied with the appearance. Therefore it is possible to consider a fixed bridge reconstruction without additional lip support.

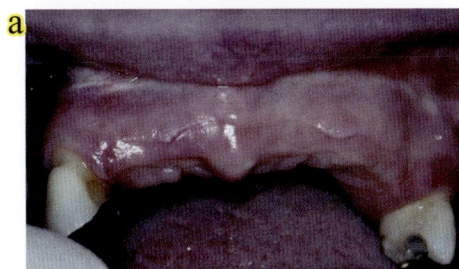

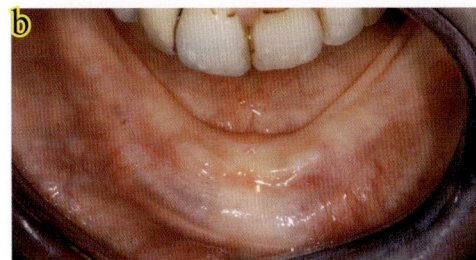

Figure 8a- The edentulous ridge in the patient shown in Figure 7. There is good ridge height and plenty of attached keratinised tissue.

Figure 8b- An edentulous mandibular ridge with moderate to severe resorption. There is a small zone of attached keratinised mucosa.

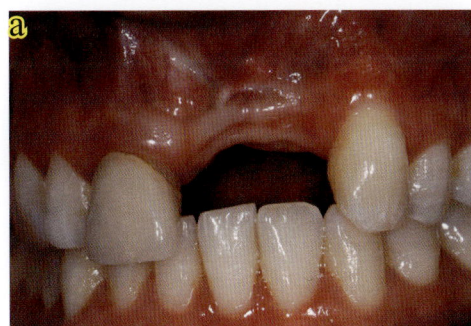

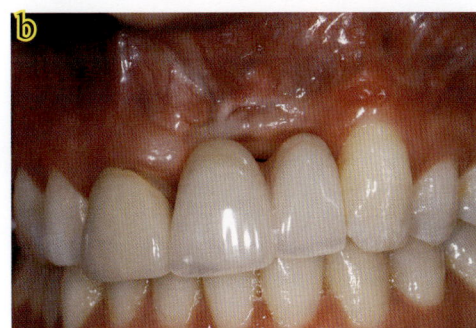

Figure 9a- Traumatic loss of the upper left central and lateral incisor has resulted in loss of ridge height and ridge thickness.

Figure 9b- The existing ridge lapped partial denture indicate that the patient would require grafting if this appearance were not acceptable.

Evaluation of the edentulous ridge

The height, width and contour of the ridge can be visually assessed and carefully palpated (*Figs.8 and 9*). The presence of concavities/depressions particularly on the labial aspects are usually readily detected. However, accurate assessment of the underlying bone width is difficult, especially where the overlying tissue is fibrous. This occurs on the palate where the tissue may be very thick and can result in a very false impression of the bone profile. Clinical techniques such as ridge mapping have been advocated but this is prone to error and the advent of high quality tomography (Chapter 5) has made it almost obsolete.

The distance between the edentulous ridge and the opposing dentition should be measured to ensure that there is adequate room for the restorative components. The angulation of the ridge and its relationship to the opposing dentition is also important. Proclined ridge forms will tend to lead to proclined placement of the implants, which could affect aesthetics and loading. Large horizontal discrepancies between the jaws, for example the pseudo class III jaw relationship following extensive maxillary resorption may not be suitable for treatment with fixed bridges.

The clinical examination of the ridge also allows assessment of the soft tissue thickness, which is important for the attainment of good aesthetics. Keratinised tissue, which is attached to the edentulous ridge, will also generally provide a better peri-implant soft tissue than non-keratinised mobile mucosa (Chapter 2). The length of the edentulous ridge can be measured to give an indication of the possible number of implants that could be accommodated. However, this also requires reference to radiographs to allow a correlation with available bone volume and the diagnostic set-up for the proposed tooth location. In edentulous ridges bound by teeth, the available space will also be affected by angulation of adjacent tooth roots, which may be palpated and assessed radiographically (*Fig.10*).

Study casts and diagnostic set-ups

Study casts allow detailed measurements of many of the factors considered in the previous section. The proposed replacement teeth can be positioned on the casts by the technician using either denture teeth or teeth carved in wax (*Fig. 11*). The former have the advantage that they can be converted into a temporary restoration, which can be evaluated in the mouth by the clinician and patient (*Figs. 5 and 7*). The diagnostic set-up therefore determines the number and position of the teeth to be replaced and their occlusal relationship with the opposing dentition.

Once the diagnostic set-up has been approved it can be used to construct a stent or guide for radiographic imaging (*Fig.12a* and see Chapter 5) and surgical placement of the implants (*Fig.12b* and see Chapter 6). The stent/guide can be positioned on the original cast and with reference to the radiographs, the clinician can decide upon the optimum location, number, and type of implants.

Implant numbers and spacing

There are a few general guidelines as to the number of implants that are required in different situations (Table 1).

Table 1

Fixed restorations:-	
Anterior teeth	*Suggested number of implants required*
One missing tooth	1
Two missing teeth	2
Three missing teeth	2 or 3
Four missing teeth	2,3 or 4
Molar teeth	
One missing tooth	1 or 2
Two missing teeth	2 or 3
Full arch bridges	
Edentulous maxilla	at least 6
Edentulous mandible	at least 4
Removable restorations:-	
Overdentures	
Edentulous maxilla	at least 4 (joined)
Edentulous mandible	2

The more teeth which require replacement, the greater the variation, especially when molar teeth are considered. For example, four missing lower incisors could be replaced quite readily with two implants supporting a four unit bridge. Four missing upper incisors could be replaced with a bridge supported by two or three implants, but four implants would be required in a spaced dentition.

Two missing molar teeth would require three standard 4mm diameter implants, or alternatively two wider diameter implants. Implants with different diameters can be chosen according to the tooth they are replacing. For example, most systems have a standard implant of about 4mm in diameter that can be used in most situations. However, replacement of single upper lateral incisors, or lower incisors, may require narrower diameter implants (eg 3.25mm) whereas a molar tooth may be replaced with an implant of 5 to 6 mm diameter.

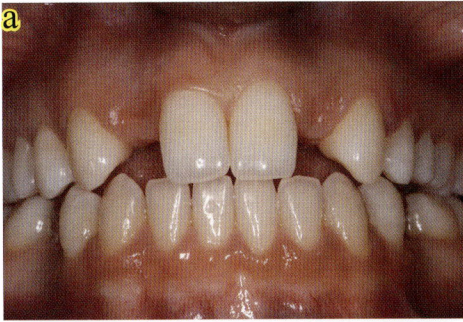

Figure 10a- A young individual who has completed orthodontics to produce a good situation for replacement of the missing lateral incisor teeth. The clinical appearance indicates good root alignment and good ridge profiles.

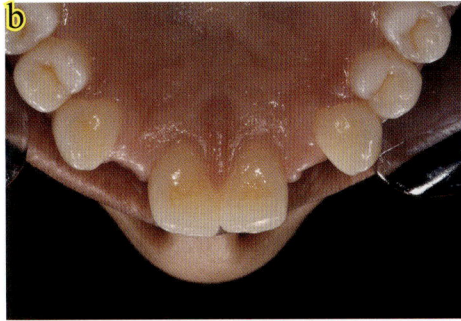

Figure 10b- An occlusal view showing adequate mesial distal space.

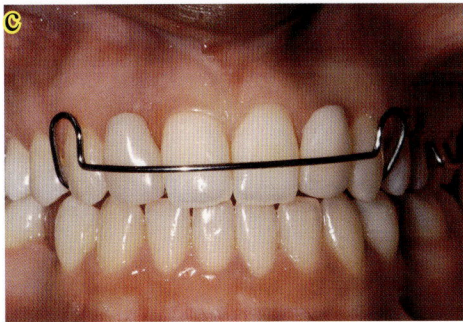

Figure 10c- The orthodontic retainer with prosthetic teeth showing good aesthetics.

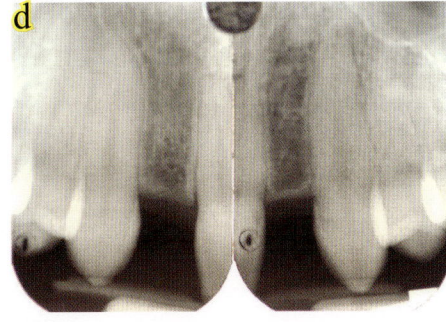

Figure 10d- Intra-oral radiographs confirming good root alignment and minimal acceptable spacing for implant placement.

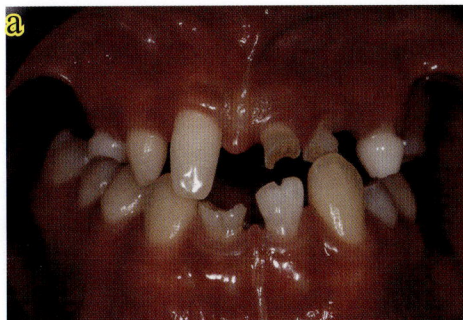

Figure 11a- A young individual with severe hypodontia and microdontia undergoing initial planning. The intra-oral appearance showing poor aesthetics and suggesting poor function.

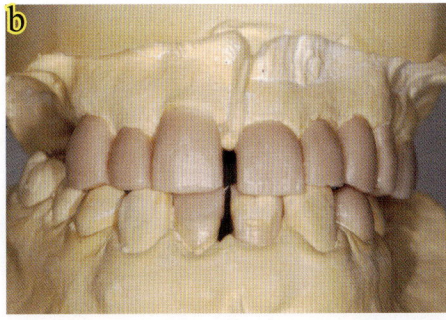

Figure 11b- A diagnostic wax up increasing the size of some teeth which are to be retained and replacing others which may be extracted.

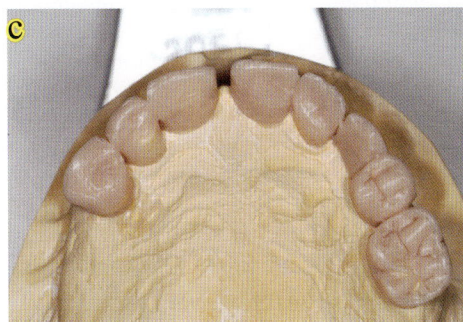

Figure 11c- An occlusal view of the same wax up.

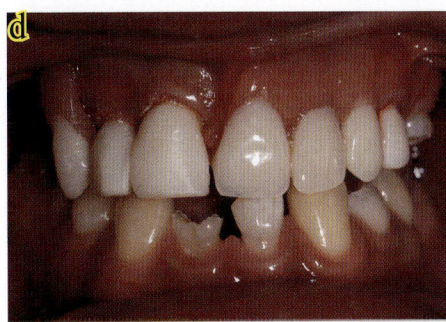

Figure 11d- The maxillary diagnostic set up has been reproduced in the mouth through composite build ups of upper right two, upper right one and upper left four and a partial denture to replace upper right three, upper left one, upper left three, upper left two. From this point further planning will be carried out to replace the denture with an implant supported restoration and manage the remaining mandibular teeth.

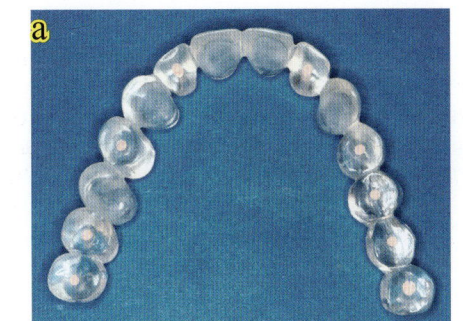

Figure 12a- An acrylic stent made from a diagnostic wax up and provisional fixed bridge. Radio-opaque markers have been placed in this stent which can be worn by the patient in place of the provisional bridge during the radiographic examination.

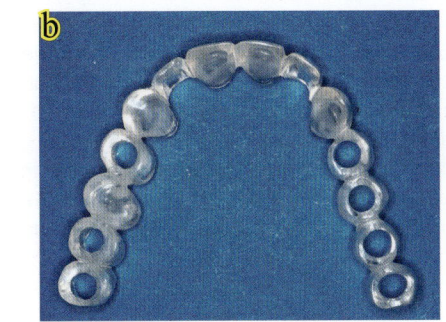

Figure 12b- The same stent subsequently adapted for guidance during implant placement.

Figure 13a- A periapical radiograph showing replacement of two premolar teeth in the upper jaw with two single tooth implants. The space is just enough to allow adequate spacing and bone between implants and between the implants and adjacent teeth.

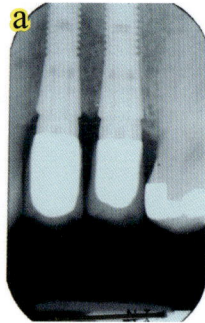

Figure 13b- The clinical appearance of the two premolar crowns. A space must be adequate to accommodate the abutments and crowns and to permit a suitable path of insertion for all components.

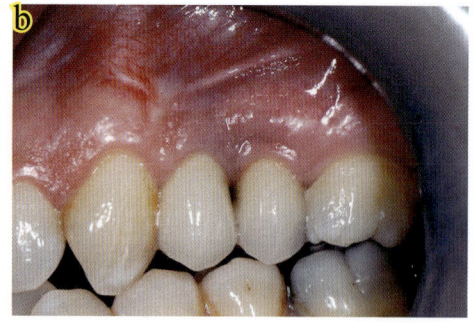

Figure 14a- Prior to orthodontics there is spacing between the incisor teeth and rotation of the premolars.

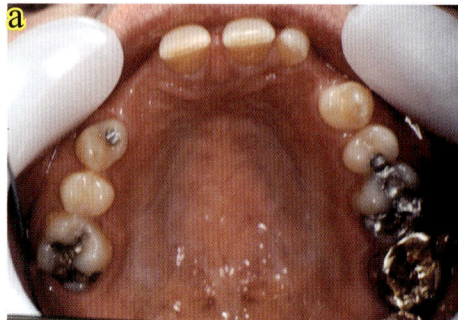

Figure 14b- Nearing completion of orthodontic treatment with closure of spacing and derotation of the premolars thereby providing better spacing for implant placement.

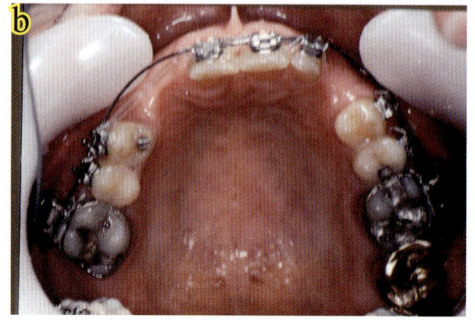

Figure 15a- A labial view of a Rochette bridge replacing the upper left lateral incisor and upper right central incisor.

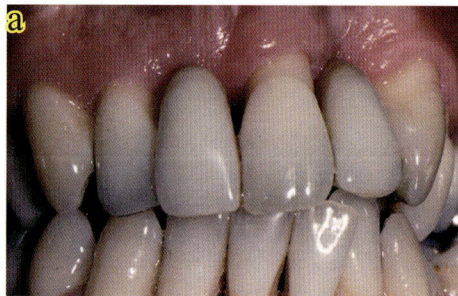

Figure 15b- An occlusal view of the Rochette bridge. Removal of composite from the retention holes should enable removal of the bridge if implant treatment is planned.

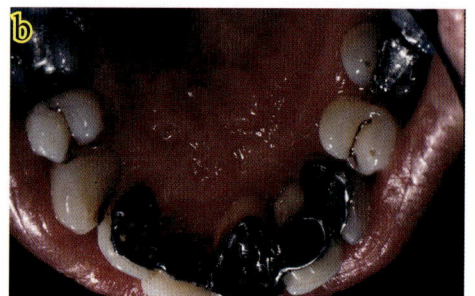

It is a great mistake to attempt to place too many implants in a given space (*Fig.13*) and, if necessary, orthodontic treatment should be used to optimise spacing (*Fig.14*). Spacing is required to provide:

- An adequate width of bone and soft tissue between implants and adjacent teeth
- For the prosthetic components not to impact on each other
- For the patient to be able to clean the prosthesis effectively.

Implants placed next to natural teeth should allow an absolute minimum of 1mm of intervening bone and preferably 2mm. It is advisable to allow a little more spacing between implant heads, ideally 3mm and no less than 2mm. This is because in many systems the abutments are larger than the implant heads, and the restoration is often designed so that it increases in diameter to establish a good emergence profile. Connection of narrower abutments than the implant head allows for more soft tissue space and has been termed "platform switching".

With all these factors competing for space it is easy to see how the soft tissue and oral hygiene may be compromised if implants are placed too close together.

The bone volume that can accommodate the proposed diameter and length of implant has to be determined radiographically. Implants should be selected to ensure optimum initial stability, but are seldom longer than 15mm. In many instances the clinician is limited by the need to avoid damage to important anatomical structures, such as the inferior dental nerve. The assessment of length should allow an adequate safety margin, particularly as most drills are designed to prepare the implant site slightly longer than the chosen implant.

Provisional restorations

In the majority of treatment plans the provisional restoration is an essential component. It helps to establish the design of the final reconstruction and is used by the patient throughout the treatment stages. The following provisional restorations are used:

- Complete denture
- Partial denture
- Adhesive bridgework
- Fixed bridgework

Complete dentures are used as a provisional restoration for edentulous patients. There is a period (at least 1 week) following surgical placement of implants when the denture wear may be limited. This avoids early loading of the implants and allows adequate reduction of post surgical oedema to take place, facilitating proper adaptation of the denture. In general bone grafting and ridge augmentation procedures should not be carried out unless the denture can be left out for a considerable period after surgery.

Partial dentures can be used for anterior and posterior saddles. They are simple and inexpensive to construct. Acrylic dentures allow easy adjustment to accommodate any changes in tissue profile following implant placement and when the transmucosal abutments are fitted.

Adhesive bridgework is most commonly used as a provisional restoration in the replacement of single teeth or small spans in anterior regions. A single tooth replacement is normally retained by a single adjacent retainer, whereas the replacement of multiple teeth requires more abutments. Provisional retainers should be easily removable and, therefore, the Rochette rather than Maryland design is recommended (*Fig.15*).

Fixed bridgework retained by full coverage restorations may be the treatment of choice for patients having extensive treatment who are not prepared to undergo a period of time without a fixed restoration. This assumes the presence of a sufficient number of teeth to support the provisional or transitional bridge. It also enables ridge augmentation procedures to be carried out without the risk of transmucosal loading and the associated micromovement affecting the healing. The bridgework may have to remain in place some considerable time with frequent removal and replacement. Abutment teeth must be adequately prepared to allow for the casting of a metal framework of sufficient strength and rigidity and for the acrylic/composite facings. Allowance should be made for the fact that the bridge will have to be modified following abutment connection.

Treatment order

Deciding on the treatment order may be very straightforward in some circumstances and in others extremely difficult, particularly for those cases involving transitional restorations.

A traditional plan may include the points listed in *Table 2*.

Table 2.	Traditional Plan
•	Examination – clinical and initial radiographic
•	Diagnostic set-up, provisional restoration and specialised radiographs if required
•	Discussion of treatment options and decision on final restoration
•	Completion of any necessary dental treatment including: extraction of hopeless teeth; periodontal treatment; restorative treatment; new restorations and/or endodontics as required
•	Construction of provisional or transitional restorations if required
•	Construction of surgical guide or stent
•	Surgical placement of implants
•	Allowing adequate time for osseointegration
•	Prosthodontic phase

Conclusion

Treatment planning for implant restorations may at first appear complicated. It is imperative to consider all treatment options with the patient, and during detailed planning it may become apparent that an alternative solution is preferred. In all cases the implant treatment should be part of an overall plan to ensure the health of any remaining teeth. Once the goal or end point has been established it should be possible to work back to formulate the treatment sequence. The cost of the proposed treatment plan is also of great relevance, and this may therefore place limits on treatment options.

Radiographic techniques

Radiographic examination is a central part of implant treatment from the planning phase to the long-term evaluation of treatment success.

Standard dental radiographs allow the clinician to make an initial assessment of the bone levels available for implant treatment, but as 2-dimensional images they give no indication of bone width. In combination with clinical examination they may provide enough information to plan treatment without resorting to more complex imaging techniques. Tomographic examinations can give cross-sectional and 3-dimensional images. In addition to providing information about bone quantity they also provide some indication of the bone quality available, notably the thickness of the cortices as well as a measure of the density of the cancellous bone.

A standard classification of bone quantity and quality has been devised and is useful to describe the degree of alveolar resorption present (*Fig.1*) although the quality is often a subjective assessment at the time of surgery. Radiographs are also used during treatment and provide an assessment of peri-implant bone levels and long-term maintenance.

The Dental Panoramic Tomograph (DPT) is often the radiograph of choice (*Fig.2*) and gives the clinician an indication of:

- The overall status of teeth and supporting bone
- Those sites where it is possible to place implants using a straight-forward protocol
- Those sites where it is unlikely that implants can be placed without using complex procedures such as grafting
- Those sites where it is inadvisable to recommend implants
- Anatomical anomalies or pathological lesions

They provide an image within a predefined focal trough of both upper and lower jaws and as such give a reasonable approximation of bone height, the position of the inferior dental neurovascular bundle, the size and position of the maxillary antra and any pathological conditions that may be present. They are therefore an ideal view for initial treatment planning and for providing patient information as they present the image in a way that many patients are able to understand. Most are narrow beam rotational tomographs, which use two or more centres of rotation to produce an image of the dental arches. Some areas may not be imaged particularly well but this can be minimised by ensuring that the patient is positioned correctly in the machine and that the appropriate programme is selected. The radiation dosage of a DPT is approximately 0.016 to 0.026 mSv. In contrast, a periapical accounts for only about 0.001 to 0.002 mSv. The DPT does provide more information about associated anatomical structures than periapical radiographs but with less fine detail of the teeth. It should be remembered that all DPT's are magnified images (at around x 1.3 for conventional film based machines). Distortion also occurs in the antero-posterior dimension reducing their usefulness when planning implant spacing and numbers.

The information provided by a DPT can usefully be supplemented using other standard extra-oral and intra-oral radiographs. For example, the lateral cephalogram can give more detail of the morphology of both jaws close to the midline, and this can be useful when planning overdenture treatment (*Fig.3*). Standard occlusal views may also aid in assessing the bone morphology in the lower jaw. Should further information be required following the screening examination, then the appropriate tomographic examination is made.

Conventional tomographic programmes are available on many DPT machines. Tomographic sections are normally 2mm or 4mm in thickness (*Fig 4*). The image produced includes adjacent structures that are not within the focal trough, which therefore appear blurred and out of focus. Because the scan sections are thicker and fewer the overall patient dose is less than a CT scan. The amount of detailed information provided is

Figure 1a- A classification of ridge resorption described by Lekholm and Zarb (1985). Redrawn from Lekholm U, Zarb G. Patient selection and preparation in Tissue Integrated Prosthesis, Branemark P I, Zarb G A, Albrektsson T (eds), pp199-210. Quintessence, 1985.

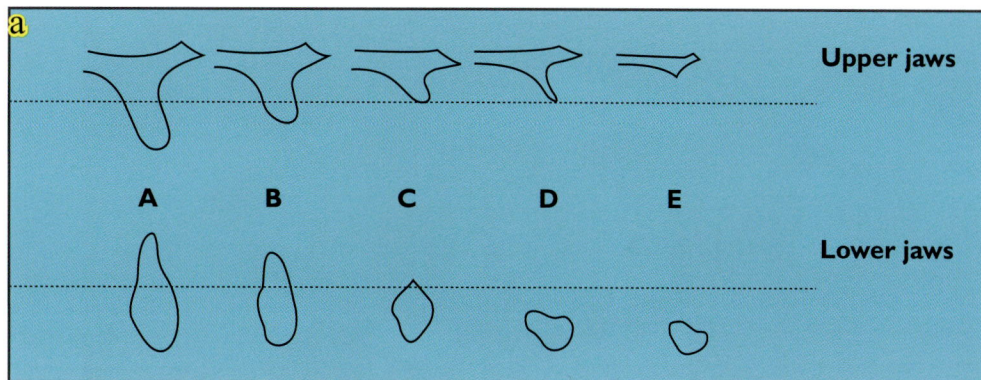

Figure 1b- Bone quality is on a four point scale: Type 1 is mainly cortical, Type 2 is a dense cortex and cancellous space, Type 3 is a thinner cortex and less dense cancellous bone, Type 4 has a very thin cortex and sparse bone trabeculae in the medullary space.

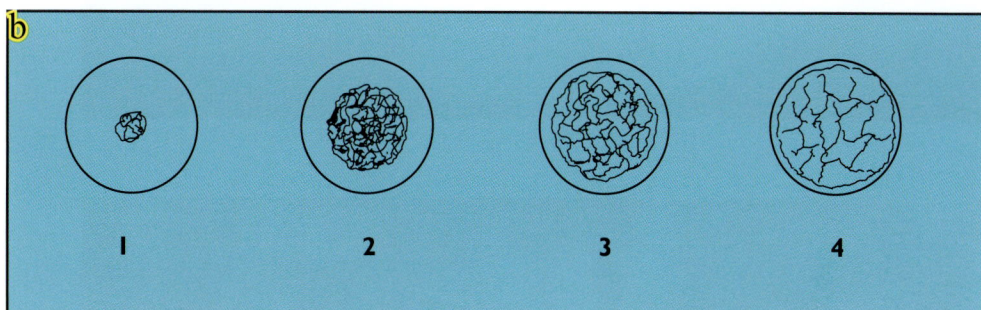

considerably less than a CT scan but is usually sufficient for less complex cases.

Radiography for single tooth replacement or small bridges in individuals with little bone loss can normally be accomplished by intra-oral radiographs taken with a long cone paralleling technique (*Fig 5*). However it must be remembered that an overall evaluation of the mouth should be made for a full assessment of treatment needs. Image quality is of the utmost importance and it should be ensured that all relevant anatomical structures are shown on the image being used and that any allowances for distortion of the image are made. This is particularly important when assessing available bone height above the inferior dental canal and when working close to other important anatomical structures.

In order to facilitate planning using images at different magnifications, overlays depicting implants of various lengths and diameters at the corresponding magnifications can be superimposed directly on the radiograph (*Figs 5b,c*). These provide a simple method of assessing implant sites and implant placement at different angulations.

Radiographic stents

In order to optimise the information provided by more advanced radiographic techniques, it is helpful to provide information about the planned final restoration. A stent, which mimics the desired tooth set-up, is constructed and radiographic markers (e.g. gutta percha, amalgam) placed within it (*Fig.6a*). Alternatively, if the patient has a suitable acrylic denture, radiographic markers may be placed within

occlusal or palatal cavities cut in the acrylic teeth. The denture can also be replicated in clear acrylic to provide the radiographic stent. A radiopaque marker can be placed in the position and angulation of the planned prosthetic set-up. Thus for a screw retained prosthesis the marker would indicate the access hole for the screw retaining the restoration. Alternatively the relation of the bone ridge to the proposed tooth set-up can be shown by painting the surface of the stent with a radiopaque medium (e.g. Temp Bond) or by incorporating barium sulphate within the acrylic (*Fig.6b*). The choice of radiographic marker is important in that it should be visible on the radiographic image but not interfere with the scan. When using Computerised Tomography (CT), metal markers should be avoided as they can produce scattering on the image. Stents are particularly useful in the edentulous patient as they also serve to stabilise the position of the jaws while the radiographs are being taken, and can also provide the radiographer with an occlusal plane from which to orientate the axial scans.

Computerised tomography (CT scan)

CT scans provide the clinician with the most detailed images currently available. Their use is often limited to more complex cases such as full arch maxillary reconstructions, bilateral posterior mandible imaging or to assess whether patients require extensive grafting procedures (*Fig.7*). CT uses x-rays to produce sectional images as in conventional tomography. High resolution images are achieved by initially scanning in an axial plane keeping

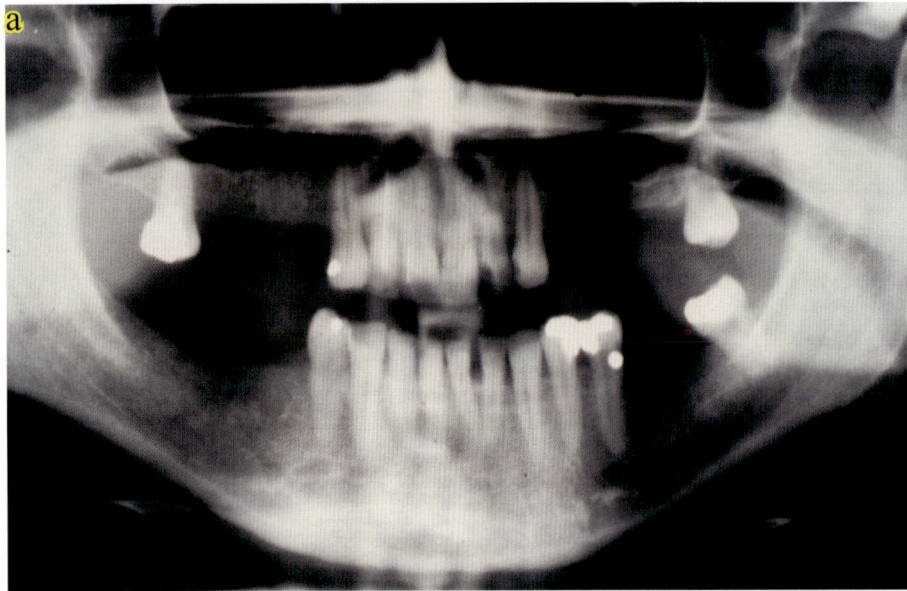

Figure 2a- A dental panoramic tomogram of a partially dentate individual who wished to be treated with implant retained prosthesis. This initial screening radiograph suggests that there is sufficient bone height above the inferior dental canal in the lower right jaw and below the maxillary sinuses.

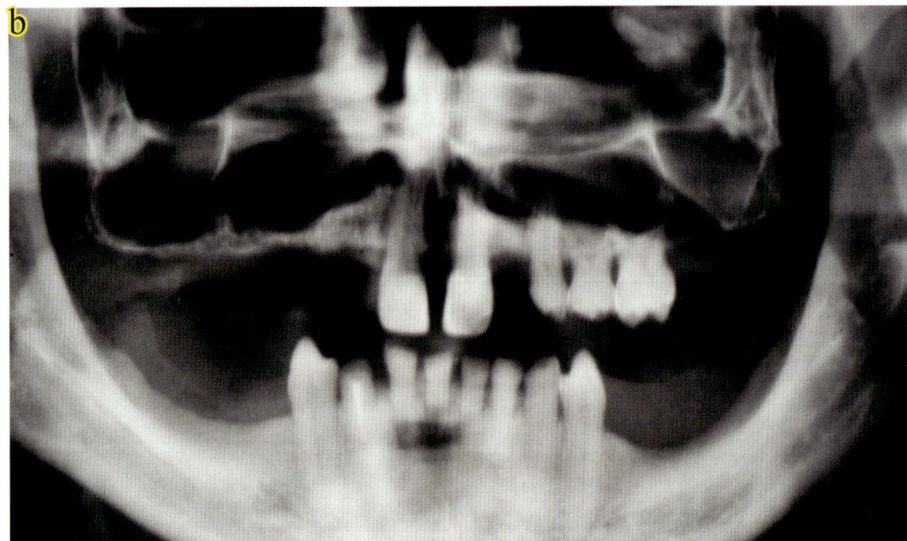

Figure 2b- A dental panoramic tomogram of a patient with hypodontia. It clearly shows very little bone height in the right maxillary edentulous region. This area is only treatable following extensive bone grafting. The only significant bone mass in the upper jaw is in the premaxilla.

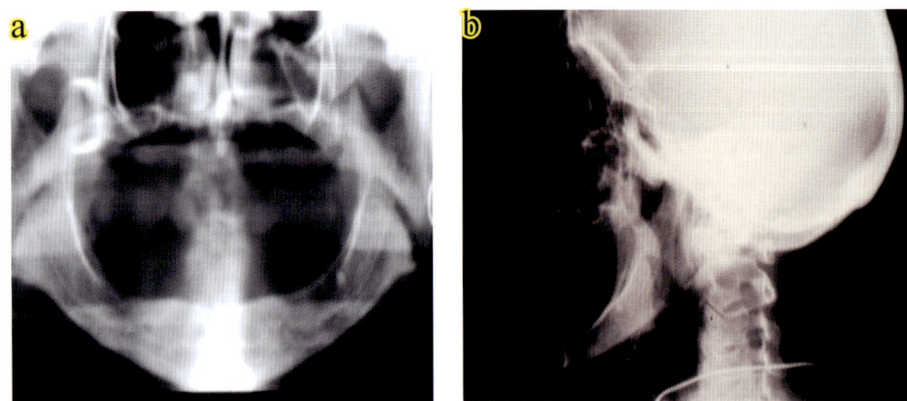

Figure 3a- A dental panoramic tomogram of an edentulous individual with good bone height in the mandible, particularly in the symphyseal region (Class C). There is extensive resorption in the maxilla (Class E). The mandible is treatable with implants and the maxilla would require extensive grafting.

Figure 3b- A lateral skull view demonstrates the ridge profile of both upper and lower jaws in the midline.

Figure 4a- A section of a dental panoramic tomogram showing an edentulous space in the right mandible clearly depicting the inferior dental canal and mental foramen.

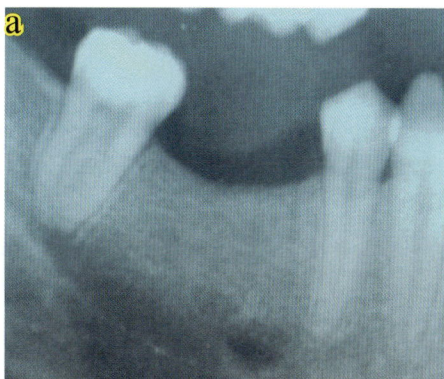

Figure 4b- A cross sectional tomographic slice in the region of the menial nerve. The mental foramen is visible as a discontinuity in the buccal cortex. The ridge profile is readily discernable.

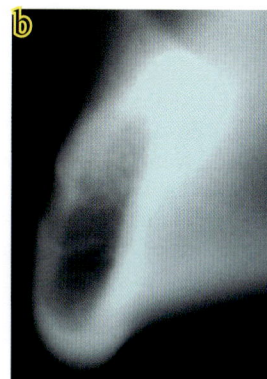

Figure 4c- Dental panoramic tomogram with the patient wearing a removable denture with three radiographic markers placed in the cingulum area of the teeth.

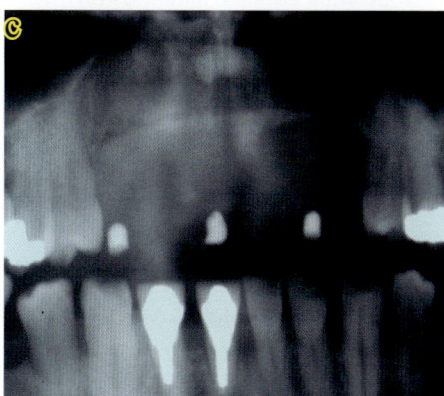

Figure 4d- A cross sectional tomographic slice of the edentulous ridge in the region of one of the tomographic markers which is visible in the bottom left of the figure. A transparent implant template of the appropriate magnification has been placed over the ridge to help decide upon suitable implant dimensions.

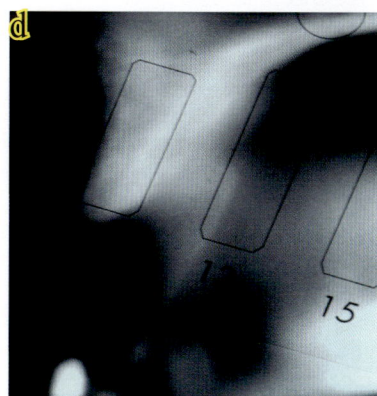

Figure 5a- A periapical radiograph of an upper right lateral incisor space with a measuring scale indicates that there is 6 mm space between the adjacent roots.

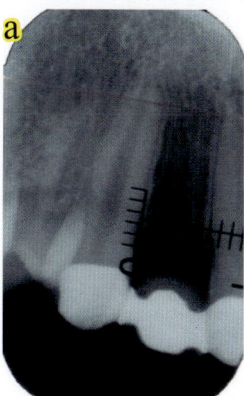

Figure 5b- Shows a superimposed implant profile of a 13 mm long x 3.5 mm diameter implant outline.

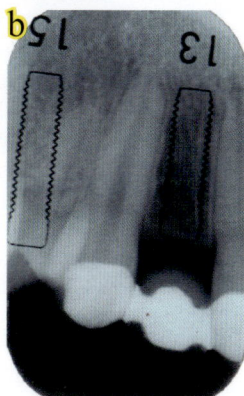

Figure 5c- This shows a 11 mm x 4 mm diameter implant outline indicating that there would be sufficient space to accommodate this diameter of implant, assuming that there is adequate bone thickness in the labial-palatal dimension.

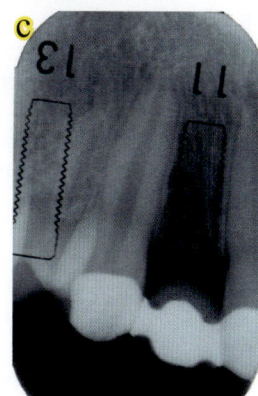

Figure 6a- An acrylic stent with radiopaque markers in the cingulum areas of the lateral incisors and the occlusal aspects of the posterior teeth. This type of stent is good for planning screw retained restorations. This stent can also be converted to a surgical guide.

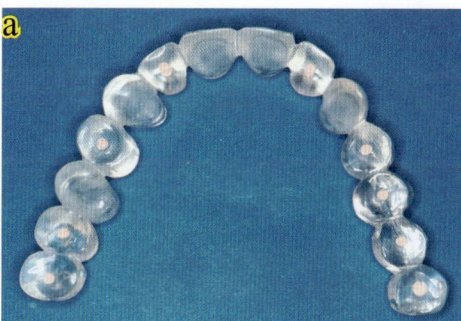

Figure 6b – A tomographic section of the maxilla in a patient wearing a radiographic stent with the outline of the tooth covered with a radiopaque marker. Superimposition of an implant transparency can assess the position and angulation of the implant in relation to the tooth outline.

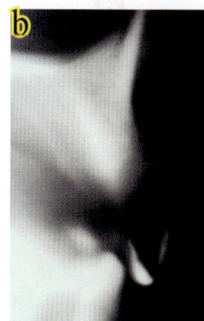

the sections thin and by making the scans contiguous or overlapping. The large number of sections in a high resolution scan of a jaw approximates to a radiation dose of 0.3 to 3 mSv. New generation cone beam scanners have lower radiation doses and have an increasing application in imaging for dental implant planning. The scans should be limited to the area of interest and avoid radiosensitive tissues such as the eyes.

Images can be produced as:

- Standard radiographic negative images on large sheets.
- Positive images on photographic paper often in book form.
- Images for viewing and manipulation with computer software.

Whatever the presentation format, it is of great importance to align the scan properly. In dentate subjects this is normally parallel to the occlusal plane. In edentulous subjects the mandible may be scanned parallel to the lower border and the maxilla parallel to the floor of the nose. Poor alignment will result in the cross-sectional slices not being in the same direction as the proposed implant placement (see radiographic stents).

Figure 7 illustrates the reformatted images that can be produced including:

- Sections in the same plane as the original slices (*Fig. 7a*).
- Images in the same plane as a conventional DPT, but at different depths (*Fig. 7b,e*).
- Cross-sectional images of the jaw at right angles to the original plane of slice, numbered consecutively and radially around the arch. These are the most useful images (*Fig. 7c,d,f*).

Heavy metals will produce a scatter-like interference pattern if they are present in the slice under examination and the interference will therefore appear in all the generated sectional images. Extensive interference can be produced by large posts in root canals or heavily restored teeth where the plane of examination passes through such a tooth as well as an area of critical interest. Consideration should be given to removing the offending metal prior to examination if appropriate in the overall treatment plan.

The various scan images can be measured for selection of implant length and diameter. The nominal magnification of the images is 1:1. A scale is usually incorporated alongside the various groups of images and the real magnification can be determined from this. A correction factor can then be applied to measurements taken directly from the films.

In contrast to hard copies of the scans, one of the advantages of the computer-based image software programs (eg Simplant) is that it is possible to produce images of implants (and their restorative components) which can then be 'placed' within the CT scan (*fig 8*). This enables the clinician to evaluate the relationships between the proposed implants and the ridge morphology, other anatomical features and adjacent teeth. When used in conjunction with a radiographic stent the possibility of reproducing the orientation envisaged at the planning stage is greatly increased. This has been developed to very high levels of sophistication using a combination of radio opaque diagnostic set-ups, CT scans and stereolithic modelling. Using these techniques it is possible to provide:

- 3D models of the jaws.
- Accurately fitting drill guides to assist the surgeon in placing the implant in the same position as that planned with the computer software.
- Fabrication of fixed prostheses that can be fitted directly to the implants at the time of placement.

This rapidly developing area is of particular benefit in management of the more complex cases.

Perioperative and follow-up radiographs

Intra-oral radiographs may be used at the time of implant placement to allow visualisation of drills or direction indicators and their relationship to adjacent teeth or anatomical structures. During the prosthetic phase it is essential to ensure full seating of components and frameworks (*Fig.9*). In implants systems with a flat head or external connection the seating of abutments may need to be checked with radiographs. In these instances it is essential that radiographs are taken at 90 degrees to the long axis of the implant under examination and it is therefore recommended to use long cone parallel radiographs. Only a relatively small deviation from the correct angulation may make the radiograph unreadable. Correct angulation is easy to check when using threaded implants as the thread profile is clearly seen when the x-ray is taken at 90 degrees.

Baseline radiographs to show crestal bone levels and the state of the peri-implant bone should be taken as part of normal documentation at the time of fitting the final prosthesis. These should be repeated on an annual basis for the first 2 or 3 years to establish that the bone levels are stable. It should be remembered that some initial bone loss may occur during the first year of function with some implants but that a steady state should then be established thereafter. The interval between radiographs may be extended if the bone appears stable over the first few years of function (see Chapter 11).

Figure 7- A series of images from a patient undergoing computerised tomography of the maxilla and mandible.

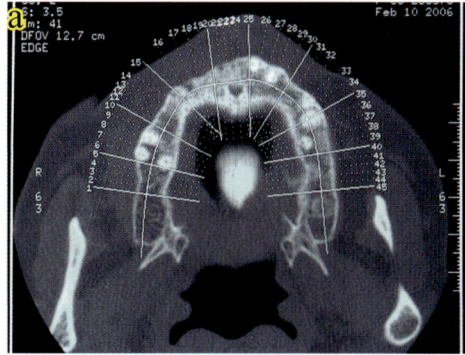

Figure 7a- A horizontal section of the maxilla parallel to the occlusal plane at a level close to the root apices. The line drawn through the middle of the arch form can be visualised as an image taken in a similar plane to a DPT radiograph (see figure 7b). The radial sections numbered 1-45 are produced as reformatted cross sectional images of the ridge as seen in figure 7c and 7d.

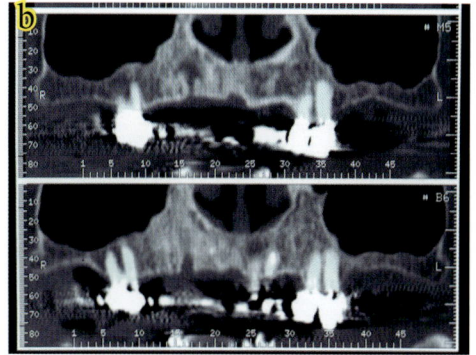

Figure 7b- This shows reformatted images in a similar plane to a DPT radiograph but at two different depths within the maxilla.

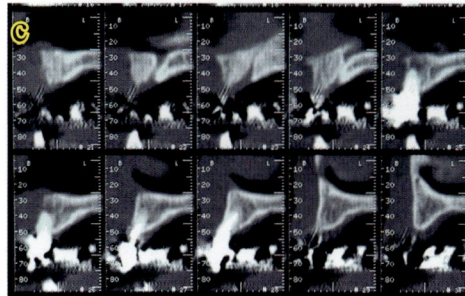

Figure 7c- This shows a series of cross sectional images of the maxilla numbered from 21 in the top left to 30 in the bottom right. The middle images in the top row pass through the incisive canal.

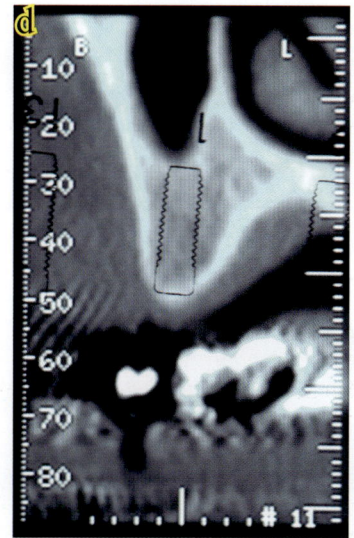

Figure 7d- Section 11 from the right molar region with a superimposed implant outline of 11 mm in length and 4 mm in diameter. The bone volume is good allowing a choice of implant position and angulation. The maxillary sinus is just apical to the implant and the nasal cavity is visible in the top right corner.

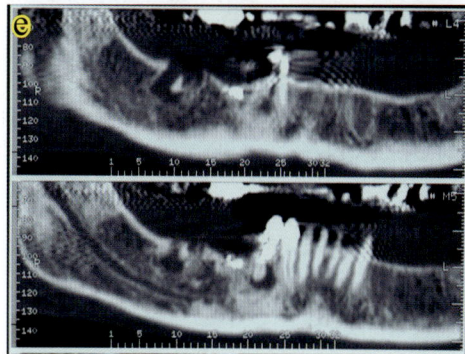

Figure 7e- Images from the mandibular scan in the DPT like format. The bottom image clearly shows the inferior dental canal as it is in this plane of section in contrast to the image above. An apical lesion is clearly visible on the lower right premolar tooth and residual sockets are still visible in the molar region.

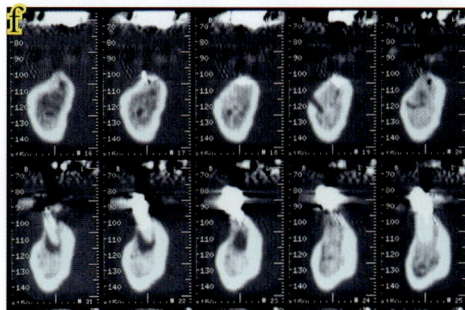

Figure 7f- Cross sectional images of the right mandible demonstrating good bone density and a readily visible inferior dental canal and mental foramen in the upper row of images. The size of the apical lesion on the lower premolar can be readily determined in the lower series of images.

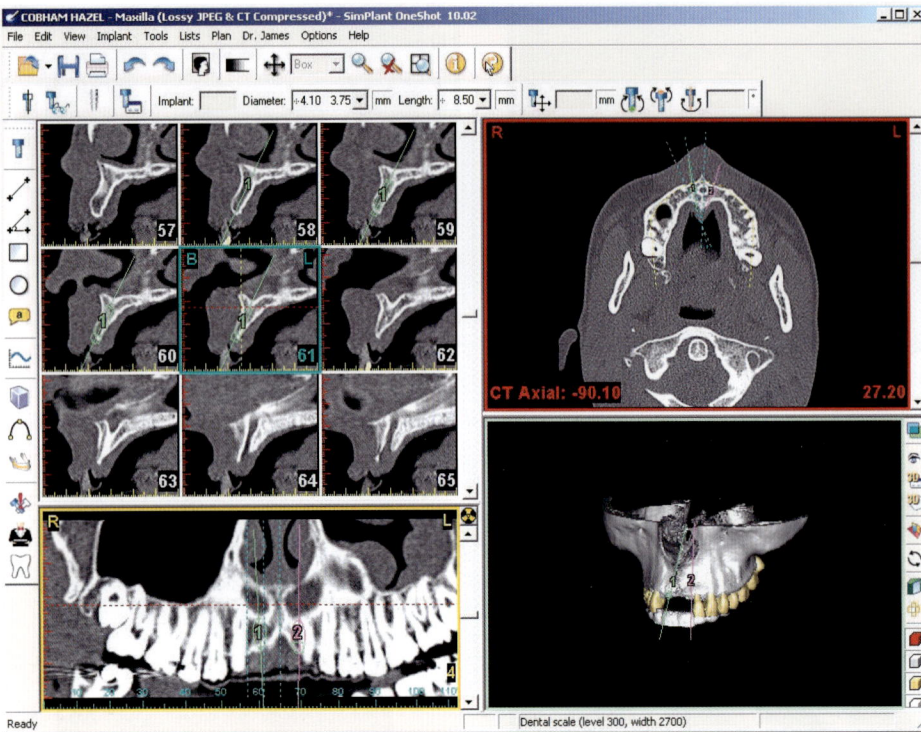

Figure 8- An example of computerised software that facilitates planning by allowing virtual placement of implants within the jaws in relationship to radiographic stents. Implants have been placed within the central incisor region and their angulation and position adjusted. The lower right image shows a very good 3 dimensional reconstruction of the maxilla and the implant positions in relationship to the stent.

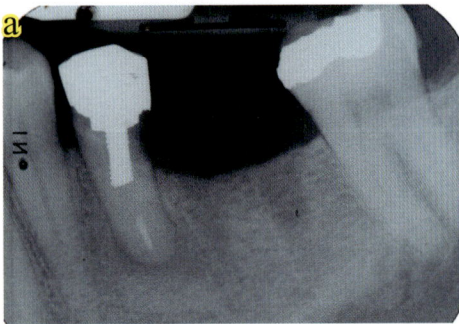

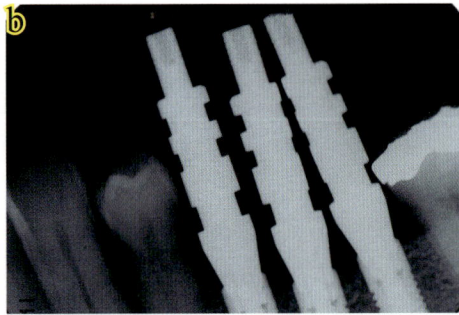

Figure 9 – A series of intraoral long cone periapical radiographs of a patient undergoing implant treatment in the left mandible.

Figure 9a- This shows a failing post crown on the lower left second premolar and an apical lesion. This tooth was subsequently extracted.

Figure 9b- This radiograph shows that 3 implants have been placed in the space and impression openings have been attached to the implants. The radiograph verifies the connection of the transfer copings and the levels of the marginal bone.

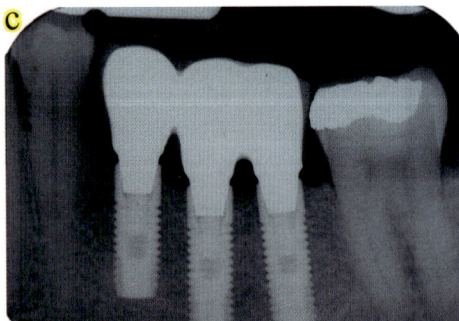

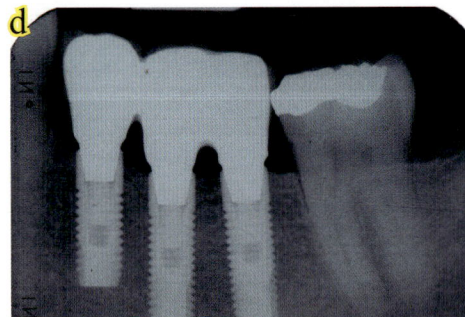

Figure 9c- A base line radiograph following fitting of the prosthesis verifies the fit of the components and bone level to assess future changes.

Figure 9d- A radiograph of the same case one year later showing maintenance of bone levels.

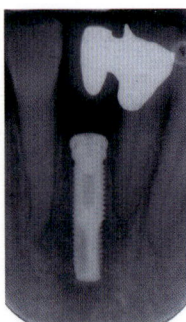

Figure 10- This periapical radiograph shows an implant which was placed approximately 4 weeks previously. An adhesive bridge provides the provisional restoration. The patient experienced discomfort and the radiograph shows an apical radiolucency around the implant. Bone resorption has occurred because of damage to the bone at implant placement. This is caused by failure to cool the bone during the drilling operation and is referred to as burnt bone syndrome.

Many of the problems that arise during treatment or once the prosthesis is in function are most readily diagnosed using standard intraoral views (*Fig 10*), these include:

- Burnt bone syndrome
- Component loosening
- Bone loss
- Screw breakage
- Implant fracture
- Adjacent endodontic lesions
- Loss of integration

These conditions will be dealt with more fully in Chapter 10, Complications and Maintenance.

Conclusion

Radiographs play an important part in the successful planning and execution of implant treatment. It is important to have an understanding of the different techniques available and their appropriate application. They are an important part of the patient's records and as such constitute a significant proportion of the medico-legal documentation of the patient. It is the responsibility of the clinician to ensure that radiographs are appropriate, readable and are reported on, retained and repeated at accepted intervals throughout treatment and follow-up.

Basic implant surgery

Implant surgery protocols differ slightly with individual systems. However, basic surgical principles are required to ensure successful osseointegration of the implant in the correct location, which allows good aesthetics and appropriate loading.

Successful implant surgery is largely dependent upon good planning and meticulous technique. The former requires an appreciation of the restorative requirements and visualisation of the desired end result of treatment, whereas the latter requires adequate surgical training and experience of the selected implant system.

The essential pre-requisites before proceeding to implant surgery are:
- The patient should be medically fit to undergo the surgery. Placement of one or two implants is equivalent to relatively minor oral surgery whereas placement of five or six implants increases the magnitude significantly. The medical history should be checked with particular reference to:

  Poorly controlled diabetes
  Blood dyscrasias
  Medications
  Irradiation to jaws
  Mucosal diseases
  Psychoses
  Substance abuse including tobacco and alcohol

- The patient should understand the procedure and be warned of any complications. They should have agreed the treatment plan, treatment schedule, costings, and given their consent.
- The diagnostic set-up, surgical stent and relevant radiographs should be available.
- The surgeon should have a clear idea of the number, size and planned location of the implants. They should be trained in the procedure and able to cope with any unforeseen circumstances.

Operative requirements

Most implant surgery can be carried out in a well equipped dental surgery. Ideally the surgery should be designed to permit surgical procedures under good aseptic conditions. The following should be available:
- Good operating light
- Good high volume suction
- A dental chair which can be adjusted by foot controls or a third party
- A surgical drilling unit which can deliver relatively high speeds (up to 3000 rpm) and low drilling speeds (down to about 10 rpm) with good control of torque
- A purpose designed irrigation system for keeping bone cool during the drilling process
- The appropriate surgical instrumentation for the implant system being used and the surgical procedure
- Sterile drapes, gowns, gloves, suction tubing etc
- The appropriate number and design of implants planned plus an adequate stock to meet unexpected eventualities during surgery
- The surgical stent
- The complete radiographs including tomographs where necessary
- A trained assistant
- A third person to act as a runner between the sterile and non-sterile environment.

Anaesthesia and analgesia

Most implant surgery can be carried out under local anaesthesia, although some patients will require sedation or general anaesthesia. The surgical time will vary greatly between different operators and cases. Short cases, for example under 1 hour for placement of one or two implants do not usually present problems with anaesthesia. Complex cases may take 2 to 3 hours and it is essential to use regional block anaesthesia (infra-orbital, palatal, inferior dental) and to supplement this during the procedure. Local infiltrations are also administered as they improve the anaesthesia and more importantly control haemorrhage. Sedation is recommended for operations of long duration eg more than 90 minutes. It is a good idea to give analgesics, such as ibuprofen or paracetamol, immediately prior to surgery.

Sterile technique

Every effort should be made to conduct implant surgery under sterile operating conditions. Chlorhexidine 0.2% is used as a pre-operative mouthwash and skin preparation circumorally. The patient is draped as for other oral surgical procedures, and drill leads should be autoclaved or covered with sterile tubing. Light handles should be autoclaved or covered with sterile aluminium foil. It is convenient to use sterile disposable suction tubing and covers. The instrument tray and any other surfaces, which are to be used, are covered in sterile drapes.

Surgical techniques for implant installation

Surgical installation of implants is facilitated by good visualisation of the bone ridge profile and meticulous preparation of the bone site to accept the implant (*Figs. 1,2 and 3*).

Anatomical considerations

The implant surgeon should be fully conversant with all anatomical structures that they are likely to encounter or that will affect implant placement, including:
* *In the maxilla*
  Air sinuses
  Nasopalatine canal
  Floor of nose and nasal spine
  Palatine and pterygoid vessels
* *In the mandible*
  Sublingual vessels
  Mental nerve
  Inferior dental nerve
  Incisive branch of inferior dental nerve
  Genial tubercles
* *Teeth*
  Position, length and angulation of roots adjacent to implant sites
* *Available bone*
  Ridge morphology
  Bone density
      Cortical
      Medullary
  Localised deformities
      Tooth sockets
      Residual cysts/granulomata

Flap design

Surgical implant placement is possible without flap elevation, and can be made more precise by using computer derived drilling guides. However, for routine implant placement full flap exposure is advocated. There are many different flap designs for implant surgery. In practically all situations a mid-crestal incision can be employed. Access and elevation of the flaps can usually be improved by the additional use of vertical relieving incisions (*Fig. 1a,b*). Relieving incisions close to adjacent teeth can be made to include the elevation of the (interdental) papilla, but some surgeons prefer to avoid raising this in case future aesthetics are compromised. Care should be taken to ensure that incision lines are not placed over structures such as the mental nerve and the palatine arteries. All incisions are made through periosteum down to bone.

Full thickness mucoperiosteal flaps are raised carefully to expose the entire extent of the edentulous ridge where the implants are to be placed (*Fig.1b*). The flaps should be elevated sufficiently far apically to reveal any bone concavities, especially at sites where perforation might occur. Important anatomical structures in the area of operation that might be damaged, such as the mental nerve, should be identified and protected.

Surgical preparation of the bone

It is essential not to allow the bone to be heated above 47^0C during preparation of the site as this will cause bone cell death and prevent osseointegration. This problem may be avoided by:
* Using sharp drills
* Employing an incremental drilling procedure with increasing diameter drills
* Avoidance of excessive speed (no more than 3,000rpm) and pressure on the drills – ensuring that the drill is withdrawn from the site frequently to allow the bone swarf to clear. This is particularly important in dense/hard bone.
* Using copious sterile saline irrigation. This can be delivered from a sterile infusion bag in a pressure cuff or a peristaltic pump. The drills can be adequately cooled by spraying the external surface of the drill. However, some systems use internally irrigated drills.

A typical sequence of drilling and implant insertion is shown in *Figures 1 and 2*. Preparation of the sites commences with penetration of the outer cortex with a small round bur followed by twist drills of increasing sizes. The drills are marked to indicate the corresponding lengths of implants. The spacing and angulation of the implant sites are checked carefully with direction indicators throughout the drilling sequence, in relation to the bone ridge, adjacent teeth, surgical stent and the opposing jaw/dentition. The angulations should be checked from different viewpoints (eg buccal and occlusal), as it is very easy to make errors when viewing from a single aspect.

Implant placement

The ideal siting and orientation of the implant is dictated by the restorative requirements, but this may have to be modified due to the existing ridge morphology and adjacent anatomical structures. Following elevation of the flaps the surgical stents should be tried in. In partially dentate cases the stent should be stabilised on adjacent teeth and provide guidance of where the planned labial faces, occlusal surfaces or cingulae of the teeth to be replaced are to be located. An example of a suitable stent is shown in *Figures 1c,d,e*. In edentulous cases it is far more difficult to provide a stable stent, as it will have to rely upon a mucosal fit in areas where the mucoperiosteum has not been raised. Some stents are designed to be stabilised using pins or screws into adjacent areas of bone.

Ideally an implant should be placed such that:
- It is within bone along its entire length. Exposure of limited areas of implant surface associated with bone defects such as dehiscences or fenestrations may be acceptable, but larger ones may require augmentation (Chapter 7).
- It does not damage adjacent structures such as teeth, nerves, and nasal or sinus cavities. It is acceptable to engage the nasal or sinus floor with a small degree of penetration (eg 1mm). An adequate safety margin of about 2mm above the inferior dental canal is recommended.
- It is located directly apical to the tooth it is replacing and not in an embrasure space.
- The angulation of the implant is consistent with the design of the restoration. This is particularly important with screw retained restorations where it is desirable to have the screw access hole in the middle of the occlusal surface or cingulum of the final restoration. Multiple implants are placed in a fairly parallel arrangement, to facilitate seating of the restoration (*Fig.3*). However most systems allow convergence/divergence of up to 30 degrees without the use of angled/customised abutments.
- The top of the implant is placed sufficiently far under the mucosa to allow a good emergence profile of the prosthesis. This is often achieved by countersinking the head of the implant (*Fig.2g*).

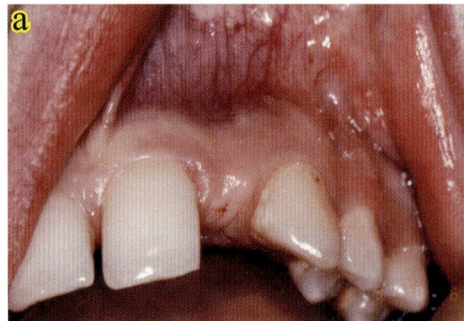

Figure 1. This series of photos shows a standard sequence of flap reflection and initial drilling protocol with the aid of a stent.

Figure 1a- The pre-operative view of the upper left lateral incisor space.

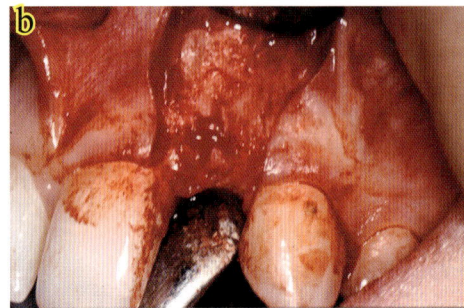

Figure 1b- A full thickness mucoperiosteal flap has been elevated to completely expose the alveolar ridge to determine its shape and whether any concavities are present. The flap has vertical labial relieving incisions, a crestal incision mesio-distally and has included elevation of the papillae to give good access to the narrow edentulous space.

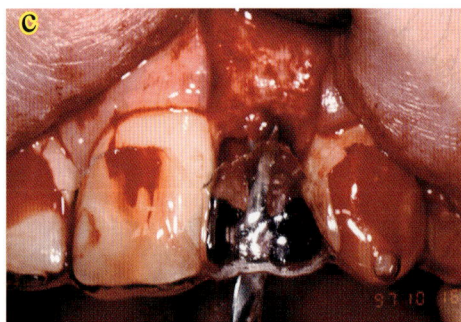

Figure 1c- A clear blow-down stent has been placed over the adjacent teeth and provides the surgeon with the position of the labial face and gingival margin of the tooth which is to be replaced. The initial preparation of the implant site is with a round bur which readily penetrates the cortex, and this is followed by a twist drill (illustrated) which determines the initial angulation and depth of the implant.

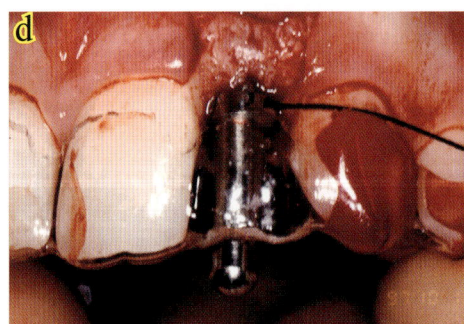

Figure 1d- A guide or indicator post is placed in the site to check on the position and angulation of the implant. Small adjustments can be made at this stage.

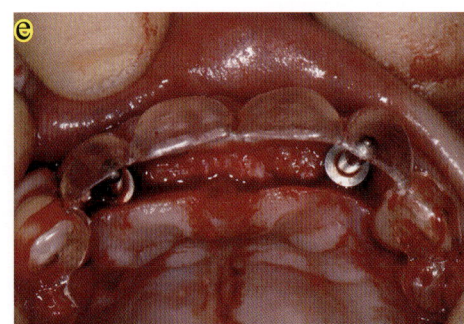

Figure 1e- A case requiring replacement of all four maxillary incisors. The stent is in place and sites have been prepared in the lateral incisor locations where direction indicators have been placed. The central incisor sites would have provided good alternative locations for the implants.

Figure 2- A series of photos to show the drilling sequence and insertion of two implants in the upper incisor region.

Figure 2a- Clinical photograph prior to surgery.

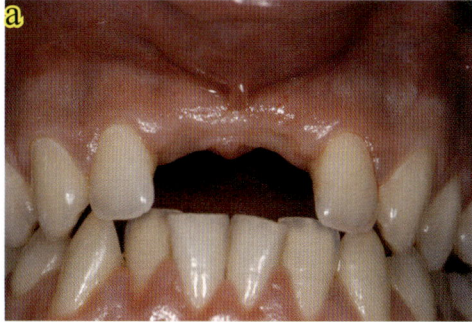

Figure 2b- Following flap reflection and initial site preparation with a round bur.

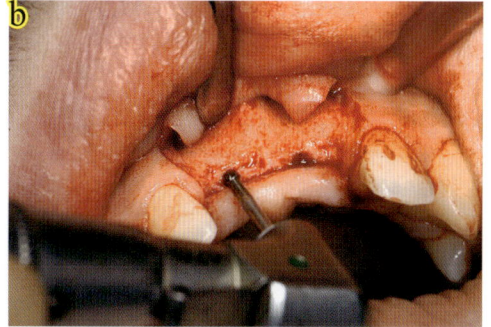

Figure 2c- Development of the angulation of the site with a narrow twist drill.

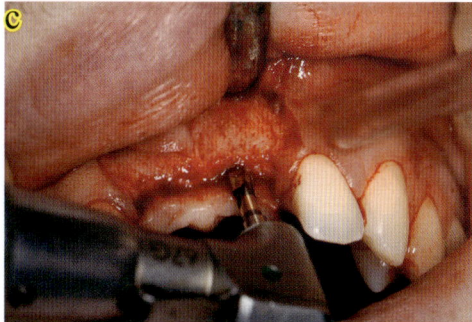

Figure 2d- A direction indicator placed in the left central incisor site and a pilot drill used to increase the size of the site on the right side.

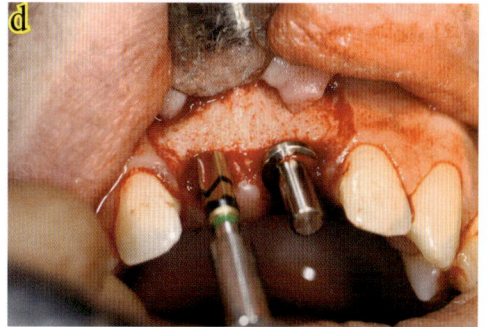

Figure 2e- A larger diameter twist drill used to the full depth of the implant site.

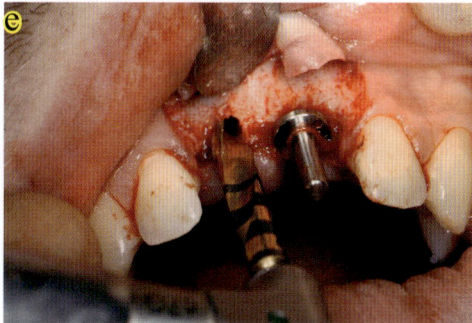

Figure 2f- An implant being inserted in the right incisor site. An implant has already been placed in the left side and the mount is still in place.

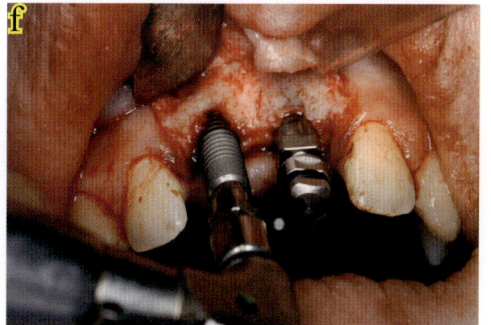

Figure 2g- An occlusal view of the implants. The left implant is placed slightly more sub crestal than that on the right.

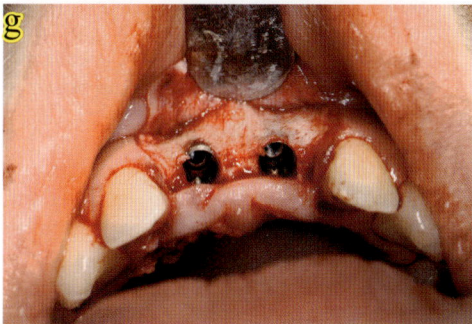

Figure 2h- Cover screws inserted into the implants

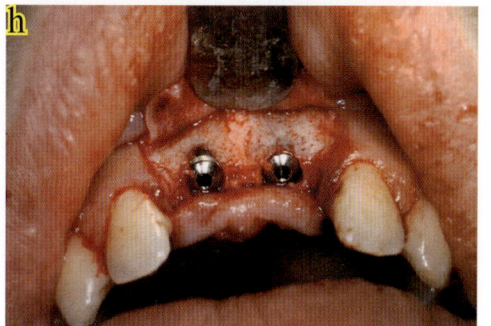

Figure 2i- Flaps sutured back to bury the implants.

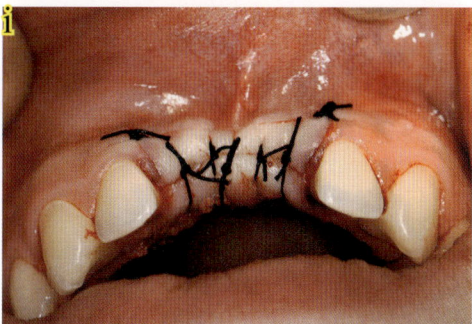

For example, it is suggested that the top of a standard diameter implant (about 4mm) when used to replace a single upper incisor tooth, should be 2 to 3 mm apical to the gingival margin of the adjacent natural tooth.

- There is sufficient vertical space above the implant head for the restorative components
- The implant should be immobile at placement. A loose implant at this stage may fail to osseointegrate
- Adequate bone is present between adjacent implants, and between implants and adjacent teeth (*Fig.2*). This should preferably be about 3mm and never less than 1mm. In some cases 1mm of bone may be acceptable implant spacing, but the abutments may have a larger diameter and therefore prevent proper abutment seating, thereby complicating the restorative procedure. A distance of 3mm will also allow better soft tissue adaptation and may allow the maintenance of an 'interdental papilla'.

The above requirements are not always easy to achieve and in many circumstances would be impossible without a properly designed stent produced from the diagnostic set up. Inevitably there are situations where a careful balance is needed between the ideal 'set up' and possible implant placement.

Implant insertion

The technique for insertion of the implant depends largely upon the system being used. In general the final bone preparation site diameter is slightly smaller than the implant. The size of the site can be adjusted according to bone quality or density. In poor quality bone the site can be made relatively smaller to produce compression of the surrounding bone on implant insertion, which will improve the initial stability. In dense bone the site has to more closely match the size of the implant. In bone with relatively poor medullary quality, where initial stability may be difficult to achieve, it may be advisable to secure the implant at each end in cortical bone (bicortical stabilisation) providing anatomical structures, length of implants and ability to provide adequate cooling allow this. The implant is supplied in a sterile container; either already mounted on a special adapter or unmounted necessitating the use of an adapter from the implant surgical kit. In either case the implant should not touch anything (other than a sterile titanium surface) before its delivery to the prepared bone site. Screw shaped implants are either self tapped into the prepared site (*Fig.2f*) or sometimes following tapping of the bone with a screw tap. Cylindrical implants are either pushed or gently knocked into place. The installation of the implants should be done with the same care as the preparation of the site by maintaining the cooling irrigation and placing the implant at slow speeds. Insertion of screw shaped implants and tapping of sites are performed at speeds of less than 20 rpm. Following placement the head and inner screw thread of the implant are protected with a cover screw (*Fig.2h*) or a healing abutment (*Fig.3d*).

The mucoperiosteal flaps are carefully closed with multiple sutures to bury the implant completely (*Fig.2i*) or to adapt the flaps around the neck of the implant/healing abutment in non-submerged systems (*Fig.3d*). Silk sutures are satisfactory and others such as PTFE or resorbables (eg vicryl) are good alternatives.

Post-operative care

After implant surgery, patients should be warned to expect:
- Some swelling and possibly bruising
- Some discomfort which can usually be controlled with oral analgesics
- Some transitory disturbance in sensation if surgery has been close to a nerve.

They should be advised:
- In many cases (particularly completely edentulous subjects) not to wear dentures over the surgical area for at least 1 week (possibly 2 weeks) to avoid loading the implants and the possibility of disrupting the sutures
- To use analgesics and ice packs to reduce swelling and pain
- To keep the area clean by using chlorexidine mouthwash 0.2% for 1 minute twice daily
- Not to smoke. This compromises healing of soft tissue and bone and may increase the risk of implant failure. Ideally patients should stop smoking for some weeks before surgery and for as long as possible thereafter.

The need for systemic antibiotics should be considered for extensive procedures, grafting and for patients with relevant systemic conditions. The original protocols recommended an antibiotic such as amoxycillin 250mg 8 hourly for 5 to 7 days, unless the patient is allergic where a suitable alternative such as metronidazole should be prescribed. Alternative regimes include administration of 3 grams of amoxycillin 1 hour before surgery, or 500mg every 8 hours for 48 hours. Treatment plans using provisional bridges have an advantage in that they do not load the implant sites and can be refitted immediately after the surgery, providing some allowance has been made to accommodate some swelling. All patients should be seen after 1 week for review, suture removal and adjustment and refitting of dentures with adequate soft linings. In some

Figure 3- A short sequence of photographs showing multiple implant placement in the lower jaw.

Figure 3a- Initial site preparation has been carried out and direction indicators are in place to check implant spacing, angulation and parallelism.

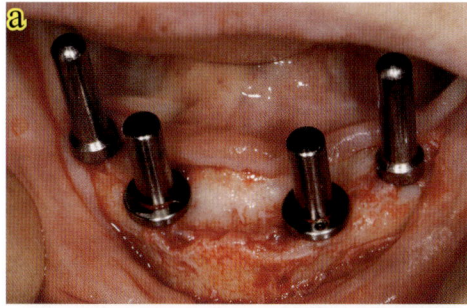

Figure 3b- The implants have been inserted and the mounts are still in place. The relationship of the mounts to the opposing dentition can be seen.

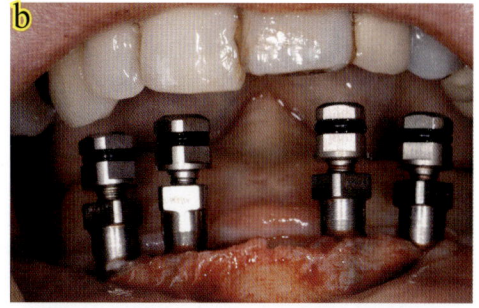

Figure 3c- An occlusal view of the implant mounts showing the implants have been placed in a curve around the jaw.

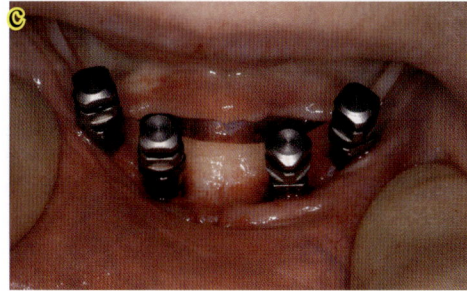

Figure 3d- Healing abutments have been placed and the flaps sutured.

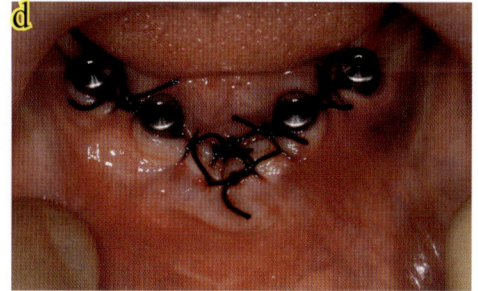

Figure 4- Small incisions have been made in the mucosa overlying submerged implants to allow removal of cover screws and placement of healing abutments.

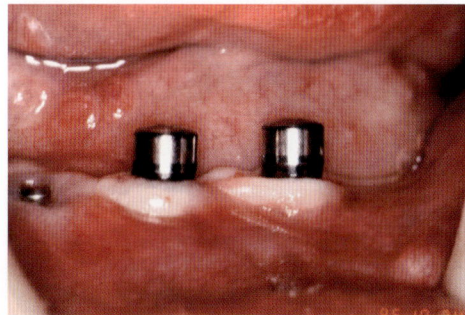

Figure 5a-A buccal flap has been raised to expose the cover screws attached to the heads of two implants. The crestal incision has been placed towards the palatal aspect so that the overlying keratinised tissue can be mobilised towards the buccal aspect.

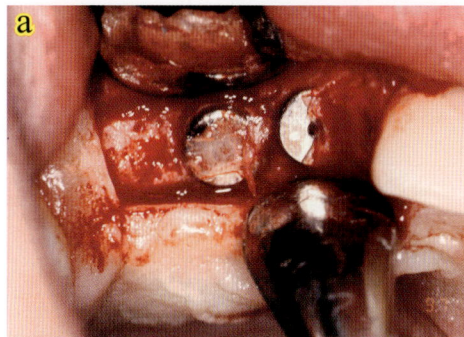

Figure 5b- The cover screws have been removed and healing abutments placed. These are simple titanium cylinders which should just protrude through the mucosa.

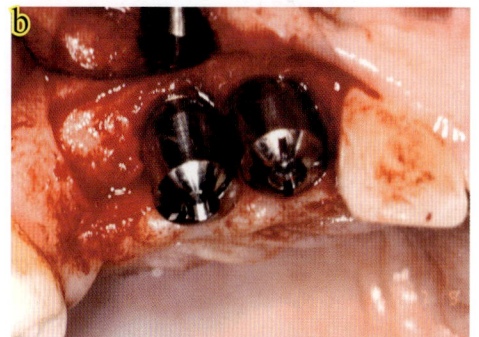

Figure 5c- The buccal flap is shaped with a scalpel to more accurately fit the healing abutments. The small pieces of tissue have been left attached rather than being removed as they can be rotated and positioned between the implant to optimise coverage of the bone.

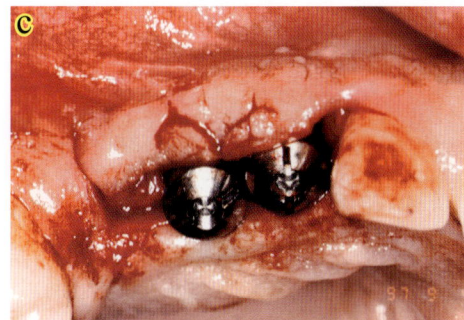

Figure 5d- The flaps have been sutured so as to fit neatly around the healing abutments.

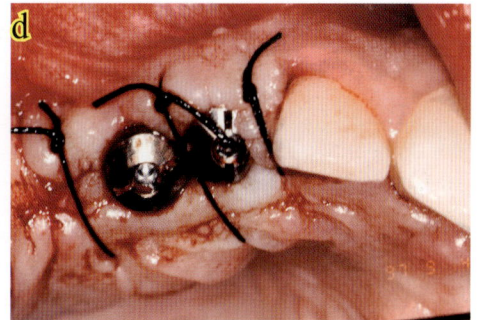

cases the tissues will not be able to accept a denture for 1 to 2 weeks. This is most likely with surgery in the edentulous mandible and with surgical flap designs that affect the sulcus shape. Patients will require regular review and change of soft liners. Exposure of cover screws through the mucosa during the early stages has little effect on the success of implants providing they are kept clean or changed to healing abutments.

Surgery for abutment connection

In non-submerged protocols (*Fig.3*), a second surgical stage is not required and prosthodontic treatment can proceed after a suitable healing period. In general, submerged implants are exposed after 2 to 3 months (original protocols recommended 3 to 6 months). Exposure of the implant at stage 2 surgery can be achieved with minimal flap reflection or sometimes making a very small incision over the implant just to allow removal of the cover screw and attachment of an abutment (*Fig.4*). In some cases bone grows over the cover screw and this necessitates greater soft tissue reflection to allow bone removal with hand instruments, burs or specially designed mills prior to abutment connection (*Fig. 5*). Healing abutments allow good mucosal adaptation and healing before selection of the abutment for the final restoration. Ideally the healing abutment should protrude about 1mm above the mucosa. It is important to check that the abutments are fully seated on the implant.

Handling of the soft tissue at abutment connection surgery should aim to preserve keratinised (and preferably attached) mucosa on the labial and lingual aspect (*Fig.5*). The position of the crestal exposing incision should serve to achieve this goal. For example, keratinised tissue overlying the implant or towards the palatal aspect can be repositioned to the buccal aspect. A number of techniques have been described to optimise soft tissue contours to produce well-formed interdental tissues and aesthetic papillae (*Fig.5c and 5d*). An overlying prosthesis will need to be adjusted to accommodate the protruding abutment. Prostheses which are designed and made with this in mind help considerably. The patient should expect some postoperative discomfort and be advised to take analgesics. They should use Chlorhexidine mouthwash until adequate oral hygiene can be re-established. The soft tissue should be allowed to heal for about 2 to 4 weeks before the restorative phase commences.

Conclusions

Implant surgery is highly technique sensitive and requires adequate training and an understanding of the restorative requirements of the proposed treatment. Control of these factors can produce a highly predictable, aesthetic and long-lasting result. In instances where there is insufficient bone and or soft tissue to allow successful implant placement and subsequent restoration, grafting and augmentation procedures will be required, and these are dealt with in Chapter 7.

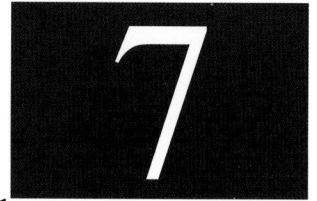

Grafting to overcome anatomical difficulties

Autogenous grafts are considered to be the most predictable for replacement of deficient bone to facilitate implant treatment. Augmentation of soft tissue may also be required to improve aesthetics and function.

The indications for employing corrective or reconstructive surgical techniques may be functional and/or aesthetic and may involve both hard and soft tissues. Sufficient bone must be present to allow placement of an implant of appropriate dimensions in a stable and correct orientation to allow construction of a successful prosthesis. Subsequently the soft tissues surrounding the implant should be able to maintain normal functional integrity and allow oral hygiene procedures. Aesthetic considerations may be relatively small involving subtle loss of alveolar ridge form or interdental papillae, but at the other extreme may involve significant skeletal jaw base discrepancies which need correction before implant treatment can commence. Before any corrective surgical procedure is attempted it is important to consider any alternative solutions. For example, potential aesthetic problems may also be overcome by using prosthetic solutions (see Chapter 9). It is important to discuss the problems and various solutions with the patient, and to explain the relative advantages and disadvantages of these approaches.

Overcoming alveolar bone deficiencies

Implant solutions

As described in Chapters 4 and 5, a full assessment of bone height and width (and quality) as well as its relationship to the proposed prosthesis is necessary to allow proper planning for implant surgery. Conventionally the aim is to have a border of 1mm of bone surrounding the implant at the time of placement. This dictates a minimum bone dimension of 6mm in both the mesial-distal and bucco-palatal direction to allow an implant of 4mm diameter to be placed. With narrower ridges the obvious alternative is to use a narrower diameter implant. While there may be merit in considering this option it is important to remember that a reduction in implant size, particularly to a diameter less than 3.5mm, can greatly reduce implant strength as well as surface area for integration/load distribution. Use of small diameter implants should there-

fore be restricted to low load situations such as replacement of missing lower incisors or upper lateral incisors. In situations where the ridge is broad but has limited height (less than 10mm), wider diameter implants up to 6mm can be used. These have a greater surface area for integration and load distribution as well as having an increased resistance to fracture. There are now a great many implant configurations to enable placement in regions with little bone volume but good long-term data on their success are lacking. Implant placement at an alternative site to facilitate treatment may also be considered, for example using the maxillary tuberosity or zygomatic buttresses for implant fixation. However, implants placed in these regions may present both surgical and prosthetic difficulties and their use should be limited to experienced clinicians.

Bone augmentation

Deficiencies in bone may be restricted to small, well defined defects involving one or more sites or may be much more generalised in their presentation affecting the entire jaw. Different techniques and materials are therefore employed to augment bone into these areas although a combination may be used to achieve the desired result.

Autogenous bone grafts

Autogenous bone remains the gold standard by which all other materials are judged. It has many advantages over the alternatives in that it is:
- Readily available from adjacent or remote sites
- Sterile
- Biocompatible/non-immunogenic
- Osseoinductive/conductive
- Easy to manipulate

It may be harvested from intra- and extra-oral sites using trephines or by taking bone blocks, chips or "scrapings". Favoured intra-oral sites include the chin, retromolar areas, and other edentulous areas local or remote to the surgical site *(Fig. 1)*. Further bone collection is possible by using surgical bone traps attached to the suction apparatus when taking grafts or preparing implant osteotomy sites. This yields an osteoconductive osseous coagulum which is easy to manipulate but care is required to avoid any salivary/bacterial contamination. Intra-oral harvesting has many merits in that the surgeon is working in an environment which is familiar, and the graft is of the same developmental origin. However, if there is a requirement for large blocks of bone an alternative site needs to be considered. Larger defects therefore require bone from extra-oral sites, the most common of which is iliac crest. While this donor site can provide large blocks of bone, the morbidity associated with this procedure must be considered. Optimisation of grafting is achieved by ensuring that the graft is stable at the time of placement and that there is close adaptation between graft and host bed. This may be achieved by compacting the bone into the available space and by direct fixation using screws or mini-plates *(Fig.2)*. Graft retention/preservation may also be improved by using GBR membranes (see below).

In an effort to overcome the morbidity of taking autogenous grafts other techniques and materials have been developed, and these are considered in the following sections.

Guided bone regeneration

One of the most popular techniques used for the treatment of localised ridge deficiencies is guided bone regeneration (GBR). This technique employs barrier membranes, which allow creation of a confined defect into which bone progenitor cells may migrate in preference to soft tissue cells, allowing bone to form within the void *(Fig.3)*. Many configurations of membranes are available. Gore-Tex^{TM} is an expanded polytetrafluoroethylene (PTFE) which was first used in periodontal regeneration. PTFE is non-resorbable and requires removal, therefore involving a second surgical procedure. Resorbable membranes overcome this problem and are widely used. They are made from animal derived sources such as porcine collagen or polymers of polylactic acid/polyglactide.

The ideal properties of GBR membranes are:
- Biocompatible to minimise any inflammatory response. Membranes which incorporate biochemical factors to enhance bone healing are under development
- Occlusive to prevent passage of cells during the healing period. Some membranes are semi permeable and allow passage of tissue fluid whereas others have been tried with are totally impermeable. Totally occlusive materials such as titanium sheets formed into the required shape have also been used
- Physical properties that allow the space under the membrane to be maintained. This may be improved by using: titanium reinforced membranes; 'tent' screws to

support the membranes; and fillers such as bone or substitutes to fill the void
- Enhance wound stability and protection of the initial clot and delicate granulation tissue. Stabilisation of the membrane may be improved by securing it with small screws/pins or the implant cover screw.

In its simplest form GBR can be used to promote bone fill of a defect before implant treatment. It can also be used to regenerate bone in dehiscences and fenestrations around implants at the time of placement *(Fig.3)*, but it must be remembered that any bone thus created does not contribute to initial implant stability and its long-term significance is currently not known.

Wound closure and stability are very important when using GBR and great efforts to maintain the vitality of the overlying soft tissues need to be made. Flaps with wound edges remote from the surgical site are recommended and wound closure without producing any tension in the soft tissues is required. Soft tissue breakdown over sites where membranes are involved can allow bacterial infection and compromised healing or failure.

Figure 1a- Grafts can be harvested using trephines. In this case the grafts have been taken from the chin region but the retromolar area is also often used.

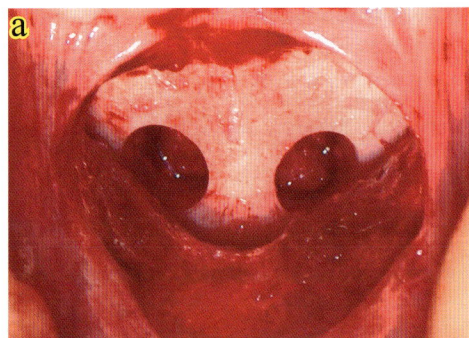

Figure 1b- A bone graft being harvested from the chin. An incision has been made below the mucogingival junction to give access to the bone apical to the incisor teeth. The block graft of cortical and underlying cancellous bone has been outlined with a fissure bur. The lingual cortex is left intact and the block can be elevated from the site.

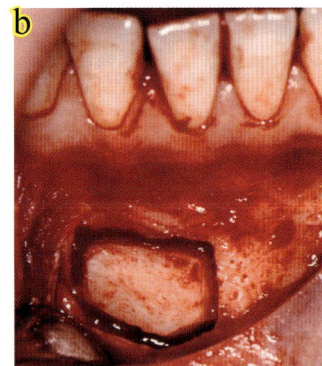

Figure 1c-A block graft harvested from the buccal and distal to the mandibular molars.

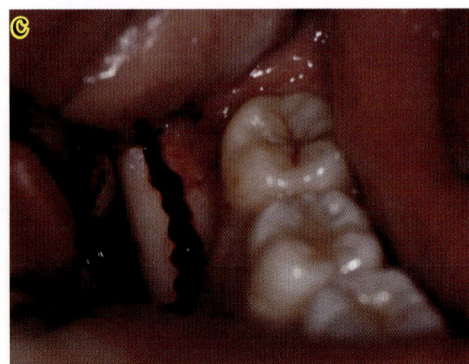

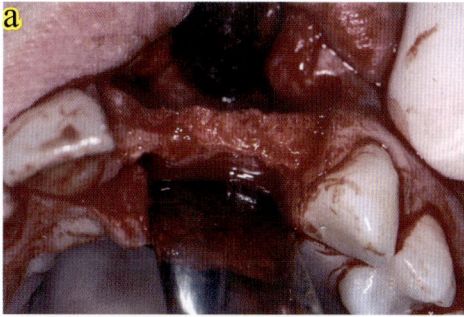

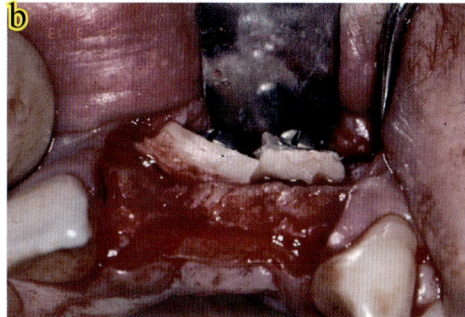

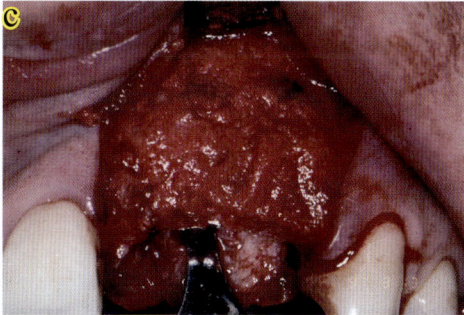

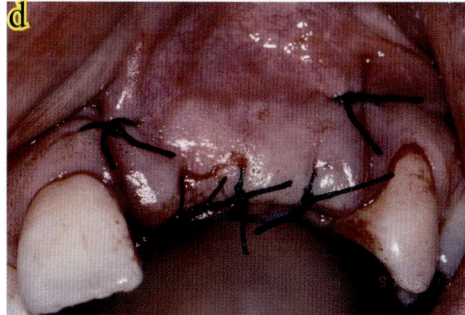

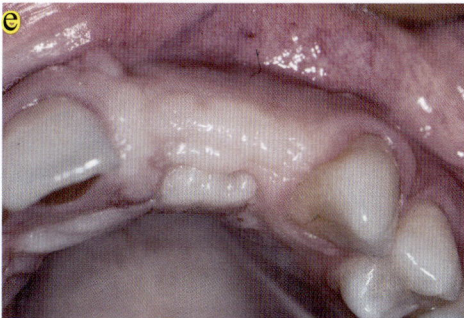

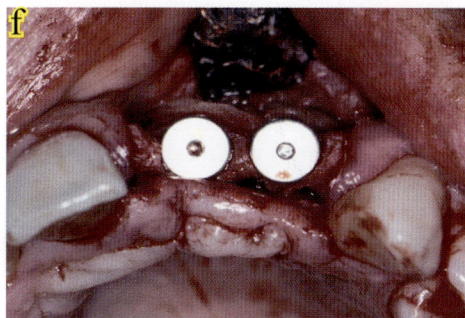

Figure 2 – A series of photos illustrating the placement of small block grafts to augment an upper incisor region.

Figure 2a- Good flap reflection to reveal the entire ridge and concave buccal surface. The crest of the ridge is under 4 mm in width.

Figure 2b- Small blocks of corticocancellous bone taken from the mandible have been secured to the buccal side of the ridge with small titanium screws.

Figure 2c- Bone coagulum collected in a trap attached to the suction at the time of bone harvesting has been used to cover the bone blocks.

Figure 2d- The flaps are closed with sutures with care to avoid any tension.

Figure 2e- The healed ridge showing improvement in contour.

Figure 2f- Successful placement of two implants into the grafted area four months later.

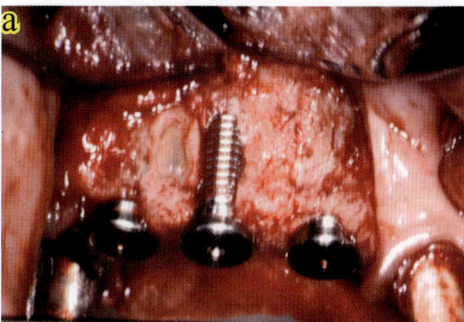

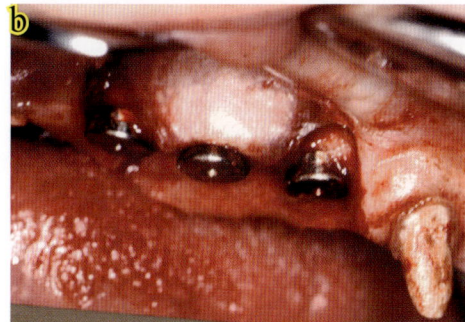

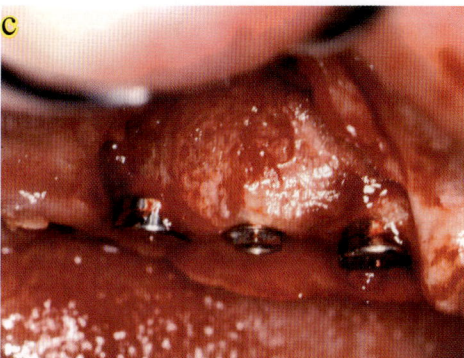

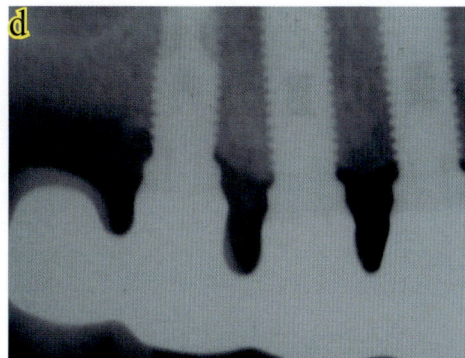

Figure 3a- Maxillary implants placed with a large dehiscence on the middle implant. The small root fragment distal to this was removed and the whole area covered with a Gore-tex membrane.

Figure 3b- Surgical exposure of the Gore-tex membrane after 7 months to remove the membrane and connect healing abutments.

Figure 3c- This shows the bone healing of the area following removal of the membrane. The dehiscence has been covered.

Figure 3d- A radiograph of the same implants following restoration.

Alloplastic graft materials

These include materials such as hydroxyapatite, tricalcium phosphate and bioactive glasses. These materials are easy to use and are commonly used as fillers on their own or in combination with autogenous bone (eg. 50:50). They provide an osteoconductive framework for bone but are not osteoinductive. Their use has been widely documented but their efficacy when used alone as grafting materials in implant surgery requires more evaluation with carefully controlled clinical trials, as is the case for many of the bone substitutes.

Hydroxyapatite is available in a variety of forms, from porous resorbable particles to dense non-resorbable and block forms. The commonly used non-resorbable HA becomes embedded in newly formed fibrous tissue and bone, and the resulting tissue combination is a less than ideal implant bed.

The new generation of bioactive glasses are an alternative synthetic bone grafting material. They are silicate glasses whose main components are sodium, calcium and phosphate in varying combinations in particulate form. They are osteoconductive as well as having bone bonding properties through corrosion of the glass when exposed to bodily fluids to produce a silica gel and a calcium phosphate surface layer. The calcium phosphate layer then recrystallises into hydroxycarbonate apatite which is able to bond to bone. This surface layer bears more similarity to the mineral component of bone than hydroxyapatite.

Allografts

Human bone material in the form of freeze dried bone or demineralised freeze dried bone (DFDB) has been used widely both in periodontology and implant dentistry. The donor bone is harvested from cadavers, processed and sterilised. A wide range of grafts are available, which may be particulate, thin sheets of cortical plate, or much larger bone blocks. They are predominantly used as a scaffold for bone repair and are resorbable but often remain as inert fragments long after placement. Despite the measures taken to ensure sterility and non-infectivity of these grafts some doubt must remain as to their absolute safety.

Xenografts

These are graft materials derived from other animal species. Some have received wide acclaim and are used to provide an inert framework for bone regeneration either alone or in combination with autogenous bone graft. Bio-Oss™ is bovine bone in which the organic component is completely removed to leave the mineralised bone architecture. This renders it non-immunogenic and presumably safe from the possibility of trans-species infection. There is a large body of literature supporting its use in a wide variety of applications.

Bone promoting molecules

The production of bone morphogenetic proteins (BMP's) are a recent advance in regenerative therapies both in periodontology and implant surgery, but high costs may limit their use. They have been used with some success in bone regeneration in the maxillary antrum when delivered in a collagen based sponge. They are also present in their natural form in demineralised freeze dried bone, which may account for the reported efficacy of this material, although the processing may inactivate the bone morphogenetic proteins. Platelet derived growth factor (PDGF) has been shown to be effective and is available commercially in some countries.

Management of localised deficiencies

Small deficiencies in the alveolar ridge may be treated using simple techniques. It is important to consider whether grafting is necessary to achieve a stable implant at the time of placement or whether it is being used to promote bone repair over exposed areas of the implant. Therefore augmentation of small defects may be considered as preparatory or perioperative procedures.

Before implant placement

Bone augmentation before implant placement is generally the preferred option. Alveolar defects should be augmented at least 3 months before implant placement but delays greater than 6 months may result in too much resorption of the graft.

At implant placement

Implant placement in thin ridges may result in incomplete bone coverage of the implant surface. The resulting defects can be described as either dehiscences involving the marginal bone or more apically located fenestrations (*Fig.3*). The clinician has to decide whether or not these require bone augmentation. This will mainly depend upon the size, location and morphology of the defect. Fenestrations are probably of little clinical significance and usually require no treatment. Grafting materials, GBR membranes or a combination can be used.

Extraction sockets

Most extraction sockets heal perfectly well without interference by the clinician. However, a large defect may be produced if the buccal plate is lost or in cases of long-standing apical or periodontal infection. These defects can be repaired using a variety of techniques including small bone grafts, GBR, or a combination of the two. It is important that any residual infection is eradicated before the implant is placed. Fortunately the removal of the offending tooth and curettage of the socket usually allows this to occur readily.

While it may be possible to improve socket infill at the time of extraction by placing graft material, an alternative is to place an implant immediately into the socket (*Fig.4*) In this situation the amount of grafting material is significantly reduced by the implant taking up most of the space (*Fig.4b,d*). A prerequisite for this technique is that sufficient bone is present to produce initial stability of the implant i.e. the graft plays no stabilising role at implant placement. Stability is normally achieved in these situations by engaging sound bone apical to the socket. With the immediate placement technique soft tissue coverage at implant placement can be difficult or impossible to achieve. Where soft tissue coverage is considered important the technique of 'delayed immediate placement' may be employed. In such situations the extraction site is left for about 4 to 6 weeks to allow soft tissue healing before an implant is placed. This period can also be useful to allow infections to completely resolve.

Management of larger deficiencies

General techniques

Larger bone deficiencies arise because of long standing progressive resorption following tooth loss and trauma, developmental anomalies, and pathological conditions (tumour resection, cysts, etc). Techniques to overcome these problems, which may involve the entire edentulous jaw, aim to improve the height and or width of the bone available as well as providing bone of sufficient quality to provide implant anchorage. Ridge resorption in the vertical plane may require grafting to allow placement of adequate length implants and to reduce the crown to implant ratio of the prosthesis. Longer implants supporting a lower profile prosthesis will reduce the mechanical demands on the prosthetic components. One of the most difficult problems is the development of a pseudo Class III jaw relation with severe resorption of the edentulous maxilla compared with the mandible. Grafting may therefore be required to provide adequate bone for implant installation and correction of the jaw relationship.

Most of the procedures described in this section are advanced surgical procedures requiring specialist training.

Onlay grafts

Onlay grafts are versatile in that they are able to augment the bone in either the vertical or lateral dimension or a combination of the two (*Fig.5*). Smaller grafts may be harvested from

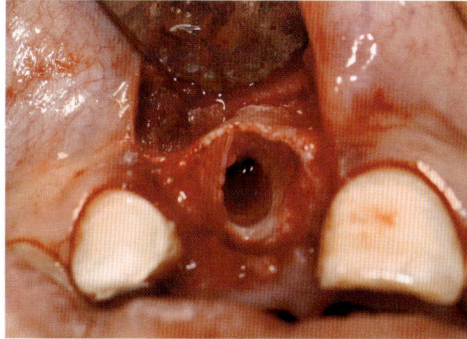

Figure 4a- Placement of an implant into an extraction socket. Flap reflection and careful extraction of the root. The socket may be gently debrided of any remaining periodontal ligament or inflammatory tissues.

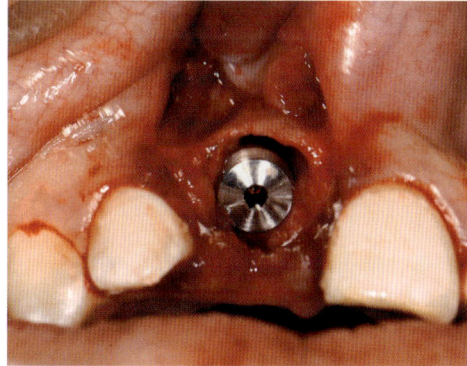

Figure 4b- Placement of an Astra Tech implant into the socket. The space between the implant and the socket wall is narrow and was left to heal.

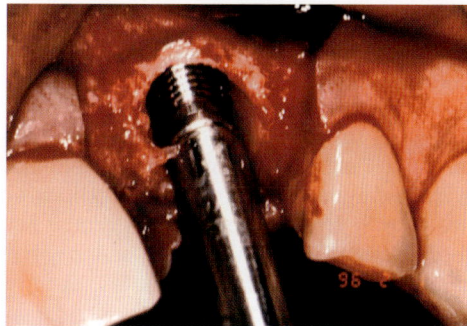

Figure 4c- Placement of a Branemark implant into a socket with a number of threads exposed.

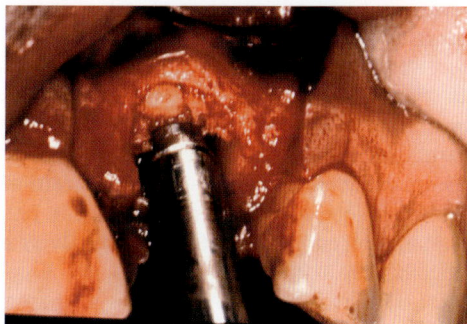

Figure 4d- The residual socket and exposed implant threads have been grafted with autogenous bone chips.

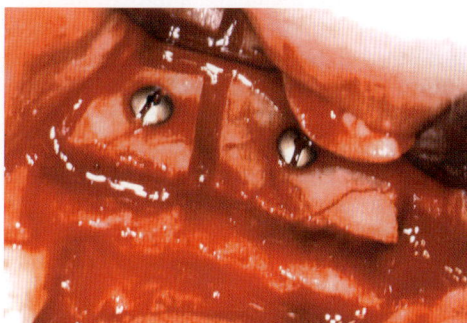

Figure 5- A thin residual alveolus exists in the posterior maxilla on both sides in this patient. Adequate volume of autogenous bone could only be obtained from an extra-oral site. In this case iliac crest corticocancellous blocks have been screwed in place to increase the thickness of the ridge. Following a healing period of 3 to 4 months implants can be placed.

the chin or retromolar area, although large cortico-cancellous grafts are usually taken from the iliac crest. Grafts should be secured to the recipient bed using miniscrews and plates or wires. The host bed is perforated with a small bur to allow blood clots to form between the two bone surfaces and to allow communication with the cancellous bone, which contains osteoprogenitor cells. Any remaining voids may be packed with cancellous bone chips to maximise the healing potential. The graft is left for 3 to 6 months before implant placement.

Ridge expansion

Lack of bone in the bucco-lingual direction may also be dealt with by using osteotomes or "site formers". These are available for most implant systems and are used instead of larger diameter drills (*Fig.6*). The site is initially prepared with a narrow diameter drill (2mm) and this is followed by careful expansion of the site with increasing diameter formers inserted to the planned depth. Case selection using this technique is critical as brittle bone may fracture in an unpredictable fashion causing further bone loss. Furthermore accurate positioning and orientation of the implants may be difficult to achieve.

Sinus lifts (sub-antral grafting)

The sinus lift or sinus floor elevation is similar to a Caldwell-Luc procedure combined with grafting of the floor of the maxillary sinus (*Fig.7*). It is a procedure that can be performed under local anaesthesia and involves carefully cutting a window in the lateral antral wall using surgical burs but retaining the integrity of the sinus membrane (*Fig.7b*). The sinus membrane is elevated to create a discrete cavity on the superior aspect of the residual alveolus, into which graft material may be inserted (*Fig.7d*). If the sinus membrane is torn and cannot be repaired with a resorbable membrane (*Fig 7c*) it is not advisable to graft particulate material although blocks of corticocancellous bone can be secured in position. The technique is commonly used as a pre-implant procedure when the residual alveolar ridge has resorbed to a point where initial implant stability is compromised (less than 5mm of available bone height). This 2-stage protocol increases the likelihood of achieving stable implants at placement and improves the overall success rate. Alternatively grafting can be performed at the same stage as implant placement (*Fig. 8*). This is normally where there is at least 5mm of residual bone height to ensure stability of the implant. The grafting can be carried out as an open sinus lift procedure as described above or as a closed procedure using osteotomes to develop the site in an apical direction (*Fig 9*).

Inlay grafts combined with maxillary osteotomies

Gross resorption of the maxilla leading to a Class III skeletal relationship can be treated using an inlay graft combined with a Le Fort I type osteotomy. This will improve the skeletal jaw relationship and available bone height while leaving the alveolar crest form unchanged. Once the Le Fort I down fracture is complete a bone inlay of predetermined thickness is placed in the void and sandwiched between the two sections and secured using mini-plates. The size of the inlay required necessitates the use of cortico-cancellous bone from the iliac crest for this procedure.

Bone deficiencies in the posterior mandible

Alveolar resorption in the posterior part of the mandible eventually reduces the available bone height above the inferior dental canal to a point where implants cannot be placed without risk of injury to the inferior dental bundle. It is important to emphasise that due consideration has to be given when planning not only for the implant length but for the fact that the drills used usually prepare the osteotomy site 1-2mm deeper than the actual implant. It is therefore imperative that the surgeon is familiar with the system and drills being used when planning surgery close to important anatomical structures.

Onlay grafts can overcome lack of height above the ID canal or alternatively the nerve bundle itself may be surgically transposed. This is a difficult technique involving deroofing the nerve and dissecting the neurovascular bundle from the body of the mandible as far distally as is required. Implants may then be placed spanning the entire height of the mandible while avoiding the nerve. This technique carries a potentially high morbidity and should be used rarely and by experienced surgeons. In the edentulous mandible it may be preferable to place multiple fixtures anterior to the mental foramen and construct a prosthesis with a distal cantilever.

Soft tissue deficiencies

Soft tissue deficiencies can give rise to both functional and aesthetic problems.

Functional problems

The soft tissue cuff around the implant abutment has to withstand oral hygiene practices and shearing forces during mastication. It is therefore desirable (but not essential) to have the implant emerging through keratinised attached mucosa. Proposed implant sites that are deficient in this tissue may be augmented by using free gingival grafts either before implant placement, at the time of implant placement, or at abutment connection. Free gingival grafts can be taken from the palate and placed on a prepared donor site, which has a good vascular supply (*Fig.10*).

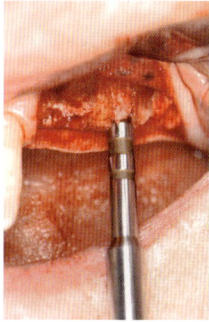

Figure 6- An osteotome being used to expand the site in a thin ridge. A narrow diameter twist drill was used prior to this wider diameter instrument which has markings indicating the lengths of available implants.

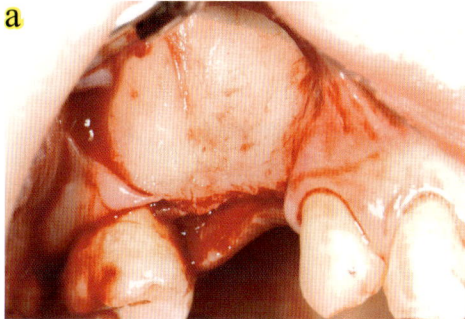

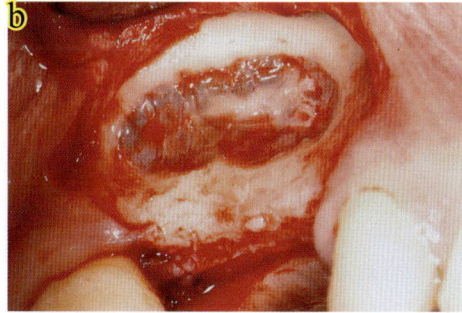

Figure 7- A series of photos demonstrating a sinus lift.

Figure 7a- Flap elevation to ensure wide exposure of the sinus wall and good coverage at completion of the procedure.

Figure 7b- The bone wall is gradually removed while attempting to preserve the integrity of the sinus membrane.

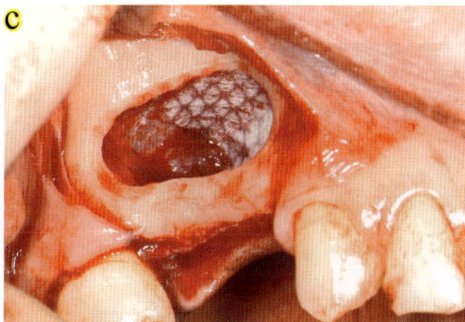

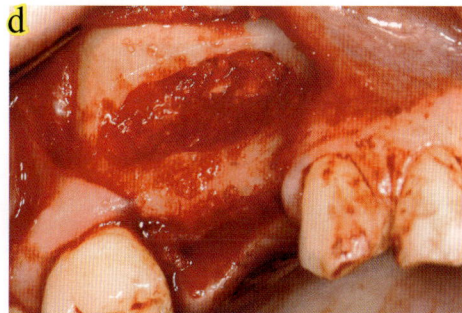

Figure 7c- The sinus membrane has been elevated carefully but a small tear has been covered with a resorbable membrane in the anterior part of the sinus.

Figure 7d- The resulting cavity has been filled with autogenous bone chips and coagulum.

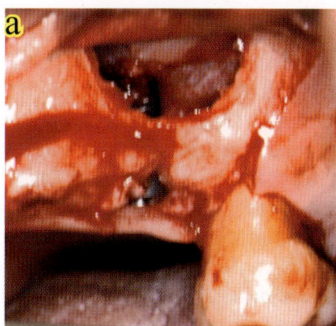

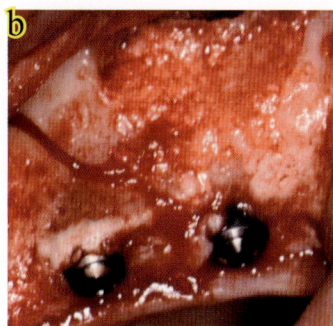

Figure 8a- Sinus grafting with simultaneous implant placement. This shows an implant secured in the marginal bone with its apex extending into the sinus and supporting a section of the buccal wall which has been elevated into the sinus cavity.

Figure 8b- The sinus cavity has been augmented with autogenous bone chips and coagulum.

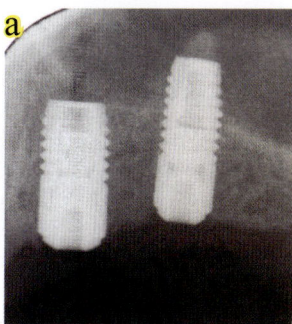

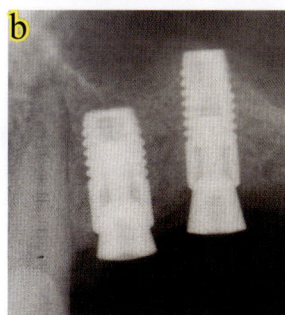

Figure 9a- Implant placement into the maxillary sinus using an osteotome technique. Radiograph immediately after placement of the implants. The distal site was developed with osteotomes to push bone apically into the sinus and keeping the sinus membrane intact.

Figure 9b- Radiograph at stage 2 surgery 4 months later showing good bone growth around the apex of the implant where it protruded above the normal bone floor.

Figure 10 a- There is complete lack of keratinised attached tissue on the buccal aspect of these two implants. The patient has experienced considerable discomfort and a free gingival graft was advised.

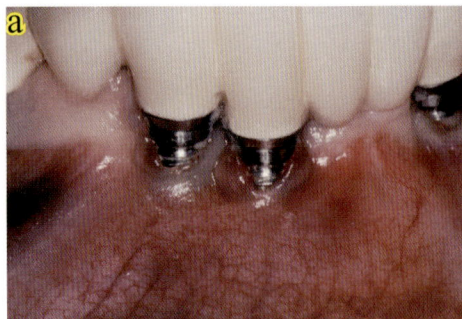

Figure 10b- A graft bed is prepared by making a split thickness dissection.

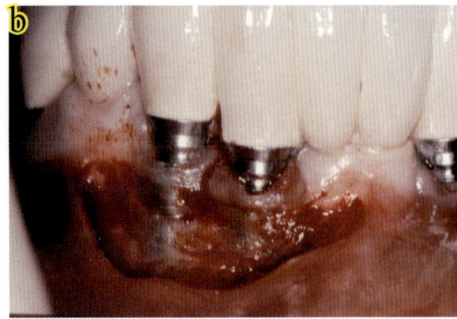

Figure 10c- A graft taken from the palate is transferred and sutured in position. This free graft initially receives nutrients from plasma exuding from the graft bed. Rapid vascularisation then occurs

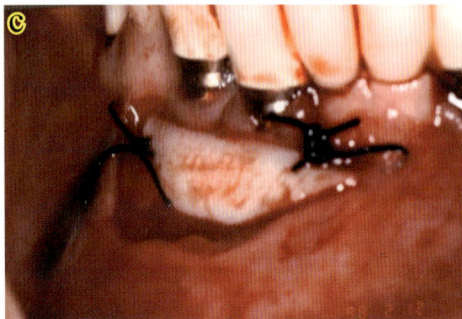

Figure 10d- The healed graft after 10 days. This will provide a zone of tissue which will be easier for the patient to maintain in health.

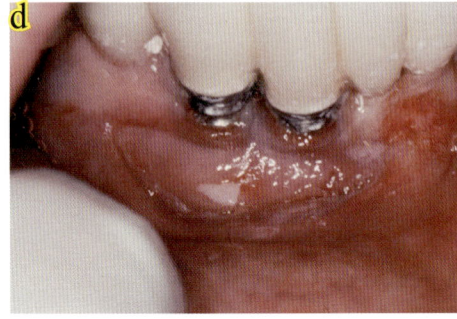

Figure 11a – A patient requiring replacement of an upper central incisor. There is a marked ridge deformity but the patient did not want to undergo grafting procedures.

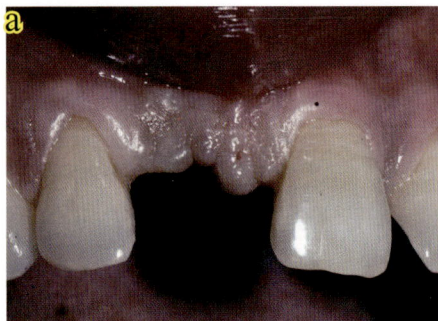

Figure 11b- The completed single tooth implant. There is no aesthetic deformity because the emergence of the crown through the soft tissue has eliminated it.

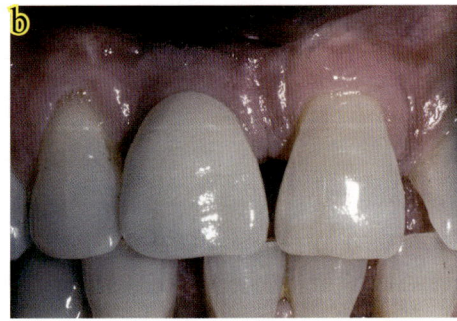

Aesthetic problems

Small defects in gingival contour may improve once the restoration emerges through the gingiva. The contours of the restorative components may provide enough support to the soft tissue to give them a perfectly satisfactory appearance without the need for grafting (*Fig. 11*). In addition remodelling of the soft tissues can continue for some time after the prosthesis has been placed.

However, larger more obvious soft tissue defects will require grafting and this is best performed as a preparatory procedure before implant placement. It can also be performed at the time of implant placement but it may be extremely difficult (or impossible) after the prosthesis has been fitted.

The ideal augmentation material is the patient's own tissue and both free gingival and connective tissue grafts can usually be used to deal with all but the most severe soft tissue deficiencies. Larger deficiencies will also require augmentation of the hard tissues. Interdental papillary regeneration has given rise to much surgical enterprise during the past few years and is desirable particularly in the partially dentate patient and around single tooth implants. Good papillary form mostly relies upon healthy gingival attachment to adjacent natural teeth (See Chapter 2). Surgical procedures to reconstruct lost papillae are unpredictable. Natural papillary remodelling occurs around single teeth implants and limited span bridges once the prosthesis has been in place for some time.

Conclusion

It can be seen that a myriad of solutions exist to overcome anatomical problems. It is important to remember the desired treatment outcome and to explore all the possible solutions. By keeping the techniques as simple and predictable as possible and using the patient's own tissue the likelihood of success increases greatly.

Basic restorative techniques

Some restorative techniques for implant supported restorations will be familiar to dentists used to providing conventional crown and bridgework. The differences and principles involved when using implants are identified.

The restorative phase of treatment starts before the implants are placed. It is essential that a clear idea of the final result should be envisaged so that the dentist and patient can appreciate any limitations or compromises that may be needed. The restorative dentist will be responsible for the fabrication of any radiographic or surgical guides that may be required to help in the surgical positioning of the implant. Provisional restorations that maintain appearance and function during implant treatment are also the restorative dentist's responsibility.

The restorative dentist familiar with routine prosthodontic techniques will recognise many of the basic procedures involved in the restorative phase of implant treatment. There is much in common: thorough examination and treatment planning, diagnostic work-up that includes tooth selection, positioning and occlusal contacts, indirect techniques with crown and bridge impression materials, accurate jaw relations and occlusal records. However, implant supported restorations also require a mechanism for attaching the restoration to the implant and this component is termed the abutment. Its selection, placement and the recording of its position with adapted impression techniques is the main difference between conventional and implant prosthodontic techniques.

The standard restorative procedure for implant restoration allows the clinician to record accurate impressions of the abutment by using machine made copings. Alternatively, impression copings are connected directly to the implant head. This is a significant advantage over tooth-borne restorations in that the copings guarantee the impression accurately relates the implant heads or abutments to one another, any remaining teeth and the soft tissue detail and subgingival margins do not need to be recorded. Replicas of the implants or abutments

are then placed into the impression which is then cast in dental stone and used to fabricate the restoration.

Provisional restorations

Before starting implant treatment a provisional or transitional restoration should be made that will be durable throughout what can sometimes be a lengthy course of treatment.

The requirements of a provisional restoration are that it should allow for the implant sites to be minimally loaded immediately after initial surgery. They should also be designed so that they are easily adapted following placement of healing abutments and subsequent implant restorative procedures. In its simplest form a provisional restoration may be a modification to an existing prosthesis but could also involve extensive fixed bridgework made with a metal framework/composite resin veneer.

Removable partial dentures should be constructed with subsequent adjustments in mind which not only include the period following surgical implant placement but also after the healing abutment and final restorative abutment are in position . If this is done with care a metal based removable partial denture can be made but usually a simple acrylic denture is easier to adapt (*Fig.1*).

For single teeth, consideration could be given to a resin bonded bridge designed so it can be relatively easily removed. A Rochette bridge with a perforated retainer is a good option (*Fig 2*). Once again, the pontic should be mainly acrylic to allow for later adjustment. Such a bridge can easily be removed and reinserted at the surgical stages, allowing the patient to remain dentate throughout treatment.

When the patient is edentulous, complete dentures should be made to allow adequate relief over the implant sites. Immediately following implant surgery a period of a week or more when dentures cannot be worn may be

Figure 1- A provisional partial acrylic denture needs to allow for adjustment when the healing abutments are placed.

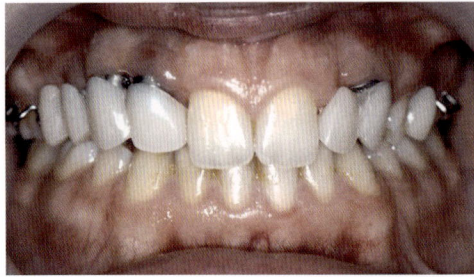

Figure 2- A Rochette bridge used as a provisional restoration.

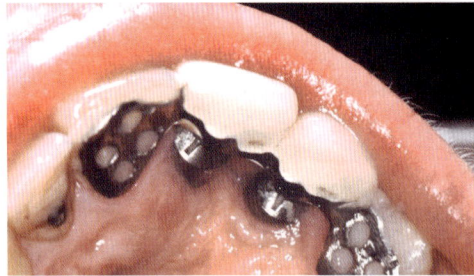

Figure 3- A full arch lower implant bridge supported on standard cylindrical abutments.

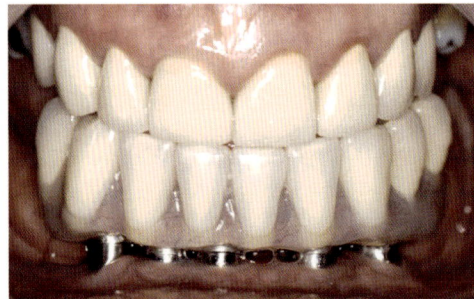

required, especially in the lower jaw. Soft lining materials such as those for tissue conditioning are used to reline the denture base. The patient should be advised to avoid biting food directly over the surgical site.

Sometimes it is not possible to adapt the provisional restoration after the abutments are placed and consideration should be given to making a provisional restoration on the implant abutments. While this may be seen as an inconvenient further step in treatment, provisional restorations can provide invaluable diagnostic information about tooth arrangement, position and shade for the definitive restoration.

If a decision has been made to restore an implant immediately upon insertion it is important that prior records have been taken to allow for sufficient laboratory work up so that a restoration can be produced at the chairside or quickly in the laboratory. Definitive abutments are best avoided and the restoration needs to be out of occlusal contact. A temporary abutment is therefore best utilised and a temporary crown constructed on this (see Fig.5b). To avoid the use of cement in the site and to facilitate easy later removal of the restoration for construction of the definitive restoration, screw retention has many advantages. With care, there is no reason why an impression of a newly placed implant cannot be taken even with sutures in place.

Abutment selection

Abutments are components that attach to the implant head and are retained to the implant by an abutment screw that extends through the abutment into the body of the implant. The abutment extends through the gingiva into the oral cavity and it provides the support for the restoration.

The simplest abutment is a titanium parallel sided cylinder that extends from the implant head through into the oral cavity by 1-2mm. From the top of the cylinder, bridgework can be made linking the abutments together (*Fig.3*). This traditional approach will produce the 'oil rig' style bridge that was pioneered by Branemark and co-workers. It is particularly useful for lower fixed bridges where appearance is not of paramount importance.

In recent years the number of abutments available for all implant systems has dramatically and confusingly increased. The main types are:

Single tooth abutments
These are designed to incorporate an anti-rotation device both at the junction of the abutment to the implant and also between the abutment and the restoration (*Figs 4 and 5*). The final restoration can be cemented or screw retained, the cemented restoration being more popular as it is more aesthetic and the angulation of the implant is less critical. Single tooth abutments for cemented restorations range from simple manufacturer made abutments which resemble conventional tooth preparations to fully customised abutments where all aspects of the abutment shape and position can be controlled by the operator either by conventional waxing and casting or utilising computer mapping and construction techniques. Abutments can be made from titanium, gold or ceramics.

Fixed bridgework abutments
These abutments are designed to be linked by the restoration to each other and so do not require anti-rotation features between the abutment and the bridge (see *Fig.8a*). The abutments are secured to the implant head in the normal way. The bridge end of the abutment is tapered to allow for different paths of insertion of the implants to be overcome by a fixed framework, which is either retained by gold screws or conventional cementation. Angled abutments are available to overcome more severe alignment problems between implants. Computer generated bridge structures can also be fabricated allowing a bridge structure to be directly screwed to the implant heads with or without abutments being present.

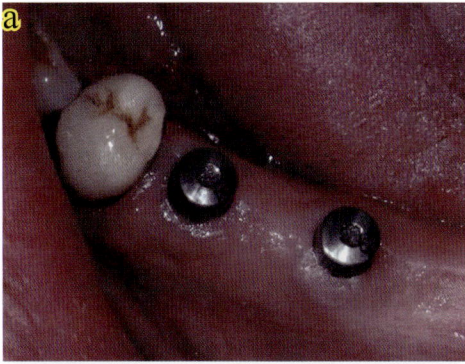

Figure 4a- Healing abutments in place for 2 missing lower molar teeth.

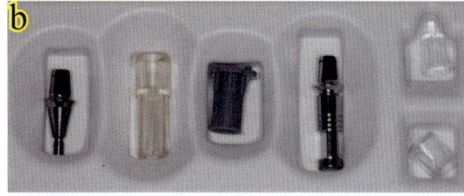

Figure 4b- The Restorative components supplied in kit form including abutment, impression coping, laboratory replica, temporary cover and burnout coping for definitive restoration.

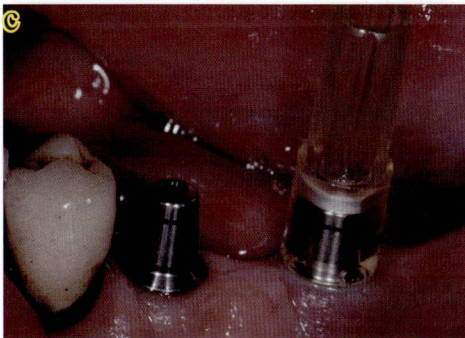

Figure 4c- The abutments are placed into position by hand.

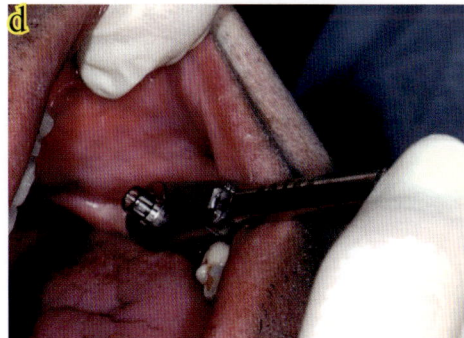

Figure 4d- Using a torque driver the correct tightening torque is applied.

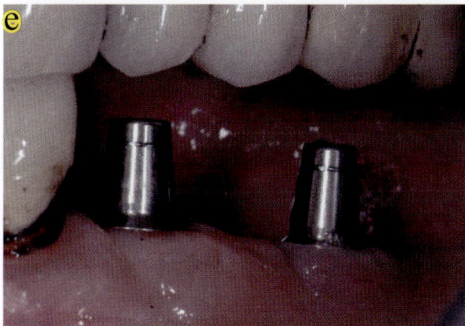

Figure 4e- Abutments in position.

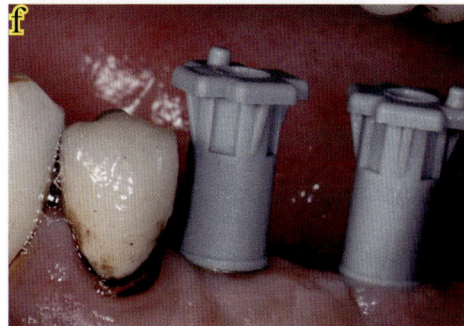

Figure 4f- Push on plastic impression copings in place.

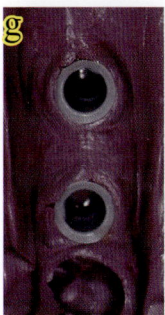

Figure 4g- Impression copings picked up in rubber base impression.

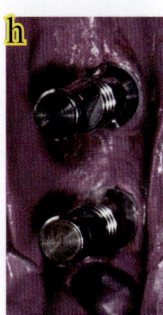

Figure 4h- Abutment replicas seated into impression copings in impression prior to casting model.

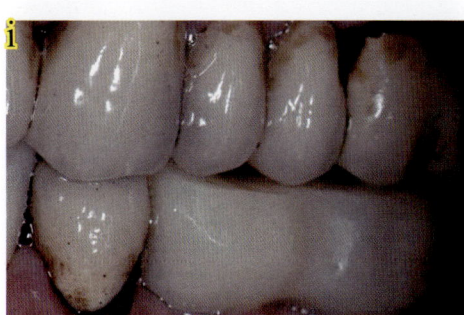

Figure 4i- Temporary cover for abutments.

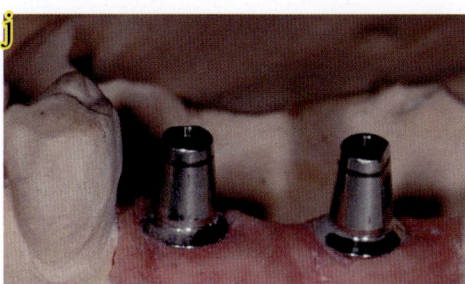

Figure 4j- Working model incorporating replicas and removable silicone gingival portion.

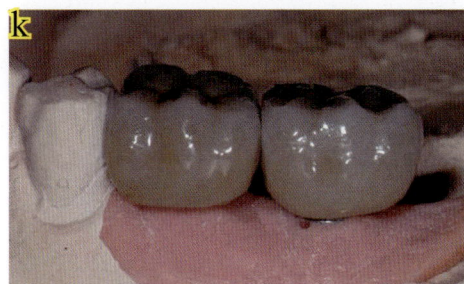

Figure 4k- Metal/ceramic crowns constructed.

Figure 4l and 4m- Crowns cemented into position. Note that access for cleaning has been obtained.

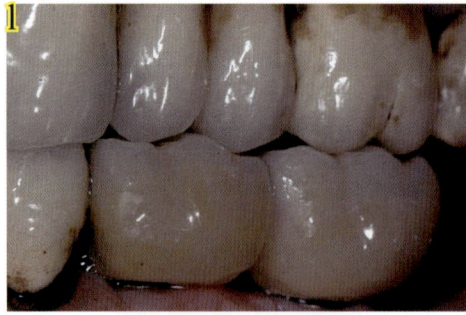

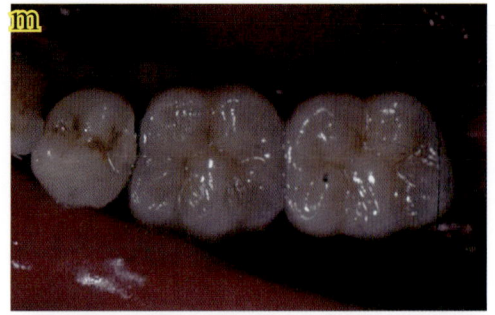

Figure 4n- Long cone radiograph post cementation to verify fit, check for excess cement and record the initial bone levels.

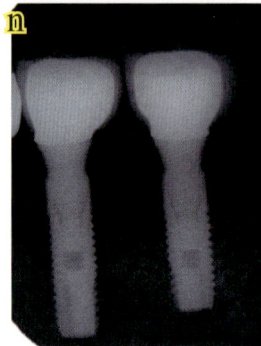

Figure 5a- Pre-treatment appearance of the right central incisor tooth to be replaced due to a root fracture.

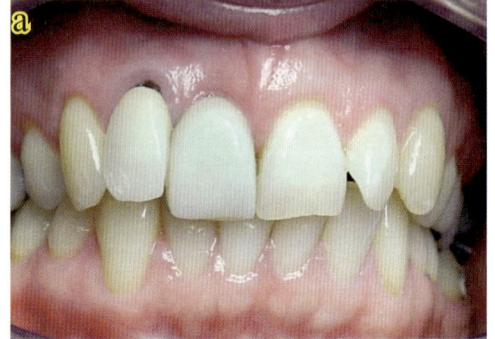

Figure 5b- . One piece screwed provisional acrylic crown on a provisional abutment.

Figure 5c- Provisional crown immediately post surgery.

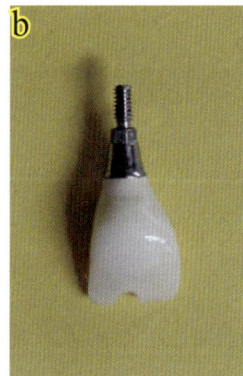

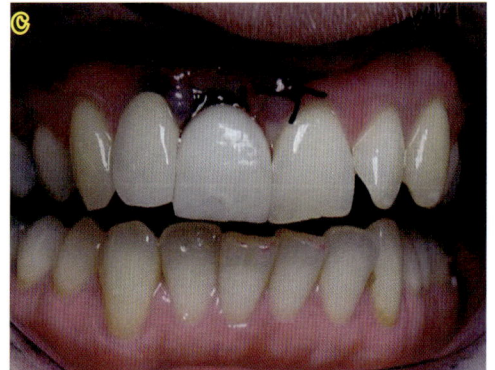

Figure 6d- 3 months later note the stable gingival margin associated with the implant crown.

Figure 6e- Healthy gingival tissue associated with the provisional crown.

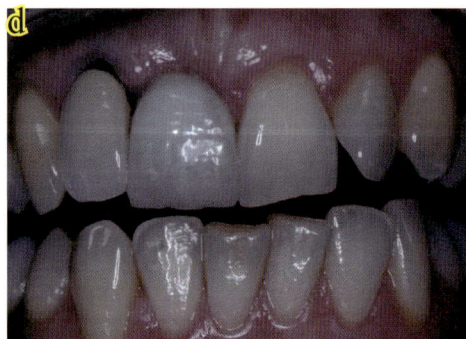

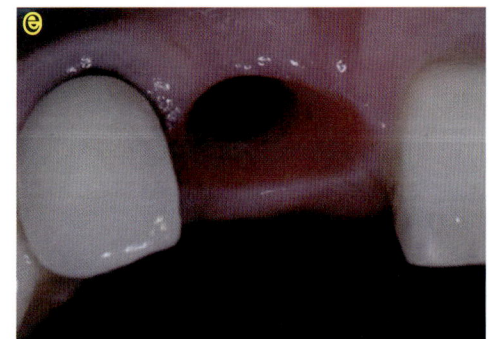

Figure 6f- Definitive abutment placed for the single tooth restoration.

Figure 6g- Cemented definitive crown.

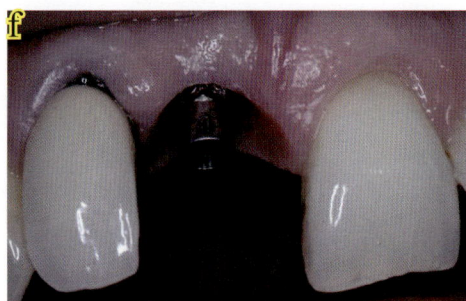

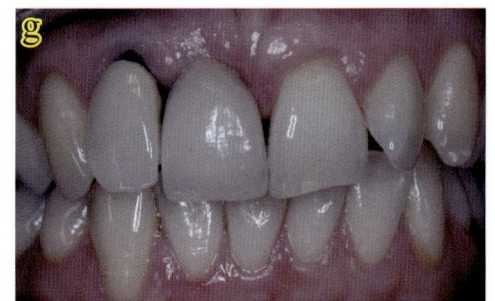

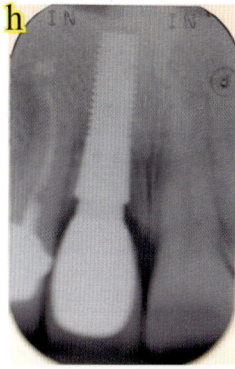

Figure 5h- Post cementation radiograph.

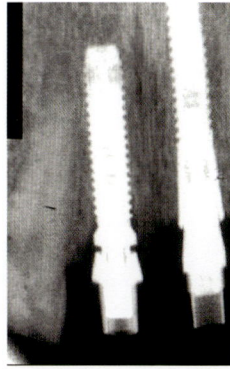

Figure 6- A radiograph demonstrating an external fit abutment that is not seated correctly and an adjacent internal fit abutment that is correctly seated.

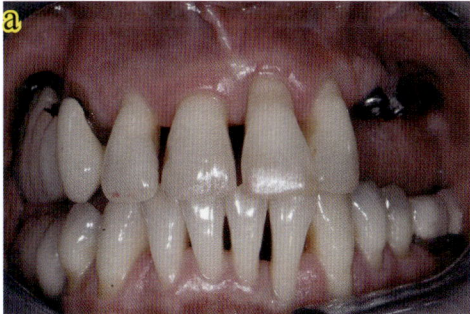

Figure 7a- Healing abutments in place for a restoration in the upper left maxilla. The patient had sinus lift bone augmentation prior to implant placement and linked restorations are indicated.

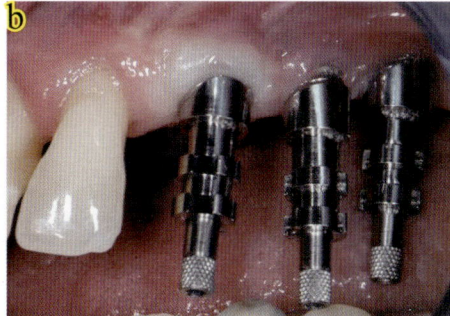

Figure 7b- Impression copings in place.

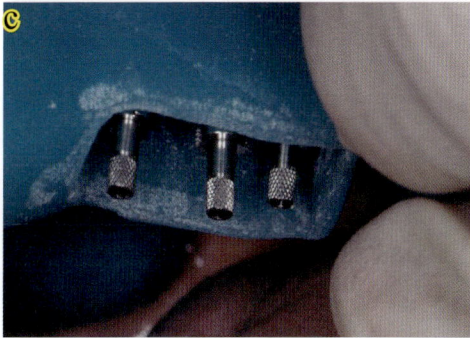

Figure 7c- Customised tray allowing the impression pins to extend through the occlusal surface.

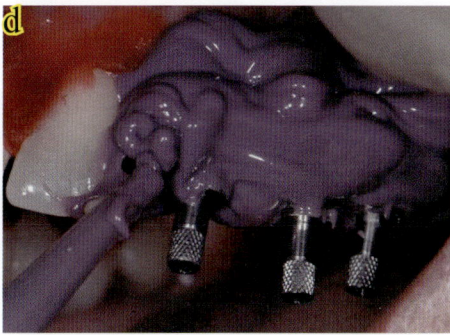

Figure 7d- Impression material syringed around the copings prior to tray insertion.

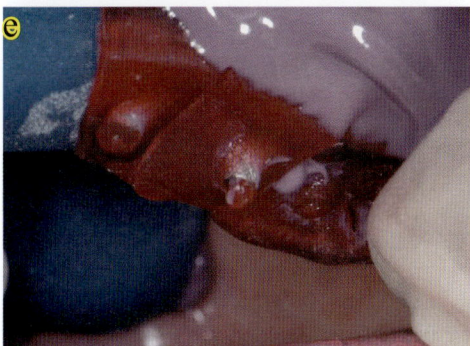

Figure 7e- Care is taken to expose the impression pin tips which are unscrewed once the material is set.

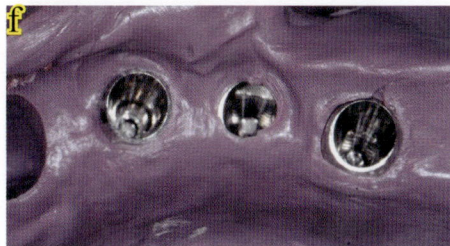

Figure 7f- The impression copings are picked up in the impression .

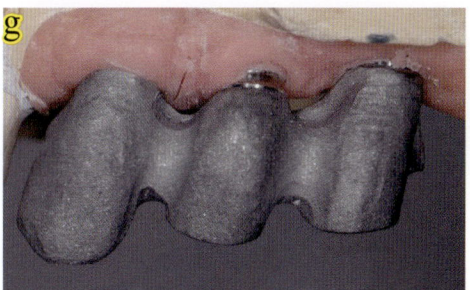

Figure 7g- A linked metal substructure fabricated on the abutment replicas.

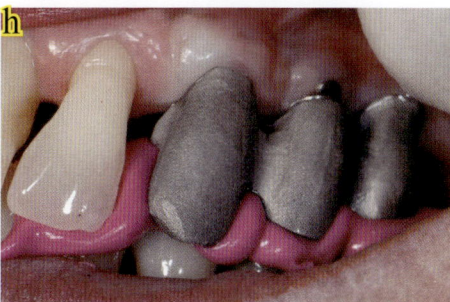

Figure 7h- The metal frame is tried in to check the fit and an occlusal record taken.

Figure 7i- The completed metal/ceramic restoration.

Figure 7j- The holes for the bridge screws emerge on the occlusal aspect and will not be visible.

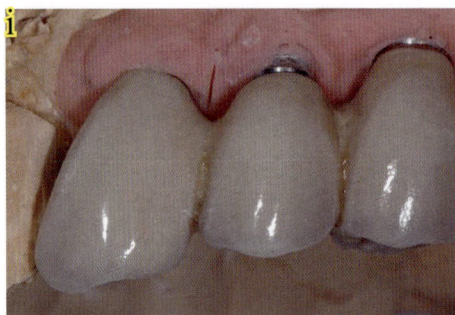

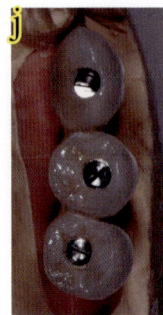

Figure 7k- The completed linked restoration in place.

Figure 8a- Conical bridge abutments in place for a lower screw retained bridge.

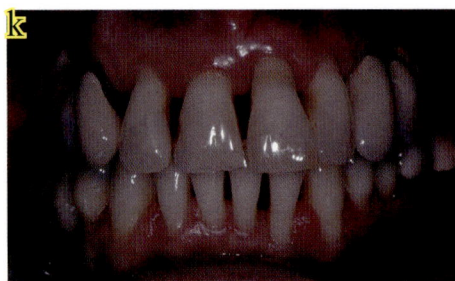

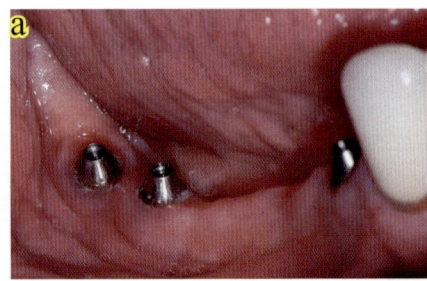

Figure 8b- Reseating impression copings placed on the distal abutments due to difficulty in access.

Figure 8c- The impression records the position and shape of the impression copings. Note the mesial abutment has been recorded using a conventional pick-up technique.

Figure 8d- The impression copings attached to the laboratory abutment replicas have been re-seated into the impression.

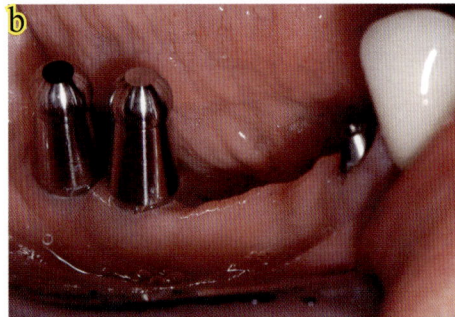

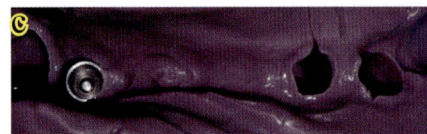

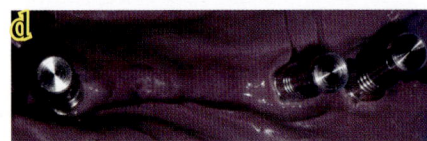

Figure 9a- Master model for a full jaw lower implant restoration. A detachable gingival mask allows access to the subgingival implant replicas.

Figure 9b- A wax occlusal rim securely positioned onto the implant heads allows stability for occlusal registration.

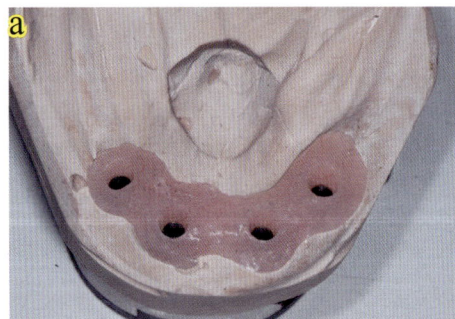

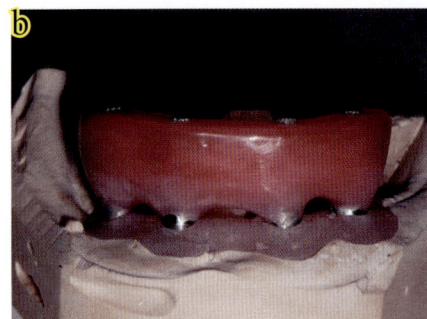

Figure 9c- The wax rim has a rigid acrylic frame supporting the wax.

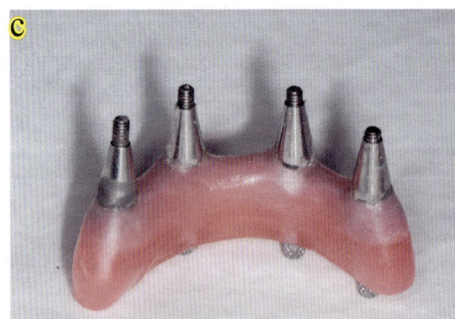

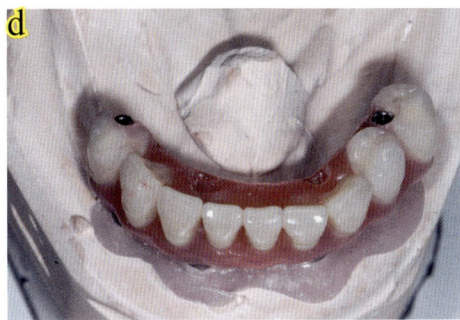

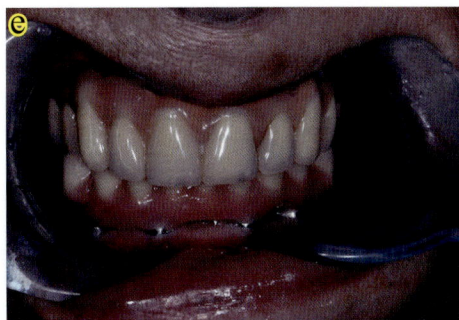

Figure 9d & e - The same acrylic frame supports acrylic teeth for a try-in.

Overdenture abutments

Either ball attachments or magnets can be used which are incorporated into the abutment or several implants can be linked together with a bar onto which a denture can be retained by clips. Abutments have to be selected dependent upon the available space within the denture. This is dealt with in more detail in Chapter 10.

Abutment length

Armed with the knowledge of which abutment type is to be used, an appropriate length of abutment can be chosen. The healing abutment is unscrewed and the height of soft tissue from the rim of the implant head to the gingival margin measured with a periodontal probe or manufacturers device. If possible and where necessary, the abutment is selected so that the margin for the restoration is placed 1-2mm subgingivally, at sites where appearance is important.

Seating the abutment

Once the appropriate abutment has been selected it is then seated onto the implant head. It is essential that full seating is ensured and as the abutment-implant junction is commonly subgingival, checking with an intra-oral radiograph may be needed particularly with systems that do not have an internal connection (*Fig.6*). When full seating has been verified, the abutment screw can be tightened to the manufacturer's recommended level of force using a torque wrench (*Fig. 4d*).

Protective caps are available to cover the abutments once they have been placed and the provisional restoration will need to be adjusted to accommodate the additional components *(Fig.4i)*. Alternatively the abutment can be removed at the end of each appointment and the healing abutment replaced onto the implant. In this situation final screw tightening is delayed until the final placement of the restoration.

Impression taking

The aim of an impression for implant restoration is to record the implant positions in a master working cast (*Figs. 7 and 8*). Many techniques have been described and materials used in making impressions. While there is no consensus on any one way of making the impression, whichever method is used, it should be done with an understanding of the technique and the properties of the impression material. Impression materials should be resilient enough to be removed from undercuts without distortion and rigid enough to allow for accurate seating of components into the impression and to prevent movement of components during pouring of the impression in dental stone.

A stock tray should be adequate for single tooth implant impressions or short span bridges. For more extensive or difficult cases a custom tray may be indicated for the final impression to ensure an optimal thickness of impression material for dimensional stability around all of the impression copings (*Fig.7c*).

There are many choices of impression technique. The standard approach is an impression made of the implant head or abutment using a transfer impression coping.

There are two types of implant transfer impression coping: pick-up and re-seating copings.

The pick-up impression coping

This is used with an open faced impression tray. The tray allows access to a retaining screw that secures the impression coping to the implant or abutment. The retaining screw should extend 1-2mm above the impression tray opening. Impression material is syringed around the impression copings first and then the tray is seated in the mouth (*Fig.7d*). After the impression material has set and before removing the tray, the retaining screw is unscrewed leaving the pick-up impression coping inside the impression. The implant laboratory replica is then attached to the coping before pouring the impression with dental stone (*Fig.4h*). For a single tooth, an impression can be made with a plastic push on coping that fits snugly over the abutment and can be picked up in a rubber base impression as above(*Figs.4f* and *g*).

The re-seating impression coping

This is used with a conventional impression tray and syringing technique and the coping remains in place on the implant after the impression material has set and the impression removed from the mouth (*Fig.8*). The transfer coping is then unscrewed from the implant and attached to the laboratory replica outside the mouth and the coping/replica is re-inserted into the impression before pouring with dental stone. This technique is useful in clinical situations where there is limited space to allow for screwdrivers to undo the long retaining screws of the pick-up technique.

Laboratory techniques

Many of the laboratory techniques for implant restorations are essentially the same as for conventional prosthodontic treatment. Working casts are made using precise replicas of the implants or abutments. The casts incorporating replica implants can be used to select appropriate abutments. Machine-made gold cylinders that fit the abutments accurately can be incorporated into conventional framework wax-ups and then cast in a suitable precious gold alloy. Casts are normally made with a flexible silicone rubber gingival cuff, which is removable from the cast, allowing the dental technician to make sure that there is an accurate fit of the abutment/restoration in the subgingival region and to help visualise and create emergence crown contours and profiles that are consistent with the gingival margin (*Figs.4j* and *9a*).

Implant supported bridges can either be made using conventional metal ceramic techniques or using denture teeth set in acrylic resin or using laboratory composite materials attached to a suitably designed metal framework. Choice of material will depend on a number of factors, not least restorations in the opposing dentition and any tendency towards parafunctional grinding habits. Increasingly alternatives to gold alloys have been sought to reduce expense and increase accuracy by avoiding large castings. Titanium frameworks can be milled from solid beams and zirconia ceramic frameworks produced by sophisticated manufacturer techniques are available.

Jaw relation registration

Conventional jaw relation records are made for single tooth and short span bridgework. The same principles for establishing occlusal plane, freeway space and recording the retruded position are applied to extensive bridgework or edentulous treatments with the advantage that bases for occlusal rims can be secured firmly to the abutments (*Fig.9*).

The gold cylinders are fixed into a cold cured or light cured resin bar and a wax rim attached. This also allows the clinician to check the accuracy of the working cast and any misfit can be corrected by sectioning the acrylic bar and rejoining with an autopolymerising resin .

Try-in appointment

From the records of the previous appointment the laboratory are able to fabricate a try-in using acrylic teeth set onto the resin bar or by waxing up the entire set-up (*Fig.9e*). This can then be used to check the appearance and occlusion as well as phonetics and cleansibility of the final restoration. It is best to check all of these features before the final framework casting is made for any longer span bridges. Single tooth restoration and short span bridges are normally produced directly from the impression stage and do not require try-in appointments.

Framework try-in

For long span bridges it is important that the final framework is tried in the mouth before the final fit appointment. It is desirable to have a passive fit of the framework onto the abutments (*Fig.7h*). For screw retained bridges this is best checked by placing the framework in the mouth secured by only one retaining screw. It should seat fully with no obvious spring or discrepancy. Discrepancies in fit require sectioning of the bridge and repair with an autopolymerising resin to allow repouring of the master cast and the soldering/laser welding of the framework. If the framework is passive the remainder of the screws should be inserted and tightened sequentially to check that no tension is produced in the bridgework. If the framework has been soldered/welded it is important to repeat this appointment to check the fit once more. A similar technique is required for extensive bridges that are to be cemented. Try in of the abutments and a passive fit for the framework are just as desirable as for screw retained bridges.

Restoration insertion

If all other procedures have been performed correctly the fit appointment should be reasonably straightforward. However, the application of acrylic or porcelain can produce stress within the framework, which may affect fit, and the procedures for framework try-in should therefore be repeated to check the final fit. The occlusion and appearance need to be checked and the patient given appropriate oral hygiene instruction. The bridge screws can then be progressively tightened in sequence in an order that will not produce stress within the bridge.

Abutments screws are tightened to manufacturers recommendations e.g. 15 to 35 Ncm. Bridge screws are tightened to 10Ncm and provisional restorations are placed in the screw access holes with cotton wool or gutta percha protecting the screw heads.

A provisional cement such as Temp bond is normally used for initial cementation of cemented restorations. The quality of fit of implant restorations is such that the temporary cement can normally be cut with small amounts of modifier or Vaseline to ensure that the restoration can be removed before final cementation. It is important to use just enough cement to coat the inner aspect of the casting but not too much to compromise seating of the restoration or expression of excess cement subgingivally. Provisional placement of implant restorations is a highly desirable aspect of treatment as it allows the patient to live with the restoration functionally and aesthetically and still allow for modification if necessary before final placement.

Occlusion

For single tooth restorations or limited span bridges, occlusal contacts need to be examined in light and heavy contact. It should be remembered that the implant is in effect ankylosed and so will not move under occlusal contact when compared with a tooth. If the restoration was made so that it was in full contact under initial occlusal contact, then once pressure was applied the implant restoration would take the full load and possibly be overloaded. In initial occlusal contact therefore the implant restoration should be in enough contact to lightly mark occlusal indicator paper but should not hold shim stock. As pressure is exerted by the patient so the implant restoration can come to hold shim stock.

It is important that the restoration is not totally out of occlusion because the risk is that there may be uncontrolled overeruption of the opposing teeth resulting in a loss of occlusal stability and occlusal interferences.

In eccentric jaw movements the ideal is to have no more than light contact on the implant retained restoration. Where possible, immediate disclusion on a natural canine is preferable. When anterior teeth/canines are involved in the restoration attempts should be made to provide occlusal contacts over multiple teeth and implants.

For fixed extensive or full arch bridges the aim is simultaneous contact on anterior and posterior teeth in centric relation with anterior group function and multiple contacts in eccentric jaw movements (no canine guidance).

Follow-up appointment

At the follow-up visit the occlusion and oral hygiene should be checked. The temporary restorations over the screw holes are removed and the screws checked for tightness. Some loosening is acceptable at this stage and ¼ turn of the screw may be required to achieve full seating of the screw. If more than ¼ is required it is possible that an error in fit or occlusion is present and will require adjustment. Once happy that the screws have remained tight, the access holes can be filled with the composite resin after covering the screw head with cotton wool or gutta percha. Accurate

long cone periapical radiographs should be taken to confirm the final fit and record the marginal bone height for future comparison.

Conclusion

Attention to detail during the prosthetic phase of implant treatment can produce highly aesthetic restorations which will continue to function at a high level over many years. The treatment planning phase is essential to make sure that the prosthodontic treatment is kept as straightforward as possible. Many of the shortcomings of conventional dentistry are avoided because of the use of manufactured components. However failure to observe the basic rules of conventional and implant dentistry can lead to problems, which may be difficult and expensive to overcome.

More advanced restorative techniques

Many alternative techniques are available to ensure the best possible outcome for an implant restoration.

Great importance has already been placed on the need for very careful planning prior to embarking on implant treatment in order to try and obtain the best possible outcome. Unfortunately there are situations where a less than ideal implant position has been achieved either by design, perhaps to overcome an anatomic problem, or because of an error at the surgical stage. It is easy to blame the surgical stage for later prosthodontic problems but in the real world, even with surgeons who have a lot of experience, there are many factors which can affect the final position of the implant which cannot be identified until the time of operation. If the surgeon and prosthodontist are working as a team it is essential that the surgeon has been provided with as much information as possible, such as stents, and is aware of 'second choice' implant sites if the prime site proves to be unusable. The worst possible scenario is for the implant to be placed in the easiest site without regard to the final restoration. Even movement of the implant by 1-2mm can have a dramatic effect on outcome with restorations at the front of the mouth (*Fig. 1*).

Patients may feel that an implant will restore them to their original appearance. They must therefore be informed that because of soft and hard tissue loss there may be an element of compromise involved (*Fig. 2*). If implants are placed in a difficult restorative position there are a multitude of alternative prosthodontic solutions available.

What are the potential problems?

Most problems can be overcome with strict attention to the guidelines given in Chapters 3 and 4, such as the use of diagnostic dentures and wax-ups followed by surgical stents. Most importantly, patient expectations should be realistic with an accurate presentation to them prior to treatment of what can be achieved and what the end result is likely to be.

Implant positioning

Errors in mesio-distal spacing may result in implants which are too close or distant to adjacent teeth or implants. If implants are too close it may be difficult to contour the restoration to allow for adequate oral hygiene or produce an aesthetic tooth shape (*Figs.3 and 4*). It can also be difficult to fit abutment components and take impressions as there are minimum dimensions for components (*Fig. 5*).

Alternatively, widely spaced implants may require oversized crowns or placing narrow double pontics, which may be unaesthetic. It should be remembered that different implant and abutment diameters can be selected and the particular width of the tooth to be replaced should be compatible.

Problems may result from the angulation of the implant, either in relation to other implants or to the desired position of the final restoration. This may occur because the shape of the remaining alveolar ridge has dictated the implant angulation or perhaps the patients' natural teeth have a curved contour, in particular a marked angle between crown and root (*Fig. 2a*).

The vertical space between the implant head and the opposing dentition may be limited and conventional components may not fit. In addition the interalveolar relationships may create a discrepancy between implant position and desired tooth placement. For example, the Class 2 div 2 incisor relationship may call for the use of angled components or where significant alveolar resorption has occurred on one arch but natural teeth remain in the opposing jaw .

Patient expectations and appearance

Patients who have worn dentures with a labial flange are used to the appearance of a restored gingival and alveolar contour, and may be dis

Figure 1a- A case with 3 missing incisor teeth. The implants have been placed evenly in the space but are too close to one another. The abutments for a cemented bridge have been placed.

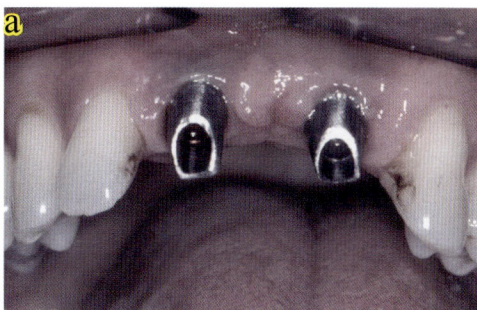

Figure 1b - The resulting bridge has a poor gingival contour. The implants should have been placed closer to the adjacent teeth.

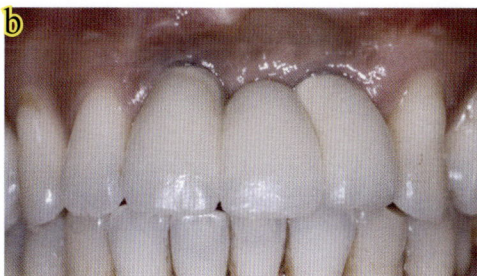

Figure 1c- A similar case with implants in a compromised position.

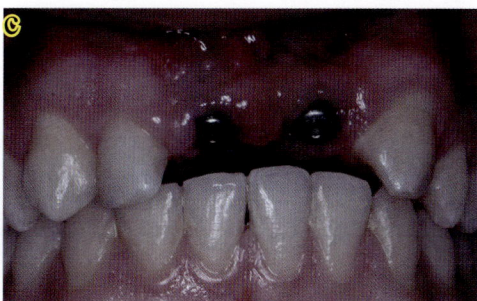

Figure 1d- The fully customised abutments have repositioned the long axis of the bridge supports in a more favourable position. The gingival replica has been removed to gain access to the sub-gingival margins.

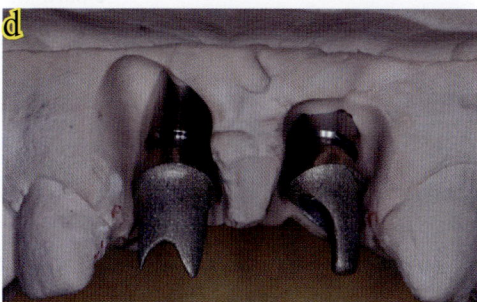

Figure 1e- The resulting bridge has a reasonable appearance but is still slightly compromised.

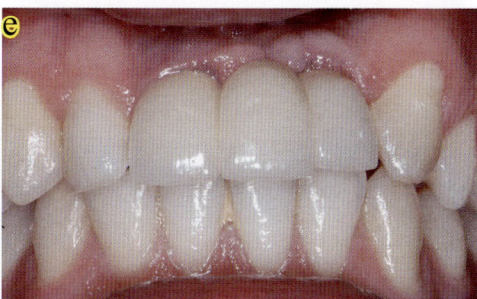

appointed if this does not exist in their new restoration.

Implant treatment is complex, lengthy and expensive, and patients often become more demanding with time during their treatment and significantly more critical than they would have been with a simpler restoration provided in less time. Beware the patient who says at the start that the appearance is not important. When restoring a tooth in the upper anterior region many patients will demand a good result, not just of the tooth shade but also of the whole tooth/gingival complex, such as the gingival margin and the interdental papilla.

Function and speech

It is rare for implant supported restorations not to provide good function even in a difficult restorative situation, however sometimes the treatment will focus problems onto existing teeth or previous restorations which may have been satisfactory before. In contrast, speech can often be affected with upper anterior restorations. This is normally transitory but may be persistent if bulky components are used which overcontour the palatal surface (*Fig. 6*) .

Excessively large embrasure spaces combined with a loss of interdental papillae may result in air and saliva being expressed which upsets some patients. The so called 'black triangle' caused by a missing gingival papilla can be reduced by over building the gingival width of the new tooth or the use of gingival coloured porcelain or acrylic but care must be taken to allow access for cleaning. Alternatively, gingival augmentation surgery may be considered.

Presence of existing teeth

In general, it is recommended that implants should not be joined to natural teeth with a fixed restoration. However, it may be necessary or desirable to include natural teeth into an implant reconstruction, perhaps because insufficient implants could be placed and the extra support of a sound tooth could help (*Fig. 7*). In some cases a sound tooth occupies space between edentulous areas and can be incorporated into the new restoration, although some clinicians would prefer to extract the tooth.

Retaining teeth can help aesthetics by preserving alveolar form. Teeth can be incorporated into a restoration using gold copings or precision attachments, however the degree of support provided by teeth in such a restoration is debatable. As the implants are essentially ankylosed it is likely that the teeth contribute little support which sometimes shows as infra-eruption or submergence.

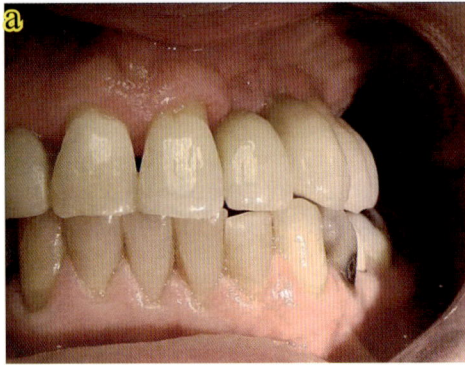

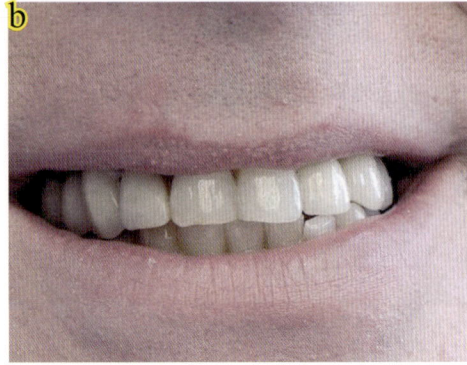

Figure 2a- Due to ridge resorption there is a steep emergence from the gingiva of the implant crowns replacing the missing lateral incisor, canine and premolar teeth.

Figure 2b- On maximum smiling this does not show.

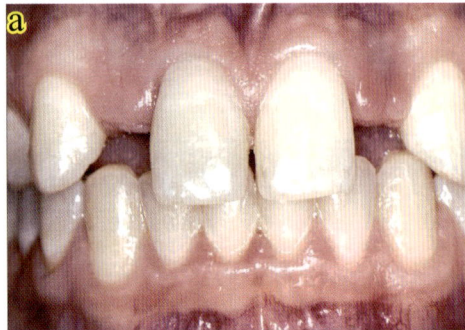

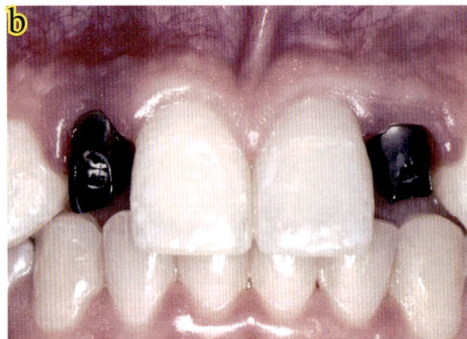

Figure 3a- Missing upper lateral incisors where the width if the space is only 5mm.

Figure 3b- Narrow width customised abutments in place.

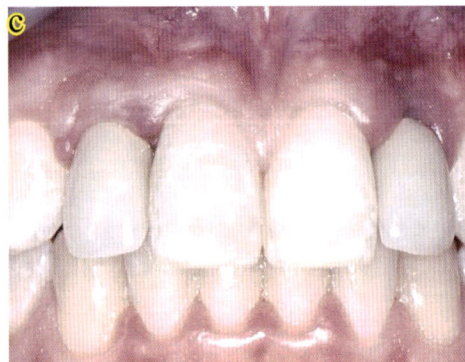

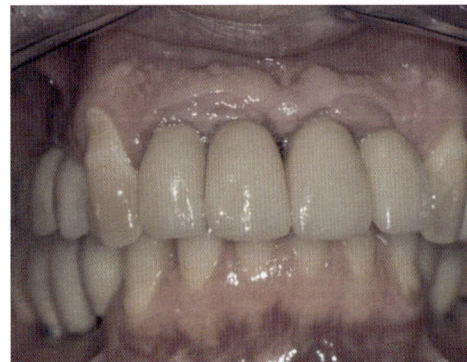

Figure 3c- Crowns immediately after insertion. There is limited space for gingival tissue and cleaning may be difficult.

Figure 4a- Four anterior crowns placed in a resorbed ridge that is not wide enough for four implants.

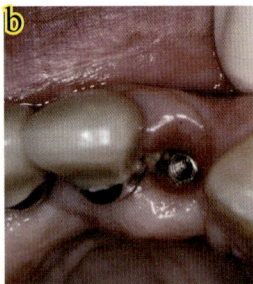

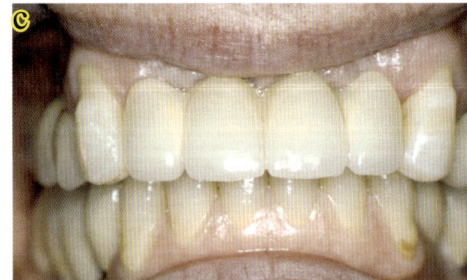

Figure 4b- On removal of the crowns the difficulty in cleaning and lack of space for the gingiva is evident.

Figure 4c- The case re-treated utilising only the two central implants supporting a four tooth bridge. The distal implants were buried.

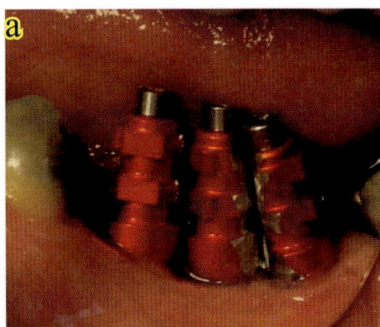

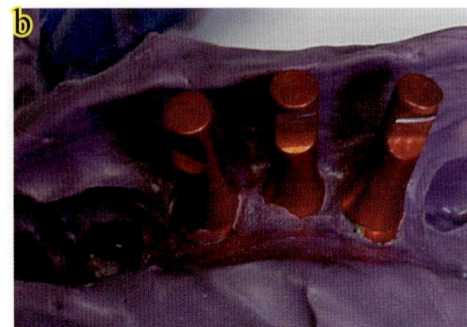

Figure 5a- Impression copings need to be adjusted due to convergence so that they do not touch.

Figure 5b- The impression with attached implant replicas demonstrate that the implants are not too close.

Figure 6a- A screw retained bridge using angled abutments resulted in a bulky palatal contour.

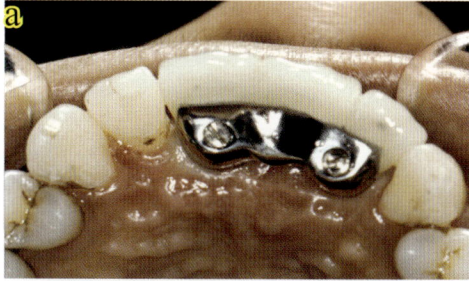

Figure 6b- The same case treated with a cemented bridge on customised abutments resulted in a more favourable contour.

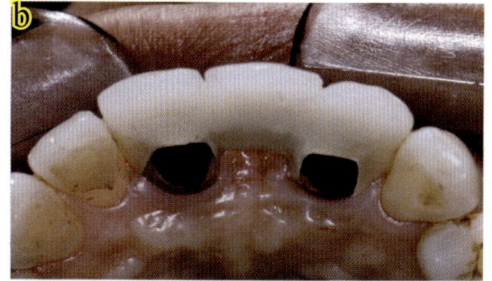

Figure 7a- Only one implant could be placed distal to the canine tooth. A gold coping has therefore been placed on the canine tooth ready for an implant to tooth fixed bridge.

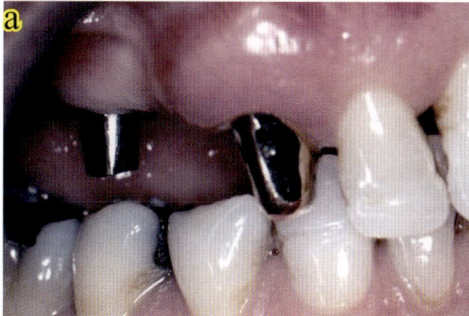

Figure 7b- The completed bridge. If de-cementation occurs the canine tooth should be protected from caries.

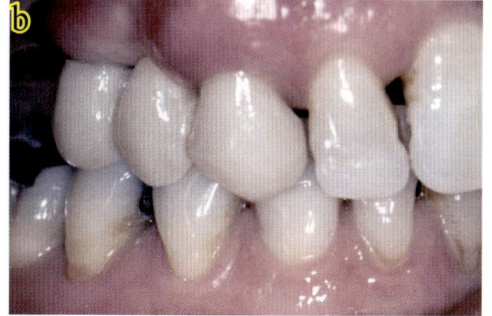

Figure 8a- A missing first premolar tooth where there is plenty of space for the implant but access is limited for the restoration. An impression coping of the implant head has been adjusted to fit.

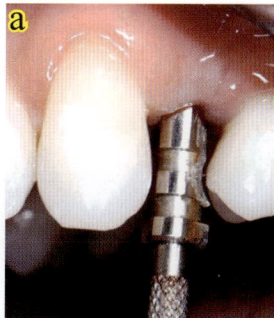

Figure 8b- A one-piece screw retained crown was constructed as a two piece construction (abutment and crown) would have been to bulky.

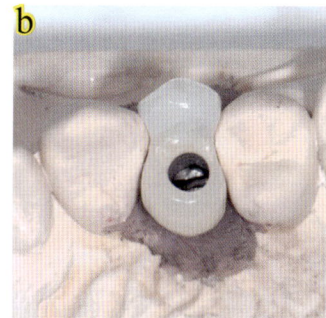

Figure 8c and 8d- The completed result. Note that composite resin has been placed in the screw access hole.- 3 months later note the stable gingival margin associated with the implant crown.

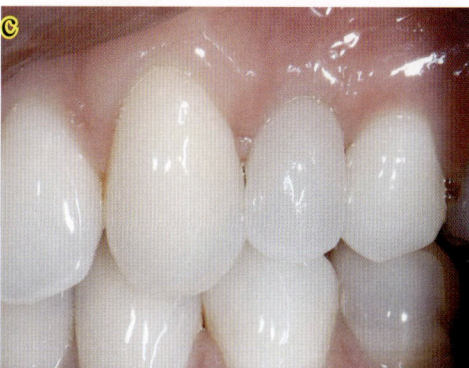

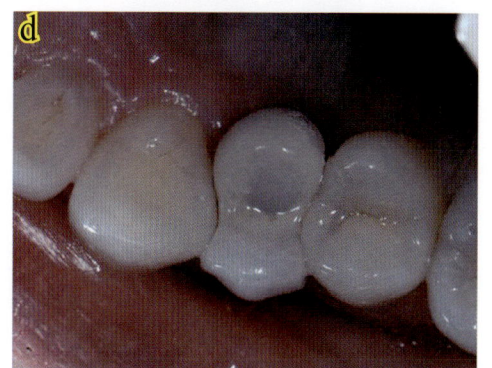

Figure 8e- The periapical radiograph.

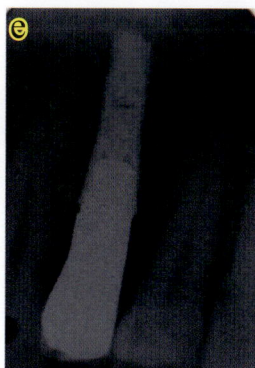

Figure 9- A diagnostic wax-up of the desired tooth position in relation to the abutments is tried in prior to metal abutment or framework construction.

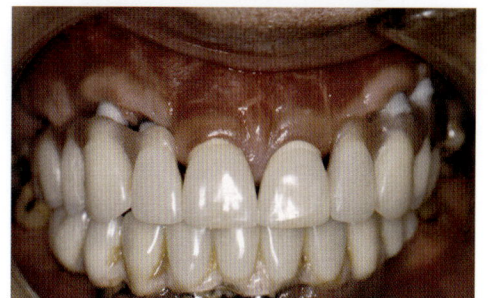

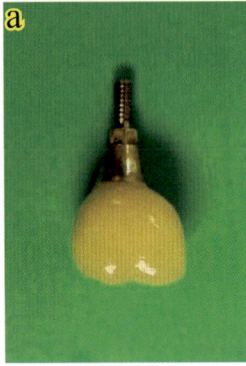

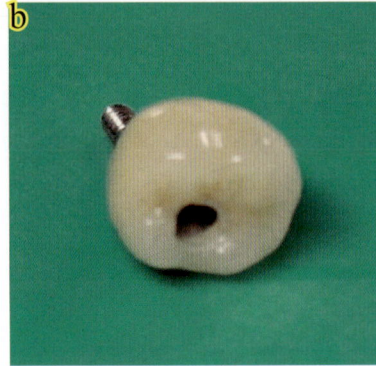

Figure 10a and 10b- A one-piece screw retained single tooth abutment and crown. The customisable abutment has been cast in bonding gold and porcelain applied directly. Note the smooth contour and occlusal screw access hole.

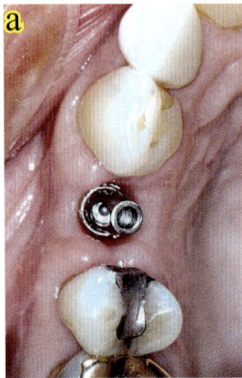

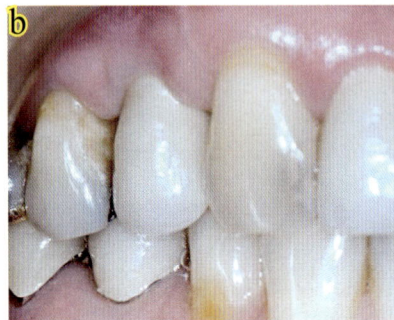

Figure 11a- A commercially made abutment for a screw retained single crown for an upper first premolar.

Figure 11b- The buccal view of the crown.

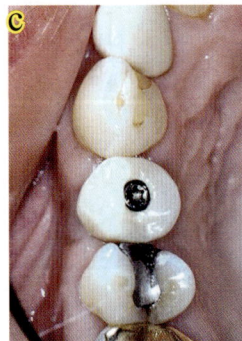

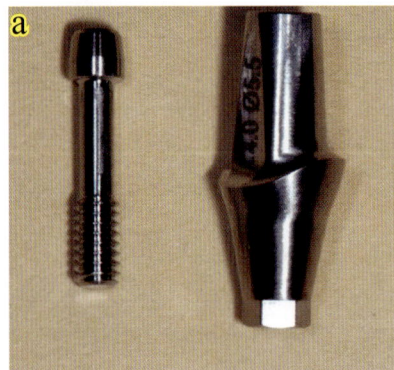

Figure 11c- The occlusal access hole can be filled with composite resin on completion.

Figure 12a- A manufactured single tooth abutment with some incorporated anatomical contours.

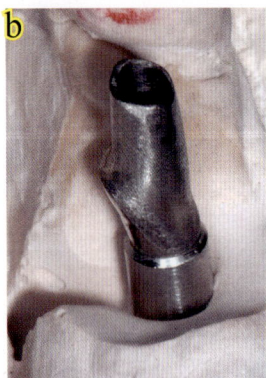

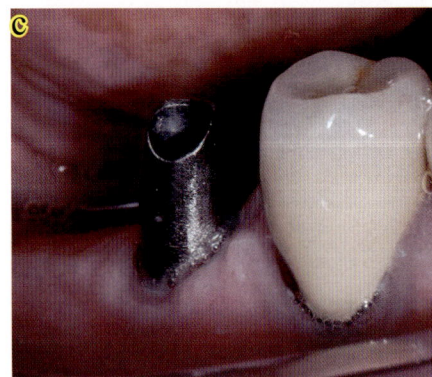

Figure 12b - On the cast this can be modified to reposition the gingival margin and change the taper and occlusal height.

Figure 12c - The abutment tried in. Note the labial gingival margin has been placed just sub-gingival.

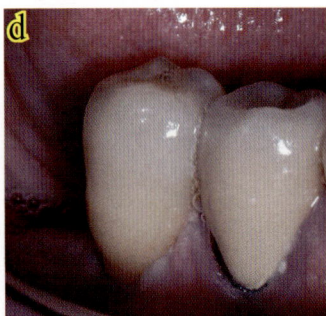

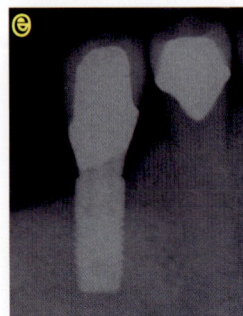

Figure 12d- Clinical appearance of the crown.

Figure 12e- The radiograph of the completed crown.

Special techniques

Traditional restorative techniques for implant restorations involve choosing the abutment, placing it and then taking an impression. This approach is fine if the case is straightforward and the implants are in the ideal place. If however there is a problem, identifying this too late can result in having to change abutments or repeating laboratory work, which can be expensive and time consuming. Alternative techniques are therefore available to overcome this.

Implant position impressions (head of fixture impressions)

Rather than take impressions at the abutment level, most manufacturers produce impression copings that record the exact position of the implant in relation to adjacent teeth and soft tissues. Impression copings are attached to the implant using guide pins and a 'pick-up' technique is employed as discussed in Chapter 8.

Following attachment of an implant analogue, a model can be produced which, with a soft tissue mask, will allow the operator and technician to choose the ideal abutment and technique for the case.

For single teeth and short span bridges this working cast is considered accurate enough to proceed with construction of the restoration using the actual abutment screwed onto the model.

Diagnostic frameworks

Following impression taking, rather than proceeding with the definitive framework, which may dictate tooth position early on, it is often desirable to have a full diagnostic try-in using acrylic and wax. The simplest approach is to construct an acrylic partial denture based on the implant position. More accurately, the bridge cylinders can be linked together with acrylic or light cured composite and the tooth contours waxed on top, or denture teeth placed in wax to produce the possible end result (*Fig. 9*) . This also allows the clinician to check the accuracy of the cast. Any problems with fit can be rectified by sectioning the try-in and rejoining.

The trial restoration can then be tried in the mouth for the patient to see and any adjustments carried out. The agreed result can be returned to the laboratory and a putty mask taken to ensure the definitive restoration copies it. The framework can be made to properly support the tooth position by cutting back from the wax teeth.

Most manufacturers now produce temporary cylinders that can be used for provisional or diagnostic restorations. These directly screw onto the implant without the need for a conventional abutment and allow even more flexibility in the decision making until all of the potential problems have been identified. They are particularly useful in complex transitional cases.

Screwed or cemented restorations

Traditional techniques were developed to construct short or long span bridges using premade components that were cast together and held in place with gold screws. Conventional cemented techniques are more frequently used in single tooth implant restorations, although screw retention may provide a good alternative for posterior single tooth restorations (*Figs. 10 and 11*). The significant advantage of easy retrievability and an excellent marginal fit of pre-made screwed components is very attractive (*Table 1*).

In the same way that conventional abutments can be chosen, prepable abutments can be chosen for height, width and angulation. These can be placed on an implant position model and trimmed to mimic tooth preparations (*Fig. 12*). Alternatively, fully customised abutments can be made using conventional waxing and casting techniques with burn-out or precious metal templates to fit the implant head (*Figs. 13* and *14*). A particular advantage is the ability to choose abutments that correspond to the width and contour of the tooth to be replaced. Although abutment preparations can be carried out in the mouth, normally only final finishing is recommended and the bulk of the work is carried out in the laboratory.

Cemented restorations

As already described, prepable and customised abutments which allow conventional crown and bridgework are supplied by most manufacturers and are chosen so that the gingival margin for the final restoration can be placed just subgingivally in the labial and proximal areas. A natural emergence angle can be developed and the soft tissue modified with a provisional restoration. This allows the soft tissue to heal around a more ideal contour. It also provides the patient with a good temporary restoration without the need to modify pre-existing temporary restorations to fit around healing abutments.

Some manufacturers produce custom abutments to follow an in-built angulation between implant and restoration. There is some scope for adjustments of the angulation with standard prepable abutments but this is limited by the need to retain bulk around the screwhole for the abutment screw.

Much has been written in the literature about the need for a passive fit for any casting that is screw retained. It would seem that this is an ideal that is rarely attained and its importance has possibly been over emphasised. Introducing a cement lute allows for small discrepancies in fit to be insignificant.

Normally the final restoration is only cemented with a weak cement, which allows the possibility for removal if necessary. If a strong cement is used, whilst this may ensure the restoration never loosens, it can make retrieval of the restoration impossible without damaging it. Restorations may need to be removed for many reasons including abutment screw loosening, porcelain fractures or adding further implants or pontics. Small lateral grub screws or a single conventional screwed abutment can be incorporated into the design to give the patient security that the bridge will not be suddenly displaced. Fortunately, decementation of implant restorations does not result in caries! Natural teeth incorporated into any cemented structure should ideally have a permanently cemented gold coping under the bridge structure so that subsequent bridge removal or debonding will not result in damage to the tooth (*Fig. 7*).

Screw retained restorations

Many clinicians prefer the simplicity and retrievability of screw retention and patients who have experienced the problems of failing conventional bridge work may appreciate the advantage of the dentist being able to remove and repair/modify the restoration easily. Implant positioning is however critical if the screw access hole is to be non-visible and in the ideal site.

On occasions it may be necessary to correct the position of the screw hole by selecting an angled abutment (which are available in a variety of angles). Selection is made easier using a head of implant impression and analogues tried in the laboratory. The final restoration is either based on standard abutment gold cylinders or customised superstructures. Ideally, with any screw retained restoration, fully machined and prefabricated components are preferred to ensure an accurate fit under screw tightening. With angled abutments aesthetics can be a problem unless the implant has been placed quite deeply as the abutment collar can show on the labial aspect.

Angled abutments can also create phonetic and oral hygiene difficulties because of the increased bulk of abutment (*Fig. 6a*). Difficulties can arise in correctly placing the abutments into the mouth, as they need to seat in the desired position on the anti-rotational element of the implant. A locating jig can be made to facilitate this.

Although abutments are available in a variety of collar heights, problems can arise when there is minimal occlusal height available as there is little room to place an aesthetic plug into the access hole to cover the screw.

Superficially placed implants where the collar of the head of the implant is near the surface can present major aesthetic problems. If a conventional metal abutment is used this may be visible or cause the marginal gingiva to have a grey appearance. Metal abutments are also a problem if the implant restoration is to be used with adjacent restorations such as ceramic crowns or veneers where matching the shade and optical properties is difficult. In these situations zirconia abutments are available from most manufacturers which can be highly aesthetic (*Fig. 15*). When selected for single teeth replacement they are used as prepable abutments or can be ordered from the manufacturers as customised abutments. All ceramic crowns can then be cemented and the only metal will be the implant and the abutment screw. For bridges, Zirconia frameworks that directly screw to the implants may eliminate the need for metal but they have not been tested in the long term.

Table 1: Advantages and disadvantages of screw retained versus cemeted restorations		
	Advantages	**Disadvantages**
Screw	Easy and predictable retrievability	Accurate framework required for passive fit
	Machined accurate components for fit	Implant position/angulation critical
	Screw acts as fail safe component	Potential for screw fracture and loosening
	Long term maintenance facilitated	Screw access hole may affect appearance and occlusion
Cemented	Customised abutment is highly flexible particularly dealing with angulation changes	Retrievability is variable dependent upon cement used
	Can join teeth and implants more readily	Conventional impression can lead to errors in marginal fit
	Small discrepancies in fit are filled by cement lute	Potential for excess cement subgingivally
	Comparable with 'ordinary' dentistry'	May encourage a lower standard of clinical and technical acceptability

Figure 13- A fully customised cast abutment. The path of insertion of the crown can be significantly altered from that of the implant as evident by the abutment screw orientation.

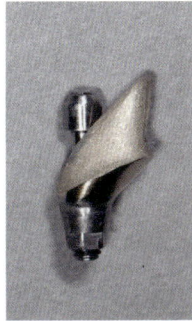

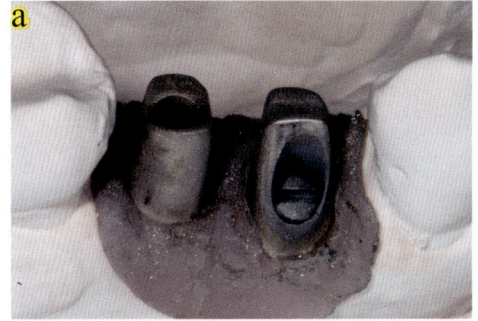

Figure 14a, 14b and 14c- Fully customised abutments used to align adjacent implants as well as develop contours and emergence similar to natural upper premolar teeth. With the soft tissue replica removed (14b) the sub-gingival margin can be accessed.

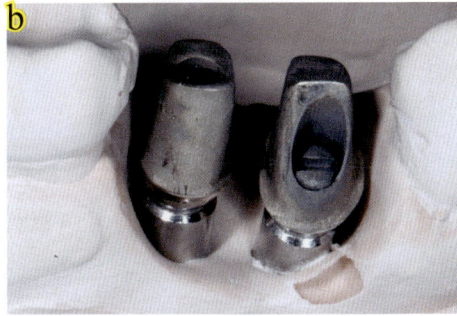

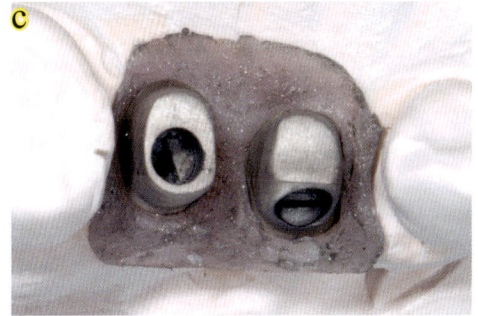

Figure 14d and 14e- The abutments are tried in. The gingival blanching on seating the abutments is normal when the emergence is being changed from a simple round healing abutment. Note the supra-gingival palatal margin for the crowns.

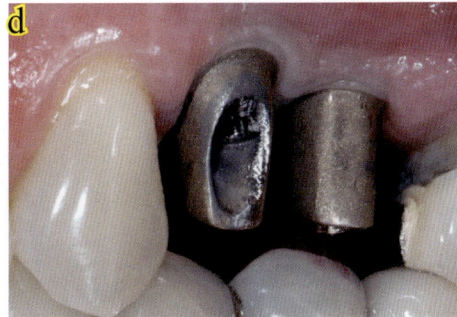

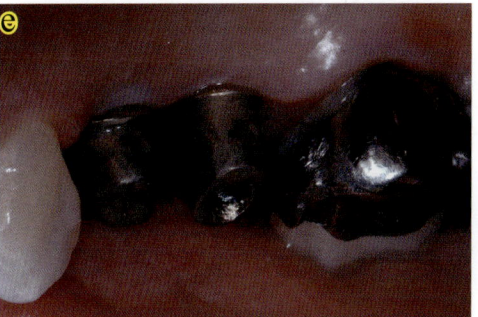

Figure 14f- The crowns on initial seating. The gingival tissue is under slight pressure.

Figure 14g- 2 weeks after cementation the gingival contour and appearance is excellent.

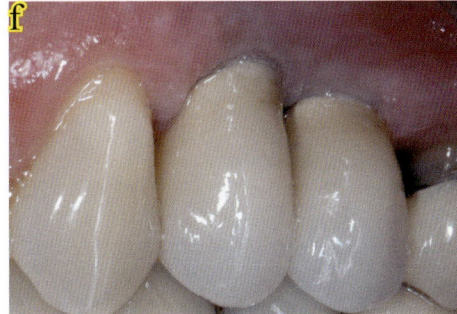

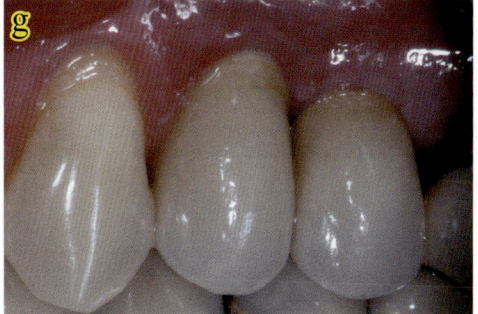

Figure 14h- The completion periapical radiograph.

Figure 15a- A missing central incisor tooth where the adjacent tooth needs a new crown. The patient has a high aesthetic expectation.

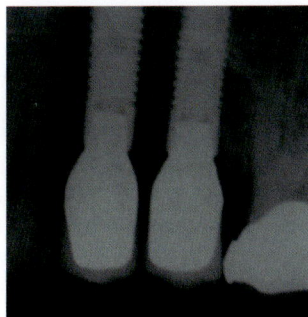

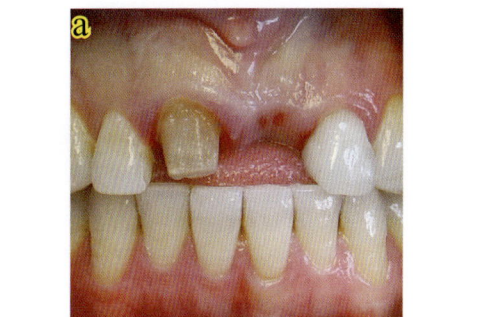

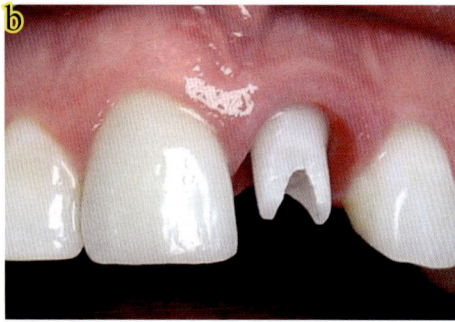

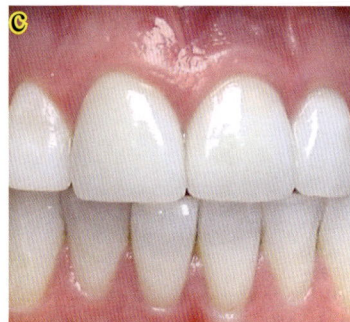

Figure 15b- A zirconia abutment has been placed to allow for all ceramic restorations.

Figure 15c- All ceramic crowns have been placed for both central incisor teeth.

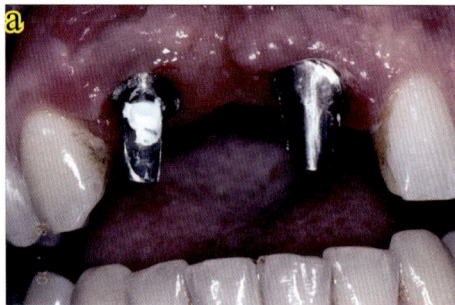

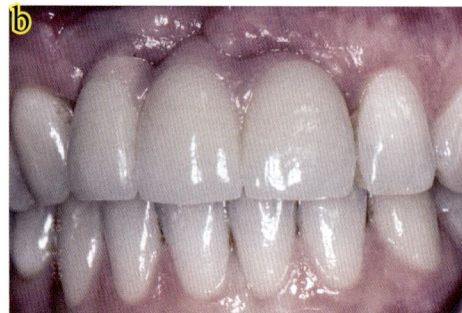

Figure 16a- Customised abutments in place where extensive bone and soft tissue loss are evident. The patient had a low smile line and did not wish to have any grafting.

Figure 16b- The bridge has the addition of pink porcelain to mask the missing gingiva.

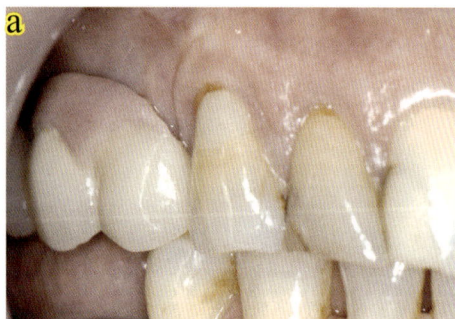

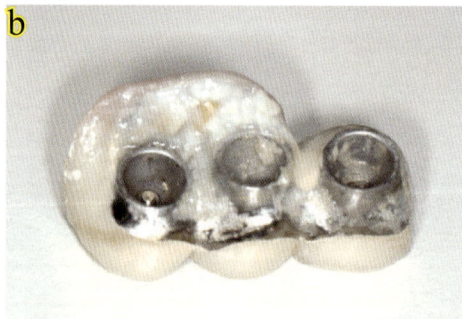

Figure 17a- A fixed buccal spoiler has been used to mask the lack of gingiva.

Figure 17b- Unfortunately this proved difficult for the patient to clean.

Replacing missing soft tissue.

Soft and hard tissue grafting techniques are often the preferred way of dealing with this problem particularly in isolated defects. However, many patients are not keen to undergo further surgery and may prefer to accept some level of compromise in the final appearance. The traditional Branemark implant supported 'oil rig' restoration approach, particularly in the upper jaw, is not acceptable for many patients although the ease of maintenance of these cases is obvious. Extension of pink acrylic, composite resin or porcelain can help (*Figs.16 and 17*), but care must be taken to ensure cleansibility. Extensions or fixed flanges (spoilers) projecting in front of abutments is a tempting solution particularly if the implant is in a poor position, but usually makes access for oral hygiene difficult or impossible. Removable flanges may not be well tolerated by patients and are difficult to maintain.

In a situation where significant amounts of tissue are missing leading to aesthetic and phonetic difficulties and the patient will not accept an implant stabilised over-denture, a milled bar linking the implants with a (patient) removable bridge superstructure retained by

locking pins can be considered. This is an elegant but complex approach with significant cost implications.

Particular problem areas

Single teeth restorations
The deeper the implant is sited the easier it is to overcome angulation and position problems and develop an ideal emergence profile. Fully customised abutments allow for the development of the emergence to be achieved by the abutment and the crown margin needs to only be 1-2mm subgingival on the labial and interproximal aspect and supragingival on the palatal. Excess cement can be a significant problem when deep margins are used as access to the excess cement is limited. Fully customised abutments also allow for the retentive element for the crown to be optimised rather than use a ready made height. This is particularly useful for long clinical crowns or areas of high load. In premolar and molar areas screw retained crowns may be considered as aesthetics are less important and have the advantage of predictable retrievability.

Short spans

The major problem with short spans is the temptation to put implants too close together leading to crowns with a poor appearance. Sometimes, if too many implants have been placed too close together, the decision has to be taken to not use one of the implants and construct a bridge using the remainder (*Fig. 4*). Where adjacent implants are to be restored with or without the need for pontics the decision often has to be made on whether to link implants together or make separate units. The decision will be made on the need to link short implants to longer ones or if it is considered a high stress area where splinted units may be beneficial. Individual units may be easier to construct and maintain, but the paths of insertion need to be considered. Providing the restorations are well contoured there should be little difference in maintaining good oral hygiene around linked or individual units.

Full arch bridges

In the upper jaw it is often best to avoid placing implants in the incisor sites so that the operator/technician can place these tooth pontics in the ideal position, not dictated by the implant position, to achieve better aesthetics. If the bone volume is adequate the canine and premolar sites are therefore to be preferred.

The difficulties of achieving a good fit for screw retention has led many to prefer the cemented approach for these long spans. It should be remembered that if multiple implants of sufficient length have been placed a potential long span bridge can often be split up into multiple smaller segments.

Conclusion

The prefabricated components available can make the prosthodontic treatment of patients with ideally positioned implants a straight-forward procedure. However, when any degree of variation from the ideal is encountered the prosthodontist can have a difficult time satisfying the patients' expectations. Implant systems should therefore be chosen with a broad range of prosthodontic components available.

In summary, start with a clear idea of the desired result and try this in the patient's mouth. By taking an impression of the implant position and relating this to the desired end result, suitable abutments can be chosen. In any complex situation it is advisable to proceed to a full try-in or a provisional implant based restoration before the super-structure is made to ensure that the abutment choice and aesthetics are correct. Above all, the surgeon should work with the prosthodontic end point in mind, to minimise the risk of an unsatisfactory aesthetic or functional restoration.

Implant Overdentures

An implant overdenture is a removable prosthesis which replaces teeth using implants to improve support, retention and stability. The denture can be partial, or more commonly complete, replacing maxillary or mandibular teeth. They have a proven track record, with published studies for this type of implant treatment spanning over 30 years. Most of this chapter will refer to complete implant overdentures rather than partial.

Indications

Implant overdentures have a particularly useful application in removable prosthodontics in those patients with severe ridge resorption such as the Lekholm and Zarb classification D or E as described in chapter 5. Other patients who can benefit are those with musculoskeletal disorders, such as Parkinson's or cerebral palsy, who may have great difficulty due to lack of the necessary muscular control required for successful denture wearing. In the partially dentate they can be helpful for those patients whose natural teeth function against a complete denture. Particularly in the case of the edentulous mandible, opposing the dentate maxilla, due to the inherent instability of the mandibular complete denture where retention is often negligible. In the opposite case of the dentate mandible opposing the edentulous maxilla, development of a "flabby ridge" in the anterior maxilla is often seen where fibrous tissue replaces bone. This is likely to be due to increased occlusal forces on the edentulous alveolar ridge. Implants used in these circumstances will provide extra support and stimulation to bone, thus potentially preventing the development of a fibrous ridge and the prosthodontic challenge this can create. As osseointegrated implants should preserve bone it is suggested that they are provided for young people who become edentulous to preserve their alveolar ridges for future denture wearing. Implants can help retain and support partial dentures particularly where there are free end saddles. However, the concept of the shortened dental arch may be more appropriate in some cases.

Another evolving field in the use of implants is to retain obturators. An obturator is a removable prosthesis used to fill a communi-
cation between the oral and maxillary and or nasal cavities. The defect in the palate may be congenital as in cleft palate or acquired following maxillary cancer surgery or more rarely trauma. Obturators provide a seal to prevent food and liquid escaping through the nose and improve speech. Retention of obturators becomes more difficult with increasing loss of teeth and increasing size of the defect. Position of the defect can also affect this particularly when it lies on or near the denture border area. Implants can have a dramatic effect on the retention of obturators but unfortunately they can cause problems in irradiated bone. Radiotherapy is a common adjunct to surgical treatment of head and neck cancer and has an adverse effect on implant survival, in addtion they can potentially increase the risk of osteoradionecrosis.

There are patients who are unable to wear upper complete dentures because the full palatal coverage that is required to achieve adequate support and retention causes them to gag or retch. In such cases an implant overdenture with a horseshoe plate and reduced palatal coverage can be provided. This can make the wearing of a maxillary complete denture an option for this group of patients, but there may be higher implant failure.

Studies have shown an improvement of quality of life for those patients who have complete mandibular dentures converted to implant retained dentures even in the absence of any physical difficulties. This has now been widely accepted and some have suggested that dentures retained by two implants should be a standard treatment protocol for the edentulous mandible.

Contraindications

A more complete list of contraindications for implant treatment is described in chapter 1. However a few factors are particularly important for removable prosthseses and the elderly for whom the majority of these will be provided. As shown by the Adult Dental Health Survey in the UK there is a declining incidence of edentulousness, but the age of becoming edentulous is increasing. Although there is no age limit for dental implant treatment, with age an increasing number of medical conditions develop requiring complex drug therapies that can compromise implant treatment. Consent is an important issue and confusion can become more pronounced with age. Patients must be able to cope with implant treatment both physically and psychologically.

Medical histories may require clarification with the patient's general medical practitioner or hospital specialist. Due to the surgery involved it is important to be aware of bleeding disorders and those on medication that increase bleeding tendency such as warfarin. Type II diabetes increases with age and if poorly controlled may increase the risk of implant failure. Osteoporosis has an increase in prevalence in the elderly population though is not a contraindication. However bisphosphonate drugs are used to treat this condition and there has been recent concern over the occurrence of some cases of bone necrosis in the jaws associated with bisphosphonate therapy, although most reports have been linked to intravenous administration used in metastatic bone cancer and multiple myeloma.

Although implant overdentures are partially implant supported, there is still an element of mucosal support. Where the quality of mucosa is severely compromised, for example bullous lesions, any dentures including implant overdentures may be contraindicated.

The state of oral health deteriorates with age with increasing levels of root caries and periodontal disease. For success in implant treatment a healthy well cared for mouth is the desirable starting point.

Fixed versus removable implant prostheses

In general fewer implants are needed to retain removable dentures compared to fixed prostheses. This can offer edentulous patients an opportunity to benefit from implants at a fraction of the cost required for fixed implant prostheses. As with all prostheses it is easier to replace soft tissue deficiencies with denture flanges especially when they are large. This may be particularly relevant in those with inadequate lip support due to the pattern of maxillary ridge resorption. A removable prosthesis also eases inspection and cleaning around the implants themselves.

As the prostheses are removable they are more accessible for repair than fixed implant retained restorations. However there is an added disadvantage of increased maintenance requirements. This is often due to the wear and fracture of the sometimes complex abutments and retainers. Denture wearers treated

with implants are able to use their teeth with renewed confidence and able to use greater forces which may not only have an effect on the implants, abutments and retaining systems but also the dentures themselves. It is essential that patients embarking on implant overdenture treatment are aware of this factor which will have time and possible cost implications. Clearly this can differ between patients but yearly reviews are generally recommended for implant overdenture maintenance.

The major advantage of the fixed implant restoration is that it is more like natural teeth. Those with a psychological problem with tooth loss are unlikely to be helped with the provision of implant overdentures. However patients who simply fear the embarrassment of denture movement can be helped with this treatment.

Protocols

The standard protocols are two implants in the mandible and four in the maxilla for implant retained overdentures. This is mainly due to the poorer quantity and quality of bone in the maxilla, but there are no good trials comparing implant requirements. Because of high reported failures of this treatment in the maxilla some clinicians recommend placing as many implants as possible! The implants should be positioned at the thickest part of the denture, in the lower canine sites and upper canine and premolar sites. They should be as parallel as possible, though there is flexibility with some of the retaining systems. In the maxilla, a bar is recommended (*Fig. 1*) to link the implants together, though where there are space constraints this can be a problem. In the mandible a bar (*Fig. 2*) can be used if the implants are in line along the ridge, although now various ball (*Fig. 3*) and locator attachments (*Fig. 4*) are more commonly used.

Figure 1- Maxillary gold bar

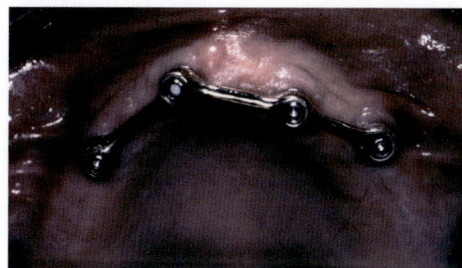

Figure 2- Mandibular gold bar

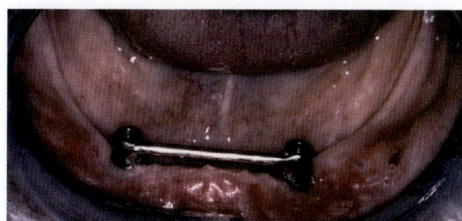

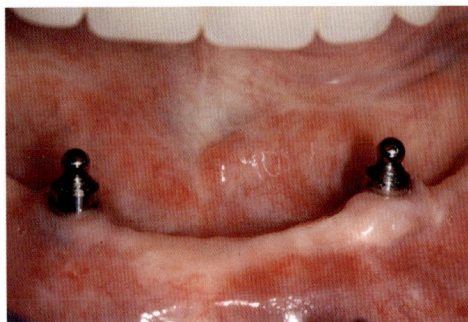

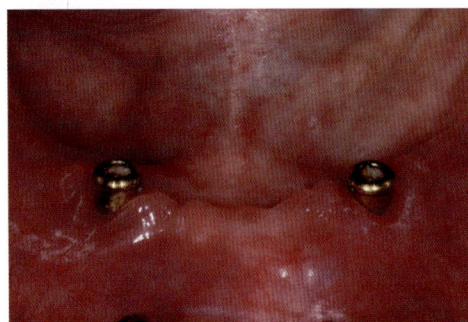

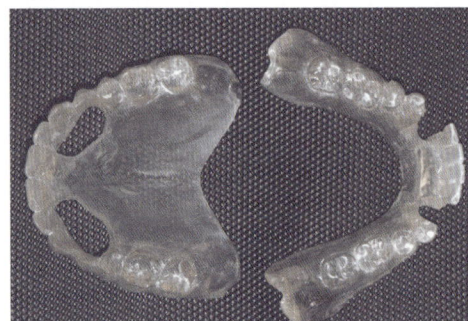

to be noted are mucosal quality, fraenal attachments, sulcus depth, tongue position and muscular influence on existing dentures. Hard tissue factors of importance are bony exostoses and tori. The quality and quantity of saliva is examined. Observation for retained roots, trauma and other abnormalities is required. The existing dentures must be examined for extension, tooth position and occlusion. General appearance, wear and denture cleanliness are also factors to note. Evidence of parafunction and clenching may be determined by examining the patient's existing dentures and or dentition. The patient's denture history may give some indication of this.

Teeth that are present must be examined. The dentate or partially dentate patient who requires extractions and in whom an implant retained overdenture is planned is more complicated. A decision will need to be made whether the patient should be made edentulous in the first instance or retention of some teeth may be an advantage during a transitional phase.

Diagnosis
In order to be satisfied that a patient will benefit from implant retained overdentures it is important to arrive at a diagnosis. Questions that must then be addressed are: Are implants desirable and will they solve the patient's problem? Is it possible to provide the patient with implant overdentures?

Tooth position
The patient must have what are deemed by the clinician to be satisfactory dentures or a trial set up is carried out before the implant overdentures are started. This is to plan the implant position and provide information on the potential space for the relatively bulky components required for overdentures. A copy of the patient's satisfactory denture or of the trial set up is made in clear acrylic and used to provide radiographic and surgical stents (*Fig. 5*). Patients with poor existing dentures may welcome the opportunity to try conventional satisfactory complete dentures before embarking on implant treatment.

Bone
Adequate height and width of bone in the correct position is necessary for implant placement in the maxilla and mandible. Height of bone can normally be assessed with a dental pantomogram (DPT), with a known magnification. A mandible of less than 7mm can be considered too resorbed for implant treatment without resorting to bone grafting. In the maxilla it is preferable to use implants longer than 7mm as short implants have a higher failure rate when used to support overdentures. Other fea-

Figure 3- Mandibular ball attachments.

Figure 4- Mandibular Locator attachments

Figure 5- Clear acrylic copy complete dentures adapted as surgical stents, cut away at proposed implant sites

Treatment planning

Assessment of the patient
As with any treatment planning patients must be fully assessed in the first instance with a complete history and examination. The nature of the dental problem must be expressed by the patient and not assumed by the dental professional. It is important to listen to patient expectations of the treatment. Problems with retained teeth and existing dentures must be explored. The denture history is important e.g. How long has the patient been edentulous? How many sets of dentures have they had made? Have they been successful? How old are their current set? In addition a full medical history and a social history are required.

Extraoral examination will include skeletal class. With existing dentures in situ an assessment of lip support, amount of visible tooth and freeway space is made. Intraoral examination to assess the extent of ridge resorption is carried out. This may be simply classified as mild, moderate or severe and any fibrous change is noted. Additional soft tissue factors

tures assessed radiographically are unerupted teeth, retained roots and anatomical features including the nasal cavity and sinuses in the maxilla and mental foramen in the mandible (which may be on the top of the ridge in severe resorption). Existing dentures and stents can be used to confirm these in relation to desirable implant position with the placement of radiographic markers. The reader is referred to Chapter 5 for more complex imaging techniques sometimes required when there is a reduced amount of bone present.

Treatment stages

Surgery

For surgical protocol the reader is referred to chapter 6 which deals with this in detail. In the mandible a decision must be made as to whether exposure of the mental nerve is required. This may not be felt necessary where the radiographs have shown the foramen to lie well distal to the canine sites. The radiographic stent can be converted into a surgical stent which is essential for correct implant placement. By limiting the flap to localized incisions (Fig. 6) surgical trauma can be greatly reduced for some of these patients. The implants are placed in the line of the arch in the thickest part of the denture. They are placed as parallel as possible angled within the long axis of the denture teeth and within the bulk of the denture base. Depending on the implant system being used single or two stage surgery is indicated. After surgery the patient is instructed to wear the denture as little as possible while soft tissue healing takes place over the first week, a temporary soft lining may be necessary. When healing abutments are placed the existing denture will require relief and reline to accommodate these.

Prosthodontics

The prosthodontic stages are similar to those for complete dentures but with the additional complication of implant connection. They are divided into the following stages.

1. Abutments and primary impressions

Once soft tissue healing has fully occurred (after about 2 weeks), the healing abutments are removed and the definitive abutments are chosen. Most have various heights allowing flexibility. A bar, studs, locators or magnets will be used to retain the denture. In the mandible studs (Fig. 3) are often used in preference to a bar (Fig. 2) which makes the laboratory work simpler and patient cleaning easier. The implants must be nearly parallel for these to be an option. The stud height is chosen so that the base emerges coronal to the gingival margin, and therefore the ball is well clear of the soft tissue. With systems where there is a standard stud height this will be fixed at the time of surgery which is limiting. An alternative system,

called locators (Fig. 4), which can be likened to a flat press stud, has the advantage of being useable with up to 40o divergence of the implants. Magnets are not effective if there is much denture movement. In the maxilla where a gold bar is being used abutments, when required, are chosen to emerge at or just below the gingival margin. The gold bar will then attach to this via screw retained gold cylinders. There are systems which allow the gold bar to be attached directly to the abutments.

Primary impressions are taken in stock trays, adapted if necessary, using alginate. The impressions are cast and outlined for the special trays which are prescribed with reference to the type of abutment and impression coping that is to be used. The position of occlusal stops are marked as required on the areas of the least displaceable mucosa.

2. Secondary impressions

At this stage the appropriate abutments are connected to the implants. If they are being left in situ they are torqued to the manufacturer's recommendation.

Secondary impressions are taken in polyether (Fig. 7) or silicone impression materials using special trays. An impression with full extension of the denture bearing area is required to ensure adequate mucosal loading and prevent overloading of the implants. Though, in the maxilla as previously discussed a horseshoe palate may sometimes be used. Where studs are used a closed tray impression technique is used, with locators impression copings are used. With a bar, impressions are taken of the previously chosen abutments or of the head of the fixture depending on the system. Either transfer copings in a closed tray or pick up impression copings in an open tray are used for this. Laboratory replicas are attached to the impressions (Fig. 8) prior to pouring the cast.

If the abutments for a gold bar are to be left in situ they will require protection with healing caps. If any of the abutments are left in situ then the dentures will require relief and reline to accommodate and protect them. Alternatively they are removed and the healing abutments are replaced.

3. Jaw relations

An advantage over conventional complete dentures is that the jaw relations can be taken on a more stable base reducing the risk of movement and inaccuracies. In the maxilla a composite link up can be attached to the abutments via modified impression screws which will confirm accuracy of the secondary impression.. With studs or locators, impression copings or the actual retention caps can be used in an acrylic base to attach to the implants, to ensure stability for the jaw relations. Wax rims can be added to composite link ups and supported on the acrylic base plates.

Information is relayed to the dental technician by adjusting the wax rims. Setting of the maxillary occlusal plane and tooth position are important with regard to lip support and tooth exposure. The centre line is then marked in the wax. The lower occlusal plane is adjusted to give an free way space anteriorly of approximately 4mm, which in the molar regions will translate to approximately 2mm. A retruded interocclusal record is taken at the desired occlusal vertical dimension using a fluid occlusal recording material (eg.silicone) which can be left attached to the lower rim. A facebow is then taken, which relates the maxilla to the condyles and horizontal plane, for a semi adjustable articulator using the upper wax rim. With a clear understanding of the patient's desired appearance, tooth shade and mould are chosen. These will be recorded with reference to the patient's previous dentures or natural dentition or other patient preference.

4.   Denture try in
The teeth should be set up on base plates in the laboratory according to the clinician's prescription. The occlusion is first checked on the articulator for maximum and even intercuspation in intercuspal position. In excursive movements a balanced occlusion is planned to ensure minimal destabilisation of the dentures in function. It is then necessary to verify this in the mouth. All the parameters described in the section on jaw relations are checked in addition to the coincidence of the retruded contact position with intercuspal position. The gold bar can also be tried in at this stage and checked for a passive fit prior to finishing of the denture.

Obviously it is essential at this stage to seek the patient's approval when any necessary changes to the teeth can be made easily.

5.   Fit and denture ease
The dentures are processed in the laboratory with the chosen matrices embedded in the acrylic. The dentures are made in acrylic though with the potential for greater occlusal forces a cobalt chromium metal base plate will give added strength.

When prescribed the gold bar is fitted in the patient's mouth. The overdentures are checked for correct extension, retention, stability, occlusion, and appearance. Adjustments may be necessary and follow up appointments are made until the patient is comfortable. It is important that the patient is educated on cleaning around their implants and denture hygiene.

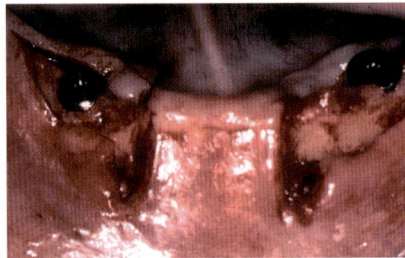

Figure 6- Mandibular stage I surgery with cover screws in canine positions in situ, showing localised flap incisions

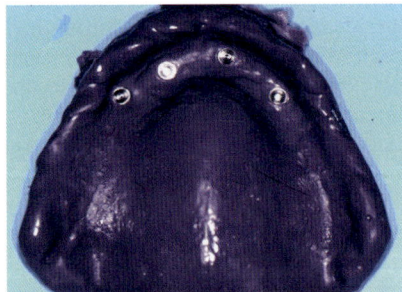

Figure 7- Maxillary secondary impression with impression copings

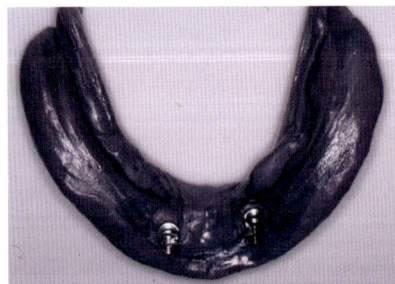

Figure 8- Mandibular secondary impression with stud replicas attached

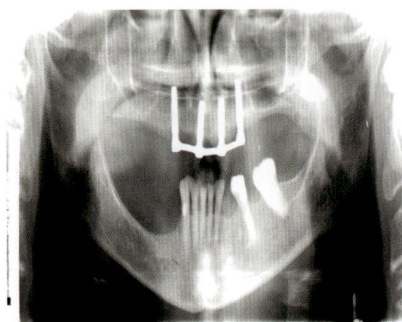

Figure 9- DPT taken at 1 year review showing gold bar and implants in maxilla

Figure 10a- Fit surface of maxillary denture with plastic inserts for gold bar retention

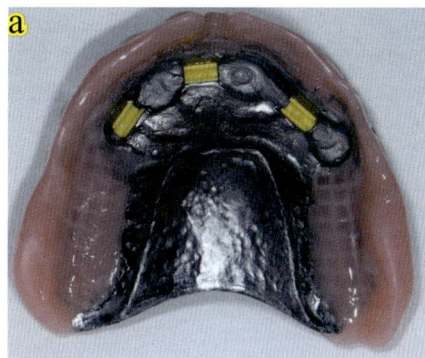

Figure 10b- Fit surface of mandibular denture with plastic inserts for locator retention

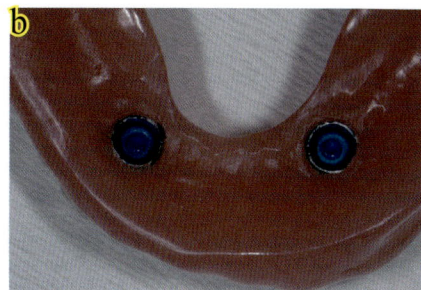

Maintenance

It is essential that all patients are forewarned of the need for maintenance prior to starting treatment. Oral hygiene should be reviewed and soft tissues examined. The bone levels around the implants are reviewed radiographically (*Fig. 9*) as described in chapter 11.

Wear and fracture of the abutments, retainers and dentures can all occur and can be difficult to manage. There seems to be no consensus on the retainer with the least maintenance although newer systems now have plastic inserts (*Figs. 10a,b*) which reduce the wear of the retainers and are more easily replaced. Most of these have several different plastic inserts which are colour coded according to the desired retention. If the implants themselves fail it may be necessary to replace them.

It is likely that yearly appointments are the minimum required for maintenance though some patients may need to be seen more often. Despite this patients will have a measurable improvement in quality of life and many will benefit greatly from the provision of implant overdentures.

Complications and maintenance

Maintenance requirements vary with the complexity of treatment provided. In well planned and treated cases, complications should be few.

The proposed success criteria for dental implant systems were described in Chapter 1. It has been suggested that longitudinal studies of implant systems should be for a minimum of 5 years (preferably prospective studies rather than retrospective), with adequate radiographic and clinical supporting data to determine the level of failure and complication rate. As described in previous chapters, failure of osseointegration of individual implants should be relatively rare, with most failures occurring during the initial healing period or following abutment connection and initial loading. Longer term complications are associated with general wear and tear, inadequate attention to oral hygiene, poorly controlled occlusal forces, poor design of prostheses or use of an inadequately tested implant system.

Maintenance requirements and complications vary widely between patients, depending on susceptibility to caries and periodontal disease in the dentate patients, complexity and type of implant supported prostheses, functional demands and the patient's ability to attain an adequate standard of oral hygiene.

Re-evaluation of the implant retained prosthesis

It is generally recommended that patients treated with implant prostheses are seen at least on an annual basis, but in many cases they will also require routine hygienist treatment at 3, 4 or 6 monthly intervals according to individual requirements. At each re-evaluation appointment the following should be reviewed:

Condition of the prosthesis/restoration

The prosthesis should be checked for signs of wear or breakage. Fixed restorations should have the cementation or screw fixation checked. This may include checking the screws which

retain the prosthesis and those which retain the abutments (see below). The occlusion should be re-evaluated, particularly where there has been occlusal wear of the prosthesis or co-existing natural dentition. In published longitudinal studies of implant systems it was necessary to remove fixed bridge superstructures to evaluate the success of individual implants. However, this is not generally recommended in normal patient follow-up unless there is suspicion that there is a problem with one of the implants. Fixed prostheses which have proved difficult to clean by the patient may require removal to allow adequate professional cleaning, which is easier with screw retained fixed prostheses than cemented types.

Removable prostheses need to be checked for retention and stability. In the case of prostheses with combined implant and mucosal support it is important to check that the implants are not suffering from overload caused by loss of mucosal support because of further ridge resorption. It has been suggested that removable prostheses often require more maintenance, in the form of adjustment and replacement of retentive elements such as clips and 'ball retainers', compared with fixed prostheses.

Screw retention and crown cementation

The screws retaining a prosthesis to the abutment are often covered with a layer of restorative material, such as composite or glass ionomer, which may need replacing. Screws which are accessible should be checked to ensure that they have not loosened. This is more likely to occur in an ill-fitting prosthesis or where high loads have been applied (see the section on Implant Component Failure).

Crown decementation of single tooth units is unusual, even in cases where a relatively weak temporary cement has been used (*Fig 1*). This is because of the close fit of the abutment

Figure 1a- A loose right central incisor crown has just been removed to reveal the hexagonal abutment. Note the health and contour of the soft tissues.

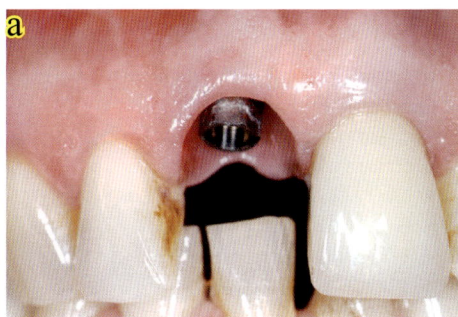

Figure 1b- The crown has been recemented and the aesthetics are good.

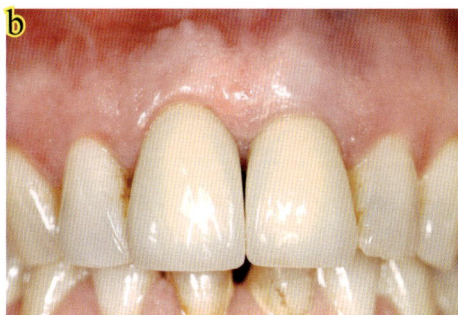

Figure 2- A radiograph of a single tooth implant replacing an upper canine. There is a large gap between the crown and the abutment because of failure to seat the crown properly during cementation. The fact that the crown did not interfere with the occlusion suggests that the original fault was failure to seat the impression coping – the crown was therefore made to fit an abutment at the wrong level.

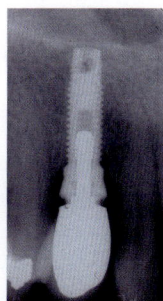

Figure 3- There is considerable inflammation in the labial soft tissues surrounding this single tooth implant replacing the upper left central incisor. The patient had suffered a severe blow to the crown which had bent and loosened the abutment screw. The resultant subgingival gap had allowed bacterial infection. The situation was corrected with replacement and tightening of the abutment screw.

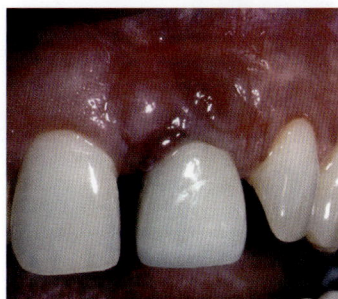

Figure 4- Marked soft tissue inflammation around a mandibular bridge. The embrasure spaces were tight and the patient found it difficult to clean.

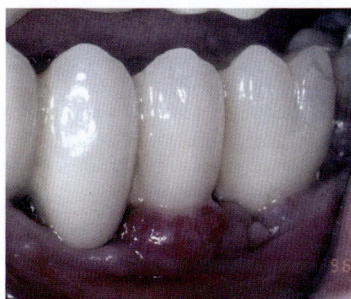

to the crown, and in some cases a high degree of parallelism between them which may make separation impossible. A more common complication is failure to seat the crown at the original cementation because of failure to relieve hydraulic pressure within the crown using a cementation vent within the crown or abutment (*Fig.2*). The resulting poor marginal fit and exposure of a large amount of cement lute may result in soft tissue inflammation because of the increased bacterial plaque retention. Venting also helps to reduce excess cement being extruded at the crown margins which can give rise to considerable inflammation, including soft tissue abscess and fistula formation. Plaque retention and development of inflammation may also be the initial sign of a loose abutment (see below).

Abutment connection

Repeated chewing cycles may produce abutment loosening and development of a gap between the abutment and implant. This complication can be largely prevented by attention to occlusal contacts and adequate tightening of the abutment screw in the first place by using specifically designed torque wrenches/hand pieces. Variations in the designs of the abutment/implant interface such as the Morse taper of the ITI system, or internal conical seal of the Astra Tech system, should reduce the incidence of this complication. Abutment loosening is more likely to occur in patients with a parafunctional activity, in situations where inadequate attention has been paid to the occlusal contacts in all excursions, and rarely when the crown has been subjected to accidental trauma (*Fig.3*). Most single tooth restorations have cemented crowns with no direct access to the abutment for screw tightening. Therefore, should this be required, removal of the crown is necessary. If a restoration is subjected to direct trauma it is preferable to have a design system where hopefully a weaker and more easily replaceable component is damaged.

Status of the soft tissue

The standard of oral hygiene should be evaluated and the presence of supragingival calculus noted (see later section on Routine hygiene treatment requirements). The mucosa surrounding the implant abutments at the emerging restorations should appear free of superficial inflammation. The transmucosal part of the implant restoration may emerge through non-keratinised mucosa, particularly in situations where there has been severe loss of bone e.g. edentulous jaws. In contrast, many restorations emerge through soft tissue which appears very similar to adjacent keratinised gingiva. There are considerable differences between the appearances of these tissues, in that the non-keratinised mucosa will appear red, possibly more mobile and will have visible blood vessels within it. Gentle pressure on the exterior surface of the soft tissue should not result in any bleeding or exudate and will produce minimal discomfort. Probing depths may be evaluated and will also depend upon the thickness of the original mucosa (see Chapter 2) and any overgrowth of gingival tissue which may have occurred. Ideally probing depths should be relatively shallow (< 4mm) with no bleeding. If increased probing depths, soft tissue proliferation, copious bleeding, exudate or tenderness to pressure are found (*Fig.4*), the area should be examined radiographically (regardless of whether radiographic re-evaluation is scheduled) to determine whether there has been any loss of marginal bone or loss of integration. In these circumstances it may be advisable to dismantle the implant superstructure to allow adequate examination of individual abutments and implants.

Radiographic evaluation

Radiographs (*Fig.5,6*) are frequently used in implant treatment to evaluate:
- Initial osseointegration
- Seating of abutments
- Fit of prostheses
- Baseline bone level evaluation following completion of prosthetic treatment
- Longitudinal evaluation of bone levels.

In all cases every effort should be made to minimise distortion and produce comparable reproducible images (see Chapter 5) to allow longitudinal assessment. Most implant systems report some bone loss in the first year following loading, followed by a steady state in subsequent years in the majority of implants. It would seem reasonable to radiograph annually for the first 2 to 3 years, then at 5 and 10 years in the absence of clinical signs or symptoms. If progressive bone loss is detected, the clinician has to decide whether this is most likely caused by bacteria induced inflammation or excessive loading (*Fig.5*). It may be very difficult to differentiate between the two, and in some circumstances the two factors may be combined.

Occlusal factors are more likely to be implicated in situations where there has been:
- A history of parafunction
- A history of breakages of the superstructure or retaining screws (or screw loosening)
- An angular/narrow pattern of bone loss
- Too few implants placed to replace the missing teeth
- Excessive cantilever extensions

Bacteria induced factors are more likely to be implicated where there is:
- A history of periodontitis
- Poor oral hygiene
- Retention of cement in the subgingival area
- Macroscopic gaps between implant components subgingivally
- Marked inflammation, exudation and proliferation of the soft tissue
- Wide saucerised areas of marginal bone loss visible on radiographs
-

This problem will be dealt with in the section on peri-implantitis.

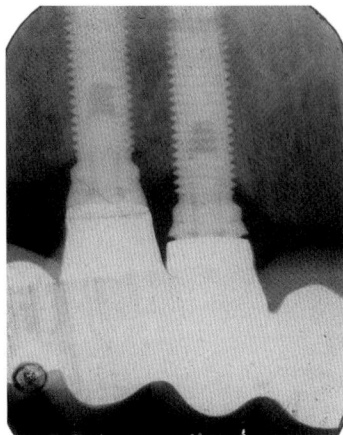

Figure 5- A Periapical radiograph of two implants incorporated in a fixed bridge showing a number of important features. In both implants the thread profiles are clearly visible confirming good paralleling technique. The implant on the left side has the bone crest coincident with the top thread and a good fit of the abutment and casting. In contrast the implant on the right side has a bone level at the second or third thread and a gap between the abutment and casting.

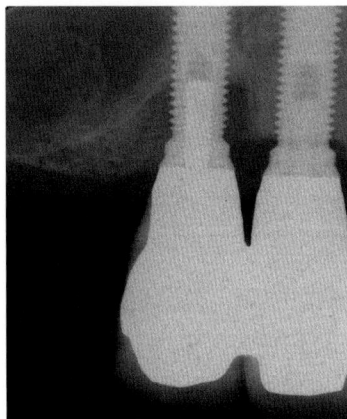

Figure 6- A periapical radiograph of two implants supporting a maxillary bridge. The abutments and castings are well seated. The bone level on the mesial implant is at the first thread but at the seventh thread on the distal implant. The bone loss at the latter implant is sorcerised and clinically there is an exudate. This could be diagnosed as a case of peri-implantitis but there has also been some evidence of occlusal overload. A distal cantilever was removed earlier following fracture of the abutment screw and replacement with a new gold abutment screw- note the abutment screw is more radiopaque in this implant than in the other one.

Routine hygiene treatment requirements

The patient's oral hygiene should be reviewed and reinforced where necessary. An individual with a healthy dentition and a single tooth implant replacement should have the simplest maintenance requirements and few, if any, complications. The patient should be able to maintain the peri-implant soft and hard tissues in a state of health equivalent to that which exists around their natural teeth, almost without professional intervention (*Fig.7*). This can be achieved with routine toothbrushing and flossing. However, in circumstances where positioning of the implant is compromised the contour of restoration may not be ideal making oral hygiene procedures more difficult. This will require modification of oral hygiene techniques to clean under the overhanging crown morphology with dental tape or super-

Figure 7a- An implant restoration replacing the upper left lateral incisor.

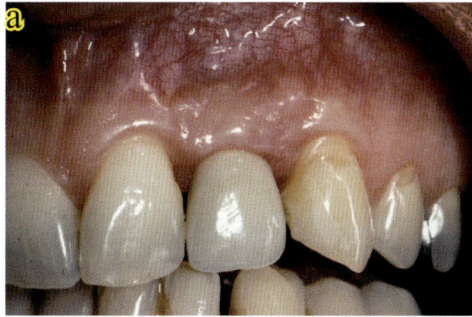

Figure 7b- The same restoration 5 years later. Note the good tissue health and improvement in the contour of the interdental tissue.

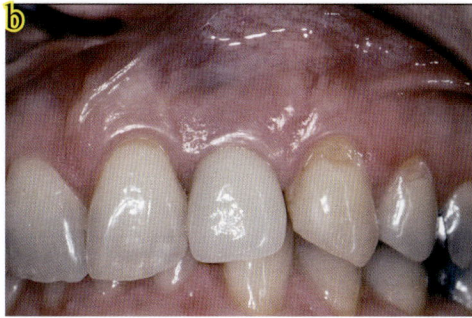

Figure 7c- Radiographic appearance at baseline showing bone levels at the top of the implant.

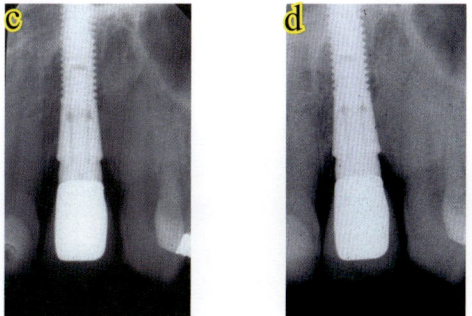

Figure 7d- Radiograph after 5 years in function showing maintenance of bone levels.

Figure 8a- Calculus will form on titanium abutments.

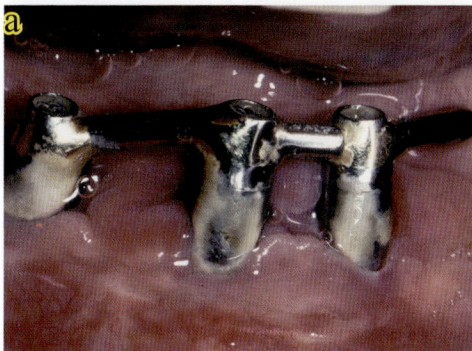

Figure 8b- Plastic scalers rather than stainless steel should be used to remove calculus from titanium surfaces to avoid damage.

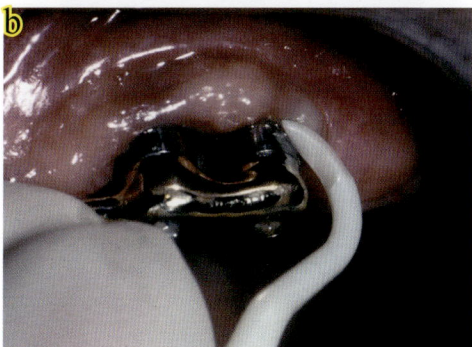

floss passed or threaded under the overhang. Single tooth restorations rarely have calculus formation on their highly glazed porcelain or polished gold surfaces. Professional scaling is not therefore normally required.

In patients with more complex fixed or removable prostheses development of readily cleansable embrasure spaces by the technician considerably facilitates patient's oral hygiene. Where calculus deposition has occurred, this should be removed. Calculus should be removed from titanium abutments with instruments which will not damage the surface (*Fig.8*). In many cases the abutments used are low profile with minimal exposure of the titanium surface subgingivally and this problem does not arise. Conventional ultrasonic instruments and steel tipped instruments are contra-indicated. Plastic tipped instruments are normally used.

Management of other specific complications

There are a number of complications which require early or urgent treatment.

Implant component failure

Retention and abutment screws which repeatedly loosen suggest either a poor fitting restoration superstructure or excessive loading. These factors require correction and proper management to avoid this complication and this is dealt with in Chapters 4 and 8. Failure to deal with these problems, particularly in patients who exhibit parafunctional activities, may predispose to screw fracture (retention screws or abutment screws) (*Figs 6 and 9*).

In many instances the fractured screw can be unwound by engaging the fractured surface with a sharp probe or using a commercially designed retrieval kit. The screw can then be replaced and due attention given to correction of the cause of the problem.

Fortunately, fracture of the implant is rare. It is more likely to occur with:
- Narrow diameter implants, particularly when the wall thickness is thin.
- Excessive load
- Marginal bone loss which has progressed to the level of an inherent weakness of the implant, often the level where wall thickness is thin at the apical level of the abutment screw.

Implant fracture is rarely retrievable, and requires either burying the fractured component beneath the mucosa or its removal. The latter can be difficult and traumatic, usually requiring surgical trephining which may leave a considerable defect in the jaw bone.

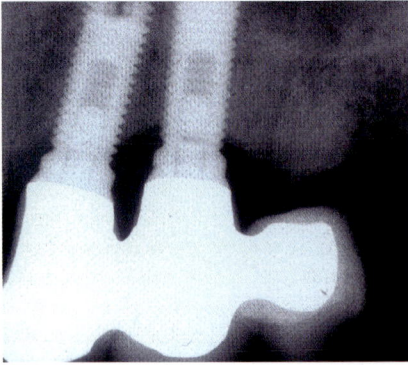

Figure 9- A Periapical radiograph of two implants used to replace three units including a distal cantilever. The abutment screw in the distal implant has fractured. The screw was replaced and the cantilever extension removed.

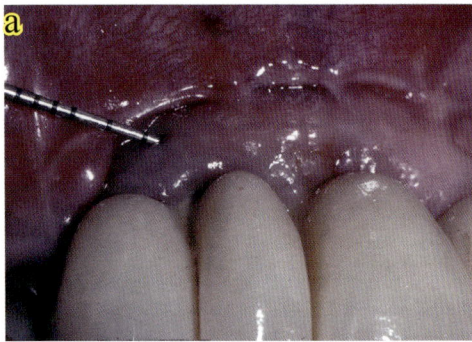

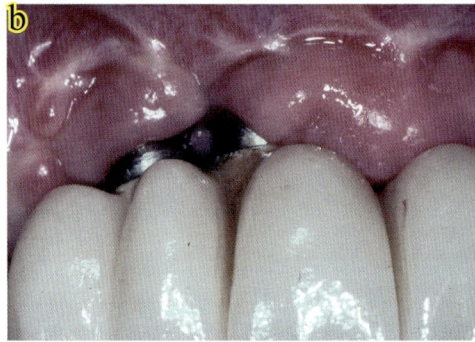

Figure 10a- This patient had repeated soft tissue abscesses and discomfort around the implant supported bridge. The probe shows a soft tissue sinus.

Figure 10b- Soft tissue surgery (as in periodontal surgery) has resulted in apical displacement of the tissue. There is an aesthetic compromise but the patient has better access to clean the under surface of the bridge and around the abutments. The original problem was caused by poor positioning of the implants in the embrasure spaces, rather than under the crowns.

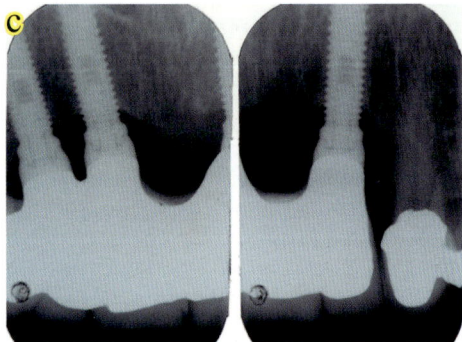

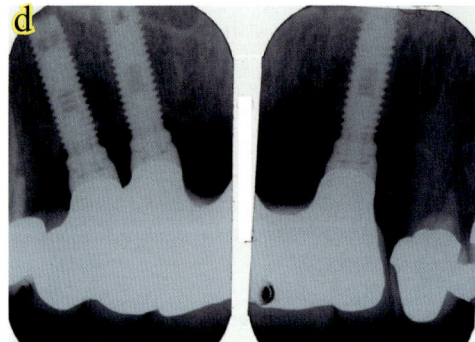

Figures 10c and 10d -Radiographs taken 7 years apart of the clinical case shown in 10a and b. Despite the early problem with soft tissue health and the poor contour of the soft tissues the bone levels had been stable over a 7 year period and they are no further apical than the second thread of the implant.

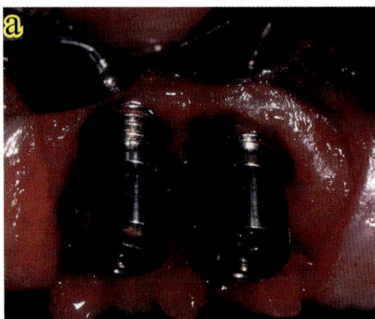

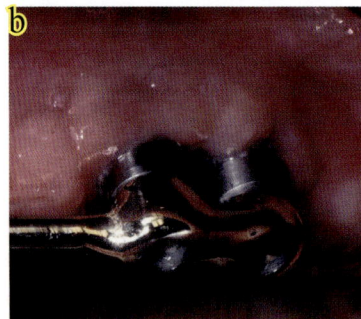

Figure 11a - Elevation of soft tissue from around two implants which had suffered from marginal bone loss and persistent inflammation. The implants surfaces were thoroughly cleaned and the soft tissue sutured at a more apical level.

Figure 11b - The flaps were placed more apically and have healed well. The patient's oral hygiene has been improved.

Soft tissue complications

Inflammation of the peri-implant soft tissues without bone loss is termed peri-implant mucositis and is akin to gingivitis. It can be corrected with attention to oral hygiene and professional cleaning. However, there are a number of instances which may require more advanced treatments including surgical correction:

- Soft tissue overgrowth
- Soft tissue deficiencies
- Peri-implantitis

Soft tissue proliferation may occur under supporting bars of overdentures. It may require simple excision if there is adequate attached keratinising tissue apical to it, or an inverse bevel resection as used in periodontal surgery to thin out the excess tissue but preserve the keratinised tissue to produce a zone of attached tissue around the abutment. In direct contrast, some patients experience considerable discomfort because of trauma from the removable denture on mobile non-keratinised mucosa surrounding the abutment. The technique of free-gingival grafting can be used to correct this problem (see Chapter 7). Soft tissue problems may arise because of poor implant positioning. Persistent inflammation or discomfort may require recontouring of the soft tissues to allow patient cleaning, and this may reveal the less than satisfactory aesthetics produced by poor planning and execution of treatment *(Fig. 10)*. In other more severe cases the only remedy may be to remove the implants or bury them permanently beneath the mucosa. Poorly designed or constructed prostheses may need to be replaced, but in some cases this would also involve correction of the implant position. A compromise solution may therefore be sought.

Peri-implantitis

Peri-implantitis is diagnosed where an inflammatory lesion produces bone loss around an implant. It is caused by bacterial colonisation of the implant surface and is managed in a similar fashion to lesions of periodontitis around teeth. The bacteria associated with peri-implantitis are those also found in periodontitis. There is some evidence of shared susceptibility. Improving oral hygiene, mechanical debridement and the use of locally delivered anti-microbials may produce resolution and stabilisation. In other cases surgery may be indicated where there is progressive loss of bone or failure to respond to simple non-surgical measures.

The keratinised mucosa should be preserved as much as possible by employing an inverse bevel incision to separate it from the underlying inflammatory tissue. Following an incision to bone the soft tissue flaps should be elevated to expose normal adjacent bone. The inflammatory tissue surrounding the implant is readily removed *(Fig.11)*. The main difficulty is adequately disinfecting the implant surface. This is more readily accomplished on a relatively smooth surface but may be almost impossible on a very porous surface such as hydroxyapatite coating. Rough surfaces require more extensive debridement than a smooth surface which may be adequately disinfected using topical antiseptic such as chlorhexidine or simple polishing. Unfortunately there are no studies that have allowed meaningful comparison of different methods of cleaning to promote resolution of the soft tissue inflammation or repair of the bone. In cases where regenerative techniques have been used and bone fill has occurred, there is considerable controversy as to whether or not the regenerated bone forms a new osseointegration with the previously contaminated implant surface.

Conclusions

Regular review and maintenance of patients are essential to maintain the health of implant supporting tissues, to prevent minor complications and measure one's own long-term success at providing this treatment. With meticulous planning, provision of treatment and use of a tried and tested system, the complication rate is low. However, it is important to realise that complications do occur and for patients to appreciate the value of long-term care.

Further Reading

1   Abrahamsson, I., Berglundh, T. & Lindhe, J. (1998) Soft tissue response to plaque formation at different implant systems. A comparative study in the dog. Clin.Oral Implants.Res. 9, 73-79.

2   Abrahamsson, I. & Soldini, C. (2006) Probe penetration in periodontal and peri-implant tissues. An experimental study in the beagle dog. Clin.Oral Implants.Res. 17, 601-605.

3   Agerbaek, M. R., Lang, N. P. & Persson, G. R. (2006) Comparisons of bacterial patterns present at implant and tooth sites in subjects on supportive periodontal therapy. I. Impact of clinical variables, gender and smoking. Clin.Oral Implants.Res. 17, 18-24.

4   Allen, P. F. & McMillan, A. S. (2003) A longitudinal study of quality of life outcomes in older adults requesting implant prostheses and complete removable dentures. Clin.Oral Implants. Res. 14, 173-179.

5   Andersson, B., Odman, P. & Carlsson, G. E. (1995) A study of 184 consecutive patients referred for single-tooth replacement. Clin.Oral Implants.Res. 6, 232-237.

6   Aparicio, C., Lang, N. P. & Rangert, B. (2006) Validity and clinical significance of biomechanical testing of implant/bone interface. Clin.Oral Implants.Res. 17 Suppl 2, 2-7.

7   Arvidson, K., Bystedt, H., Frykholm, A., von, K. L. & Lothigius, E. (1998) Five-year prospective follow-up report of the Astra Tech Dental Implant System in the treatment of edentulous mandibles. Clin.Oral Implants.Res. 9, 225-234.

8   Astrand, P., Engquist, B., Dahlgren, S., Grondahl, K., Engquist, E. & Feldmann, H. (2004) Astra Tech and Branemark system implants: a 5-year prospective study of marginal bone reactions. Clin.Oral Implants.Res. 15, 413-420.

9   Bain, C. A. & Moy, P. K. (1993) The association between the failure of dental implants and cigarette smoking. Int.J.Oral Maxillofac.Implants. 8, 609-615.

10   Bain, C. A. (1996) Smoking and implant failure--benefits of a smoking cessation protocol. Int.J.Oral Maxillofac.Implants. 11, 756-759.

11   Balshi, T. J., Hernandez, R. E., Pryszlak, M. C. & Rangert, B. (1996) A comparative study of one implant versus two replacing a single molar. Int.J.Oral Maxillofac.Implants. 11, 372-378.

12   Becker, W., Goldstein, M., Becker, B. E. & Sennerby, L. (2005) Minimally invasive flapless implant surgery: a prospective multicenter study. Clin.Implant.Dent.Relat Res. 7 Suppl 1, S-1-S27.

13   Belser, U. C., Mericske-Stern, R., Bernard, J. P. & Taylor, T. D. (2000) Prosthetic management of the partially dentate patient with fixed implant restorations. Clin.Oral Implants.Res. 11 Suppl 1, 126-145.

14   Bengazi, F., Wennstrom, J. L. & Lekholm, U. (1996) Recession of the soft tissue margin at oral implants. A 2-year longitudinal prospective study. Clin.Oral Implants.Res. 7, 303-310.

15   Benington, I. C., Biagioni, P. A., Briggs, J., Sheridan, S. & Lamey, P. J. (2002) Thermal changes observed at implant sites during internal and external irrigation. Clin.Oral Implants.Res. 13, 293-297.

16   Berglundh, T., Lindhe, J., Ericsson, I., Marinello, C. P., Liljenberg, B. & Thomsen, P. (1991) The soft tissue barrier at implants and teeth. Clin.Oral Implants.Res. 2, 81-90.

17   Berglundh, T., Abrahamsson, I., Lang, N. P. & Lindhe, J. (2003) De novo alveolar bone formation adjacent to endosseous implants. Clin. Oral Implants.Res. 14, 251-262.

18   Bragger, U., Aeschlimann, S., Burgin, W., Hammerle, C. H. & Lang, N. P. (2001) Biological and technical complications and failures with fixed partial dentures (FPD) on implants and teeth after four to five years of function. Clin.Oral Implants.Res. 12, 26-34.

19   Bragger, U., Krenander, P. & Lang, N. P. (2005) Economic aspects of single-tooth replacement. Clin.Oral Implants.Res. 16, 335-341.

20   Bragger, U., Karoussis, I., Persson, R., Pjetursson, B., Salvi, G. & Lang, N. (2005) Technical and biological complications/failures with single crowns and fixed partial dentures on implants: a 10-year prospective cohort study. Clin.Oral Implants.Res. 16, 326-334.

21   Branemark, P. I., Svensson, B. & van, Steeberghe, D. (1995) Ten-year survival rates of fixed prostheses on four or six implants ad modum Branemark in full edentulism. Clin. Oral Implants.Res. 6, 227-231.

22   Buser, D., Mericske-Stern, R., Bernard, J. P., Behneke, A., Behneke, N., Hirt, H. P., Belser, U. C. & Lang, N. P. (1997) Long-term evaluation of non-submerged ITI implants. Part 1: 8-year life table analysis of a prospective multi-center study with 2359 implants. Clin. Oral Implants.Res. 8 , 161-172.

23   Buser, D. & von, Arx, T. (2000) Surgical procedures in partially edentulous patients with ITI implants. Clin.Oral Implants.Res. 11 Suppl 1, 83-100.

24   Cardaropoli, G., Wennstrom, J. L. & Lekholm, U. (2003) Peri-implant bone alterations in relation to inter-unit distances. A 3-year retrospective study. Clin.Oral Implants.Res. 14, 430-436.

25   Cawood, J. I. & Howell, R. A. (1988) A classification of the edentulous jaws. Int.J.Oral Maxillofac.Surg. 17, 232-236.

26   Chang, M., Wennstrom, J. L., Odman, P. & Andersson, B. (1999) Implant supported single-tooth replacements compared to contralateral natural teeth. Crown and soft tissue dimensions. Clin.Oral Implants.Res. 10, 185-194.

27   Chiapasco, M., Zaniboni, M. & Boisco, M. (2006) Augmentation procedures for the rehabilitation of deficient edentulous ridges with oral implants. Clin.Oral Implants.Res. 17 Suppl 2, 136-159.

28   Cordaro, L., Torsello, F., Mirisola, D. T., V & Rossini, C. (2006) Retrospective evaluation of mandibular incisor replacement with narrow neck implants. Clin.Oral Implants.Res. 17, 730-735.

29   Dahlin, C., Lekholm, U., Becker, W., Becker, B., Higuchi, K., Callens, A. & van, Steenberghe, D. (1995) Treatment of fenestration and dehiscence bone defects around oral implants using the guided tissue regeneration technique: a prospective multicenter study. Int.J.Oral Maxillofac.Implants. 10, 312-318.

30   Davis, D. M. & Packer, M. E. (2000) The maintenance requirements of mandibular overdentures stabilized by Astra Tech implants using three different attachment mechanisms-balls, magnets, and bars; 3-year results. Eur.J.Prosthodont.Restor.Dent. 8, 131-134.

31   Davis, D. M., Packer, M. E. & Watson, R. M. (2003) Maintenance requirements of implant-supported fixed prostheses opposed by implant-supported fixed prostheses, natural teeth, or complete dentures: a 5-year retrospective study. Int.J.Prosthodont. 16, 521-523.

32   de Albuquerque Junior, R. F., Lund, J. P., Tang, L., Larivee, J., de, G. P., Gauthier, G. & Feine, J. S. (2000) Within-subject comparison of maxillary long-bar implant-retained prostheses with and without palatal coverage: patient-based outcomes. Clin.Oral Implants. Res. 11, 555-565.

33   Duyck, J., Van, O. H., Vander, S. J., De, C. M., Puers, R. & Naert, I. (2000) Magnitude and distribution of occlusal forces on oral implants supporting fixed prostheses: an in vivo study. Clin.Oral Implants.Res. 11, 465-475.

34   Ekfeldt, A., Christiansson, U., Eriksson, T., Linden, U., Lundqvist, S., Rundcrantz, T., Johansson, L. A., Nilner, K. & Billstrom, C. (2001) A retrospective analysis of factors associated with multiple implant failures in maxillae. Clin.Oral Implants.Res. 12, 462-467.

35   Ellegaard, B., Baelum, V. & Karring, T. (1997) Implant therapy in periodontally compromised patients. Clin.Oral Implants.Res. 8, 180-188.

36   Ellegaard, B., Kolsen-Petersen, J. & Baelum, V. (1997) Implant therapy involving maxillary sinus lift in periodontally compromised patients. Clin.Oral Implants.Res. 8, 305-315.

37   Eriksson, R. A. & Adell, R. (1986) Temperatures during drilling for the placement of implants using the osseointegration technique. J.Oral Maxillofac.Surg. 44, 4-7.

38   Esposito, M., Hirsch, J. M., Lekholm, U. & Thomsen, P. (1998) Biological factors contributing to failures of osseointegrated oral implants. (II). Etiopathogenesis. Eur.J.Oral Sci. 106, 721-764.

39   Esposito, M., Hirsch, J. M., Lekholm, U. & Thomsen, P. (1998) Biological factors contributing to failures of osseointegrated oral implants. (I). Success criteria and epidemiology. Eur.J.Oral Sci. 106, 527-551.

40   Esposito, M., Coulthard, P., Thomsen, P. & Worthington, H. V. (2005) Interventions for replacing missing teeth: different types of dental implants. Cochrane.Database.Syst.Rev. CD003815.

41   Esposito, M., Grusovin, M. G., Coulthard, P. & Worthington, H. V. (2006) Interventions for replacing missing teeth: treatment of perimplantitis. Cochrane.Database.Syst.Rev. 3, CD004970.

42   Esposito, M., Grusovin, M. G., Worthington, H. V. & Coulthard, P. (2006) Interventions for replacing missing teeth: bone augmentation techniques for dental implant treatment. Cochrane.Database.Syst.Rev. CD003607.

43   Esposito, M., Grusovin, M. G., Willings, M., Coulthard, P. & Worthington, H. V. (2007) Interventions for replacing missing teeth: different times for loading dental implants. Cochrane.Database.Syst.Rev. CD003878.

44   Esposito, M. A., Koukoulopoulou, A., Coulthard, P. & Worthington, H. V. (2006) Interventions for replacing missing teeth: dental implants in fresh extraction sockets (immedi-

ate, immediate-delayed and delayed implants). Cochrane.Database.Syst.Rev. CD005968.

45 Ferrigno, N., Laureti, M. & Fanali, S. (2006) Dental implants placement in conjunction with osteotome sinus floor elevation: a 12-year life-table analysis from a prospective study on 588 ITI implants. Clin.Oral Implants.Res. 17, 194-205.

46 Fransson, C., Lekholm, U., Jemt, T. & Berglundh, T. (2005) Prevalence of subjects with progressive bone loss at implants. Clin.Oral Implants.Res. 16, 440-446.

47 Frei, C., Buser, D. & Dula, K. (2004) Study on the necessity for cross-section imaging of the posterior mandible for treatment planning of standard cases in implant dentistry. Clin.Oral Implants.Res. 15, 490-497.

48 Friberg, B., Jemt, T. & Lekholm, U. (1991) Early failures in 4,641 consecutively placed Branemark dental implants: a study from stage 1 surgery to the connection of completed prostheses. Int.J.Oral Maxillofac.Implants. 6, 142-146.

49 Friberg, B., Grondahl, K., Lekholm, U. & Branemark, P. I. (2000) Long-term follow-up of severely atrophic edentulous mandibles reconstructed with short Branemark implants. Clin.Implant.Dent.Relat Res. 2, 184-189.

50 Glauser, R., Sennerby, L., Meredith, N., Ree, A., Lundgren, A., Gottlow, J. & Hammerle, C. H. (2004) Resonance frequency analysis of implants subjected to immediate or early functional occlusal loading. Successful vs. failing implants. Clin.Oral Implants.Res. 15, 428-434.

51 Gotfredsen, K., Holm, B., Sewerin, I., Harder, F., Hjorting-Hansen, E., Pedersen, C. S. & Christensen, K. (1993) Marginal tissue response adjacent to Astra Dental Implants supporting overdentures in the mandible. Clin.Oral Implants.Res. 4, 83-89.

52 Graziani, F., Donos, N., Needleman, I., Gabriele, M. & Tonetti, M. (2004) Comparison of implant survival following sinus floor augmentation procedures with implants placed in pristine posterior maxillary bone: a systematic review. Clin.Oral Implants.Res. 15, 677-682.

53 Gunne, J., Astrand, P., Lindh, T., Borg, K. & Olsson, M. (1999) Tooth-implant and implant supported fixed partial dentures: a 10-year report. Int.J.Prosthodont. 12, 216-221.

54 Hammerle, C. H., Wagner, D., Bragger, U., Lussi, A., Karayiannis, A., Joss, A. & Lang, N. P. (1995) Threshold of tactile sensitivity perceived with dental endosseous implants and natural teeth. Clin.Oral Implants.Res. 6, 83-90.

55 Hansson, S. (1999) The implant neck: smooth or provided with retention elements. A biomechanical approach. Clin.Oral Implants.Res. 10, 394-405.

56 Hansson, S. (2003) A conical implant-abutment interface at the level of the marginal bone improves the distribution of stresses in the supporting bone. An axisymmetric finite element analysis. Clin.Oral Implants.Res. 14, 286-293.

57 Hardt, C. R., Grondahl, K., Lekholm, U.

& Wennstrom, J. L. (2002) Outcome of implant therapy in relation to experienced loss of periodontal bone support: a retrospective 5- year study. Clin.Oral Implants.Res. 13, 488-494.

58 Hermann, J. S., Buser, D., Schenk, R. K., Higginbottom, F. L. & Cochran, D. L. (2000) Biologic width around titanium implants. A physiologically formed and stable dimension over time. Clin.Oral Implants.Res. 11, 1-11.

59 Hermann, J. S., Buser, D., Schenk, R. K., Schoolfield, J. D. & Cochran, D. L. (2001) Biologic Width around one- and two-piece titanium implants. Clin.Oral Implants.Res. 12, 559-571.

60 Heydecke, G., Boudrias, P., Awad, M. A., De Albuquerque, R. F., Lund, J. P. & Feine, J. S. (2003) Within-subject comparisons of maxillary fixed and removable implant prostheses: Patient satisfaction and choice of prosthesis. Clin. Oral Implants.Res. 14, 125-130.

61 Hinode, D., Tanabe, S., Yokoyama, M., Fujisawa, K., Yamauchi, E. & Miyamoto, Y. (2006) Influence of smoking on osseointegrated implant failure: a meta-analysis. Clin.Oral Implants.Res. 17, 473-478.

62 Hobkirk, J. A. & Wiskott, H. W. (2006) Biomechanical aspects of oral implants. Clin.Oral Implants.Res. 17 Suppl 2, 52-54.

63 Isidor, F. (1997) Histological evaluation of peri-implant bone at implants subjected to occlusal overload or plaque accumulation. Clin.Oral Implants.Res. 8, 1-9.

64 Isidor, F. (2006) Influence of forces on peri-implant bone. Clin.Oral Implants.Res. 17 Suppl 2, 8-18.

65 Jacobs, R., Manders, E., Van, L. C., Lembrechts, D., Naert, I. & van, Steenberghe, D. (2001) Evaluation of speech in patients rehabilitated with various oral implant-supported prostheses. Clin.Oral Implants.Res. 12, 167-173.

66 Jaffin, R. A. & Berman, C. L. (1991) The excessive loss of Branemark fixtures in type IV bone: a 5-year analysis. J.Periodontol. 62, 2-4.

67 Jeffcoat, M. K., Reddy, M. S., van den Berg, H. R. & Bertens, E. (1992) Quantitative digital subtraction radiography for the assessment of peri-implant bone change. Clin.Oral Implants. Res. 3, 22-27.

68 Jemt, T. & Lekholm, U. (1995) Implant treatment in edentulous maxillae: a 5-year follow-up report on patients with different degrees of jaw resorption. Int.J.Oral Maxillofac.Implants. 10, 303-311.

69 Kahnberg, K. E., Ekestubbe, A., Grondahl, K., Nilsson, P. & Hirsch, J. M. (2001) Sinus lifting procedure. I. One-stage surgery with bone transplant and implants. Clin.Oral Implants.Res. 12, 479-487.

70 Karoussis, I. K., Salvi, G. E., Heitz-Mayfield, L. J., Bragger, U., Hammerle, C. H. & Lang, N. P. (2003) Long-term implant prognosis in patients with and without a history of chronic periodontitis: a 10-year prospective cohort study of the ITI Dental Implant System. Clin.Oral Implants.Res. 14, 329-339.

71 Kim, Y., Oh, T. J., Misch, C. E. & Wang,

H. L. (2005) Occlusal considerations in implant therapy: clinical guidelines with biomechanical rationale. Clin.Oral Implants.Res. 16, 26-35.

72   Klinge, B. & Meyle, J. (2006) Soft-tissue integration of implants. Clin.Oral Implants.Res. 17 Suppl 2, 93-96.

73   Kramer, F. J., Baethge, C., Swennen, G. & Rosahl, S. (2005) Navigated vs. conventional implant insertion for maxillary single tooth replacement. Clin.Oral Implants.Res. 16, 60-68.

74   Kumar, A., Jaffin, R. A. & Berman, C. (2002) The effect of smoking on achieving osseointegration of surface-modified implants: a clinical report. Int.J.Oral Maxillofac.Implants. 17, 816-819.

75   Kuzmanovic, D. V., Payne, A. G., Kieser, J. A. & Dias, G. J. (2003) Anterior loop of the mental nerve: a morphological and radiographic study. Clin.Oral Implants.Res. 14, 464-471.

76   Lang, N. P., Pjetursson, B. E., Tan, K., Bragger, U., Egger, M. & Zwahlen, M. (2004) A systematic review of the survival and complication rates of fixed partial dentures (FPDs) after an observation period of at least 5 years. II. Combined tooth--implant-supported FPDs. Clin.Oral Implants.Res. 15, 643-653.

77   Lekholm, U., Grondahl, K. & Jemt, T. (2006) Outcome of oral implant treatment in partially edentulous jaws followed 20 years in clinical function. Clin.Implant.Dent.Relat Res. 8, 178-186.

78   Lindh, T., Gunne, J., Tillberg, A. & Molin, M. (1998) A meta-analysis of implants in partial edentulism. Clin.Oral Implants.Res. 9, 80-90.

79   Lindquist, L. W., Carlsson, G. E. & Jemt, T. (1996) A prospective 15-year follow-up study of mandibular fixed prostheses supported by osseointegrated implants. Clinical results and marginal bone loss. Clin.Oral Implants.Res. 7, 329-336.

80   Lindquist, L. W., Carlsson, G. E. & Jemt, T. (1997) Association between marginal bone loss around osseointegrated mandibular implants and smoking habits: a 10-year follow-up study. J.Dent.Res. 76, 1667-1674.

81   Listgarten, M. A., Lang, N. P., Schroeder, H. E. & Schroeder, A. (1991) Periodontal tissues and their counterparts around endosseous implants [corrected and republished with original paging, article orginally printed in Clin Oral Implants Res 1991 Jan-Mar;2(1):1-19]. Clin.Oral Implants.Res. 2, 1-19.

82   Makkonen, T. A., Holmberg, S., Niemi, L., Olsson, C., Tammisalo, T. & Peltola, J. (1997) A 5-year prospective clinical study of Astra Tech dental implants supporting fixed bridges or overdentures in the edentulous mandible. Clin.Oral Implants.Res. 8, 469-475.

83   Meredith, N., Book, K., Friberg, B., Jemt, T. & Sennerby, L. (1997) Resonance frequency measurements of implant stability in vivo. A cross-sectional and longitudinal study of resonance frequency measurements on implants in the edentulous and partially dentate maxilla. Clin.Oral Implants.Res. 8, 226-233.

84   Mericske-Stern, R. D., Taylor, T. D. & Belser, U. (2000) Management of the edentulous patient. Clin.Oral Implants.Res. 11 Suppl 1 , 108-125.

85   Mombelli, A., Feloutzis, A., Bragger, U. & Lang, N. P. (2001) Treatment of peri-implantitis by local delivery of tetracycline. Clinical, microbiological and radiological results. Clin.Oral Implants.Res. 12, 287-294.

86   Mombelli, A. & Cionca, N. (2006) Systemic diseases affecting osseointegration therapy. Clin.Oral Implants.Res. 17 Suppl 2, 97-103.

87   Naert, I., Gizani, S., Vuylsteke, M. & van, Steenberghe, D. (1998) A 5-year randomized clinical trial on the influence of splinted and unsplinted oral implants in the mandibular overdenture therapy. Part I: Peri-implant outcome. Clin.Oral Implants.Res. 9, 170-177.

88   Naert, I. E., Duyck, J. A., Hosny, M. M. & van, Steenberghe, D. (2001) Freestanding and tooth-implant connected prostheses in the treatment of partially edentulous patients. Part I: An up to 15-years clinical evaluation. Clin.Oral Implants. Res. 12, 237-244.

89   Neukam, F. W. & Flemmig, T. F. (2006) Local and systemic conditions potentially compromising osseointegration. Clin.Oral Implants.Res. 17 Suppl 2, 160-162.

90   Nkenke, E., Schultze-Mosgau, S., Radespiel-Troger, M., Kloss, F. & Neukam, F. W. (2001) Morbidity of harvesting of chin grafts: a prospective study. Clin.Oral Implants.Res. 12, 495-502.

91   Nkenke, E., Radespiel-Troger, M., Wiltfang, J., Schultze-Mosgau, S., Winkler, G. & Neukam, F. W. (2002) Morbidity of harvesting of retromolar bone grafts: a prospective study. Clin.Oral Implants.Res. 13, 514-521.

92   Norton, M. R. (1997) An in vitro evaluation of the strength of an internal conical interface compared to a butt joint interface in implant design. Clin.Oral Implants.Res. 8, 290-298.

93   Ortorp, A., Jemt, T., Back, T. & Jalevik, T. (2003) Comparisons of precision of fit between cast and CNC-milled titanium implant frameworks for the edentulous mandible. Int.J.Prosthodont. 16, 194-200.

94   Palmer, R. M., Floyd, P. D., Palmer, P. J., Smith, B. J., Johansson, C. B. & Albrektsson, T. (1994) Healing of implant dehiscence defects with and without expanded polytetrafluoroethylene membranes: a controlled clinical and histological study. Clin.Oral Implants.Res. 5, 98-104.

95   Palmer, R. M., Palmer, P. J. & Smith, B. J. (2000) A 5-year prospective study of Astra single tooth implants. Clin.Oral Implants.Res. 11, 179-182.

96   Palmer, R. M., Howe, L. C. & Palmer, P. J. (2005) A prospective 3-year study of fixed bridges linking Astra Tech ST implants to natural teeth. Clin.Oral Implants.Res. 16, 302-307.

97   Persson, L. G., Lekholm, U., Leonhardt, A., Dahlen, G. & Lindhe, J. (1996) Bacterial colonization on internal surfaces of Branemark system implant components. Clin.Oral Implants.Res. 7, 90-95.

98   Persson, L. G., Berglundh, T., Lindhe, J. & Sennerby, L. (2001) Re-osseointegration after treatment of peri-implantitis at different implant surfaces. An experimental study in the dog. Clin. Oral Implants.Res. 12, 595-603.

99   Pjetursson, B. E., Tan, K., Lang, N. P., Bragger, U., Egger, M. & Zwahlen, M. (2004) A systematic review of the survival and complication rates of fixed partial dentures (FPDs) after an observation period of at least 5 years. Clin.Oral Implants.Res. 15, 667-676.

100   Quirynen, M., Bollen, C. M., Eyssen, H. & van, Steenberghe, D. (1994) Microbial penetration along the implant components of the Branemark system. An in vitro study. Clin.Oral Implants.Res. 5, 239-244.

101   Quirynen, M., Peeters, W., Naert, I., Coucke, W. & van, Steenberghe, D. (2001) Peri-implant health around screw-shaped c.p. titanium machined implants in partially edentulous patients with or without ongoing periodontitis. Clin. Oral Implants.Res. 12, 589-594.

102   Quirynen, M., Mraiwa, N., van, Steenberghe, D. & Jacobs, R. (2003) Morphology and dimensions of the mandibular jaw bone in the interforaminal region in patients requiring implants in the distal areas. Clin.Oral Implants.Res. 14, 280-285.

103   Quirynen, M., Vogels, R., Alsaadi, G., Naert, I., Jacobs, R. & van, Steenberghe, D. (2005) Predisposing conditions for retrograde peri-implantitis, and treatment suggestions. Clin. Oral Implants.Res. 16, 599-608.

104   Rangert, B., Jemt, T. & Jorneus, L. (1989) Forces and moments on Branemark implants. Int.J.Oral Maxillofac.Implants. 4, 241-247.

105   Rangert, B., Gunne, J., Glantz, P. O. & Svensson, A. (1995) Vertical load distribution on a three-unit prosthesis supported by a natural tooth and a single Branemark implant. An in vivo study. Clin.Oral Implants.Res. 6, 40-46.

106   Rangert, B. R., Sullivan, R. M. & Jemt, T. M. (1997) Load factor control for implants in the posterior partially edentulous segment. Int.J.Oral Maxillofac.Implants. 12, 360-370.

107   Renouard, F. & Nisand, D. (2006) Impact of implant length and diameter on survival rates. Clin.Oral Implants.Res. 17 Suppl 2, 35-51.

108   Romeo, E., Ghisolfi, M., Murgolo, N., Chiapasco, M., Lops, D. & Vogel, G. (2005) Therapy of peri-implantitis with resective surgery. A 3-year clinical trial on rough screw-shaped oral implants. Part I: clinical outcome. Clin.Oral Implants.Res. 16, 9-18.

109   Romeo, E., Lops, D., Chiapasco, M., Ghisolfi, M. & Vogel, G. (2007) Therapy of peri-implantitis with resective surgery. A 3-year clinical trial on rough screw-shaped oral implants. Part II: radiographic outcome. Clin.Oral Implants.Res. 18, 179-187.

110   Rompen, E., Domken, O., Degidi, M., Farias Pontes, A. E. & Piattelli, A. (2006) The effect of material characteristics, of surface topography and of implant components and connections on soft tissue integration: a literature review. Clin. Oral Implants.Res. 17 Suppl 2, 55-67.

111   Salvi, G. E., Persson, G. R., Heitz-Mayfield, L. J., Frei, M. & Lang, N. P. (2007) Adjunctive local antibiotic therapy in the treatment of peri-implantitis II: clinical and radiographic outcomes. Clin.Oral Implants.Res. 18, 281-285.

112   Schenk, R. K. & Buser, D. (1998) Osseointegration: a reality. Periodontol.2000. 17, 22-35.

113   Schou, S., Holmstrup, P., Worthington, H. V. & Esposito, M. (2006) Outcome of implant therapy in patients with previous tooth loss due to periodontitis. Clin.Oral Implants.Res. 17 Suppl 2, 104-123.

114   Sennerby, L., Ericson, L. E., Thomsen, P., Lekholm, U. & Astrand, P. (1991) Structure of the bone-titanium interface in retrieved clinical oral implants. Clin.Oral Implants.Res. 2, 103-111.

115   Serhal, C. B., van, Steenberghe, D., Quirynen, M. & Jacobs, R. (2001) Localisation of the mandibular canal using conventional spiral tomography: a human cadaver study. Clin.Oral Implants.Res. 12, 230-236.

116   Sigurdsson, T. J., Fu, E., Tatakis, D. N., Rohrer, M. D. & Wikesjo, U. M. (1997) Bone morphogenetic protein-2 for peri-implant bone regeneration and osseointegration. Clin.Oral Implants.Res. 8, 367-374.

117   Simion, M., Jovanovic, S. A., Tinti, C. & Benfenati, S. P. (2001) Long-term evaluation of osseointegrated implants inserted at the time or after vertical ridge augmentation. A retrospective study on 123 implants with 1-5 year follow-up. Clin.Oral Implants.Res. 12, 35-45.

118   Tan, K., Pjetursson, B. E., Lang, N. P. & Chan, E. S. (2004) A systematic review of the survival and complication rates of fixed partial dentures (FPDs) after an observation period of at least 5 years. Clin.Oral Implants.Res. 15, 654-666.

119   ten Bruggenkate, C. M., Krekeler, G., Kraaijenhagen, H. A., Foitzik, C. & Oosterbeek, H. S. (1993) Hemorrhage of the floor of the mouth resulting from lingual perforation during implant placement: a clinical report. Int.J.Oral Maxillofac.Implants. 8, 329-334.

120   ter Brugge, P. J., Wolke, J. G. & Jansen, J. A. (2003) Effect of calcium phosphate coating composition and crystallinity on the response of osteogenic cells in vitro. Clin.Oral Implants.Res. 14, 472-480.

121   Teughels, W., Van, Assohe, N., Sliepen, I. & Quirynen, M. (2006) Effect of material characteristics and/or surface topography on biofilm development. Clin.Oral Implants.Res. 17 Suppl 2, 68-81.

122   Ulm, C., Kneissel, M., Schedle, A., Solar, P., Matejka, M., Schneider, B. & Donath, K. (1999) Characteristic features of trabecular bone in edentulous maxillae. Clin.Oral Implants.Res. 10, 459-467.

123   van, Steenberghe, D., Jacobs, R., Desnyder, M., Maffei, G. & Quirynen, M. (2002) The relative impact of local and endogenous patient-related factors on implant failure up to the abutment stage. Clin.Oral Implants.Res. 13, 617-622.

124   van, Steenberghe, D., Molly, L., Jacobs, R., Vandekerckhove, B., Quirynen, M. & Naert, I. (2004) The immediate rehabilitation by means of a ready-made final fixed prosthesis in the edentulous mandible: a 1-year follow-up study on 50 consecutive patients. Clin.Oral Implants.Res. 15, 360-365.

125   von, Arx, T. & Buser, D. (2006) Horizontal ridge augmentation using autogenous block grafts and the guided bone regeneration technique with collagen membranes: a clinical study with 42 patients. Clin.Oral Implants.Res. 17, 359-366.

126   von, Wowern, N. (1977) Variations in bone mass within the cortices of the mandible. Scand.J.Dent.Res. 85, 444-455.

127   Watson, R. M. & Davis, D. M. (1996) Follow up and maintenance of implant supported prostheses: a comparison of 20 complete mandibular overdentures and 20 complete mandibular fixed cantilever prostheses. Br.Dent.J. 181, 321-327.

128   Weber, H. P., Kim, D. M., Ng, M. W., Hwang, J. W. & Fiorellini, J. P. (2006) Peri-implant soft-tissue health surrounding cement- and screw-retained implant restorations: a multi-center, 3-year prospective study. Clin.Oral Implants. Res. 17, 375-379.

129   Wennerberg, A., Albrektsson, T., Andersson, B. & Krol, J. J. (1995) A histomorphometric and removal torque study of screw-shaped titanium implants with three different surface topographies. Clin.Oral Implants.Res. 6, 24-30.

130   Wennerberg, A., Ide-Ektessabi, A., Hatkamata, S., Sawase, T., Johansson, C., Albrektsson, T., Martinelli, A., Sodervall, U. & Odelius, H. (2004) Titanium release from implants prepared with different surface roughness. Clin.Oral Implants.Res. 15, 505-512.

131   Wennstrom, J., Zurdo, J., Karlsson, S., Ekestubbe, A., Grondahl, K. & Lindhe, J. (2004) Bone level change at implant-supported fixed partial dentures with and without cantilever extension after 5 years in function. J.Clin.Periodontol. 31, 1077-1083.

132   Wennstrom, J. L., Bengazi, F. & Lekholm, U. (1994) The influence of the masticatory mucosa on the peri-implant soft tissue condition. Clin.Oral Implants.Res. 5, 1-8.

133   Wennstrom, J. L., Ekestubbe, A., Grondahl, K., Karlsson, S. & Lindhe, J. (2004) Oral rehabilitation with implant-supported fixed partial dentures in periodontitis-susceptible subjects. A 5-year prospective study. J.Clin.Periodontol. 31, 713-724.

134   Wikesjo, U. M., Qahash, M., Thomson, R. C., Cook, A. D., Rohrer, M. D., Wozney, J. M. & Hardwick, W. R. (2004) rhBMP-2 significantly enhances guided bone regeneration. Clin.Oral Implants.Res. 15, 194-204.

135   Wright, P. S., Glantz, P. O., Randow, K. & Watson, R. M. (2002) The effects of fixed and removable implant-stabilised prostheses on posterior mandibular residual ridge resorption. Clin. Oral Implants.Res. 13, 169-174.

136   Yerit, K. C., Posch, M., Seemann, M., Hainich, S., Dortbudak, O., Turhani, D., Ozyuvaci, H., Watzinger, F. & Ewers, R. (2006) Implant survival in mandibles of irradiated oral cancer patients. Clin.Oral Implants.Res. 17, 337-344.

137   Young, M. P., Worthington, H. V., Lloyd, R. E., Drucker, D. B., Sloan, P. & Carter, D. H. (2002) Bone collected during dental implant surgery: a clinical and histological study. Clin.Oral Implants.Res. 13, 298-303.

138   Zhao, G., Zinger, O., Schwartz, Z., Wieland, M., Landolt, D. & Boyan, B. D. (2006) Osteoblast-like cells are sensitive to submicron-scale surface structure. Clin.Oral Implants.Res. 17, 258-264.

Index

CHOOSING & AUSTRALIAN

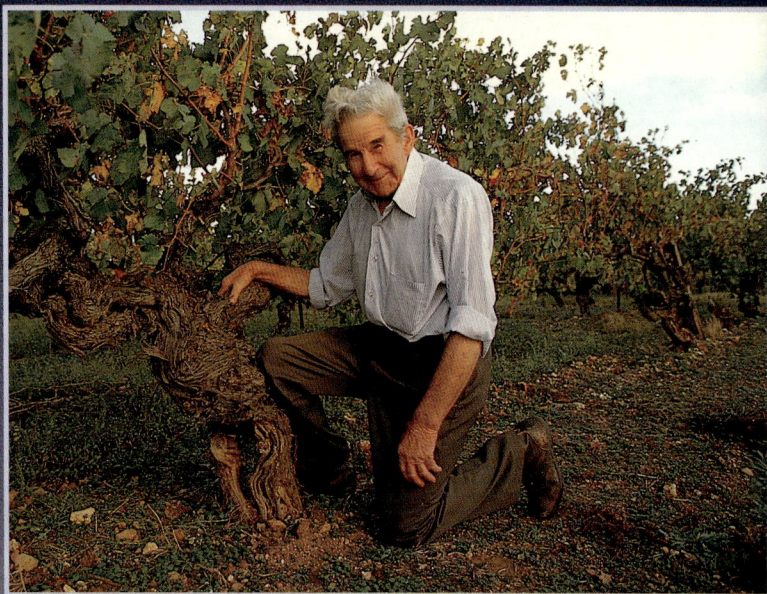

Robert Mayne

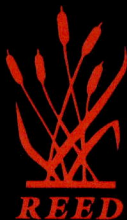

REED

The soil.

What influence does the soil have on the wine? Grapes are the complex result of the interacting influences on their growth. One of the major influences is the soil.

The following information will prove interesting to show how distinctive varietal characteristics are a result of the soil (and climate) in our different vineyards.

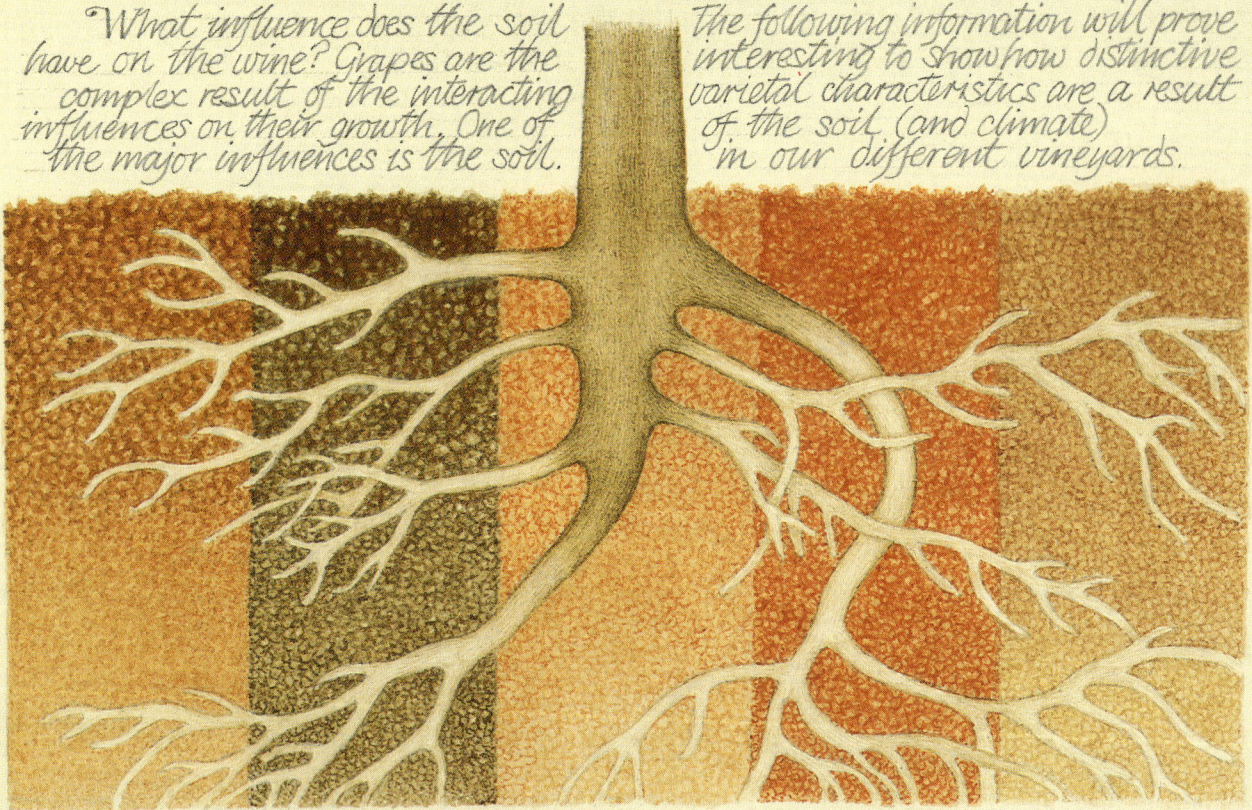

Milawa.

Soil: Alluvial, red sandy loam/clay loam, to a depth of 1200 mm, moderate to high pH.
Elevation: 155 metres.
Mean January Temperature: 23.2°C.
Rainfall: 660 mm annually.
Major Varieties: Muscadelle, Rhine Riesling, Sauvignon Blanc, Gewürztraminer, Mondeuse, Shiraz, Cabernet Sauvignon, Pinot Noir.

Whitlands.

Soil: Volcanic, brown loam/clay loam, to a depth of 2000 mm (to Kaolinitic clay), low to moderate pH.
Elevation: 800 metres.
Mean January Temperature: 19.0°C.
Rainfall: 1410 mm annually.
Major Varieties: Chardonnay, Gewürztraminer, Rhine Riesling, Merlot, Pinot Noir.

King Valley.

Soil: Colluvial, red sandy clay loam to a depth of 1200 mm, low to moderate pH.
Elevation: 360 metres.
Mean January Temperature: 20.5°C.
Rainfall: 1151 mm annually.
Major Varieties: Gewürztraminer, Rhine Riesling, Merlot, Sauvignon Blanc.

Koombahla.

Soil: Colluvial, red loam/clay loam, to a depth of 1500 mm, moderate pH.
Elevation: 300 metres.
Mean January Temperature: 21.0°C.
Rainfall: 1130 mm annually.
Major Varieties: Chardonnay, Rhine Riesling, Sauvignon Blanc, Cabernet Sauvignon, Pinot Noir, Shiraz.

Meadow Creek.

Soil: Colluvial, red brown loam/clay loam, to a depth of 1000 mm, low to moderate pH.
Elevation: 200 metres.
Mean January Temperature: 22.0°C.
Rainfall: 826 mm annually.
Major Varieties: Chardonnay, Cabernet Sauvignon, Shiraz.

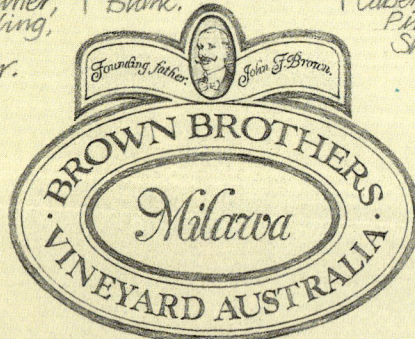

Founding father. John J. Brown.

BROWN BROTHERS
Milawa
VINEYARD AUSTRALIA

Taste the fruits of our labours.

DAVID FROST 90.

CONTENTS

PULLING THE FIRST CORK

White grapes, not yet matured, ripen on the vine. Every drop of juice has been drawn up from the ground through the stem of a grapevine before it can be transformed into wine.
Inset: *Wine can tell you things! Author Robert Mayne, with bottle to his ear, enjoys a wine festival crowning with friends.*

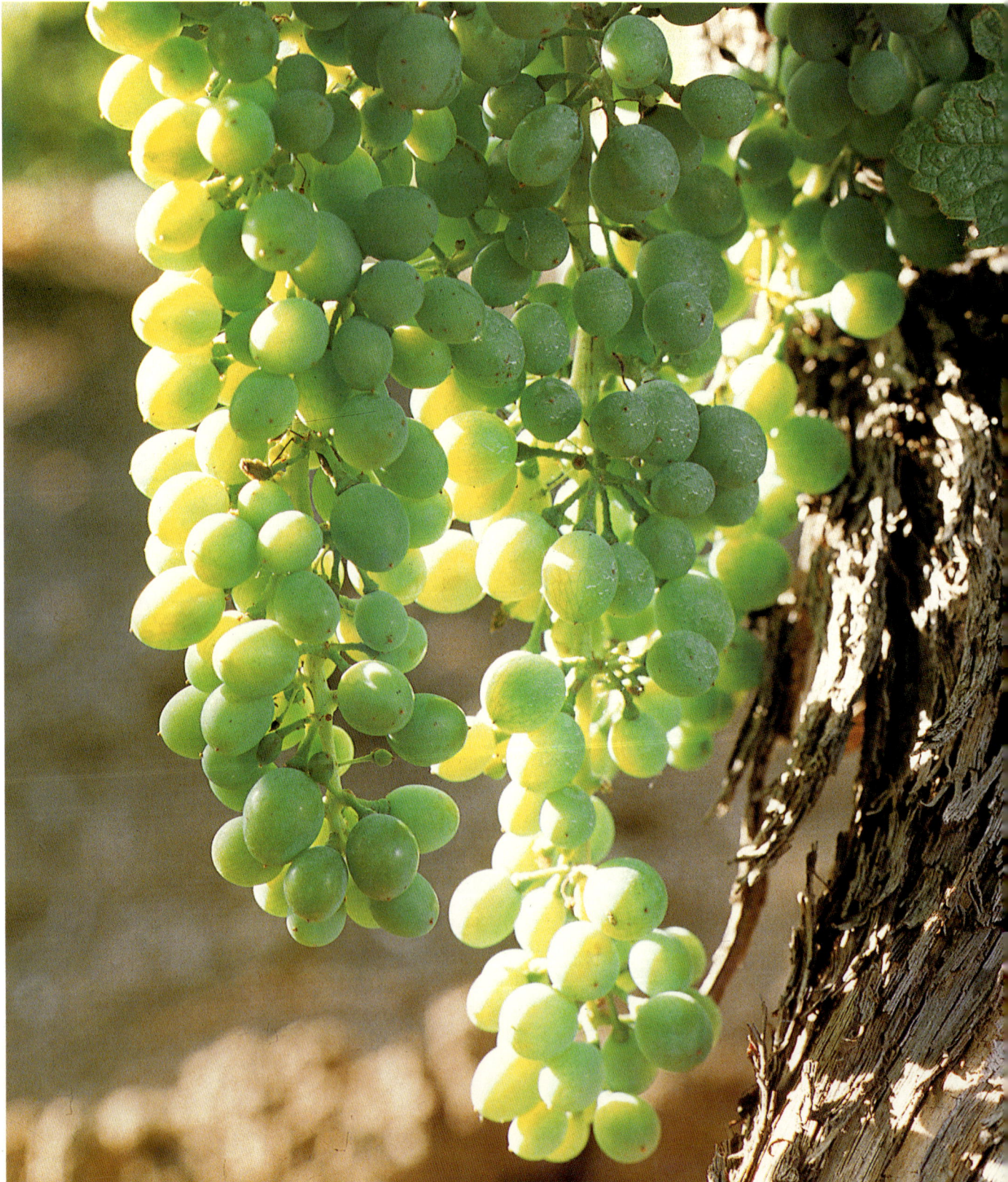

CHOOSING & ENJOYING 4 AUSTRALIAN WINES

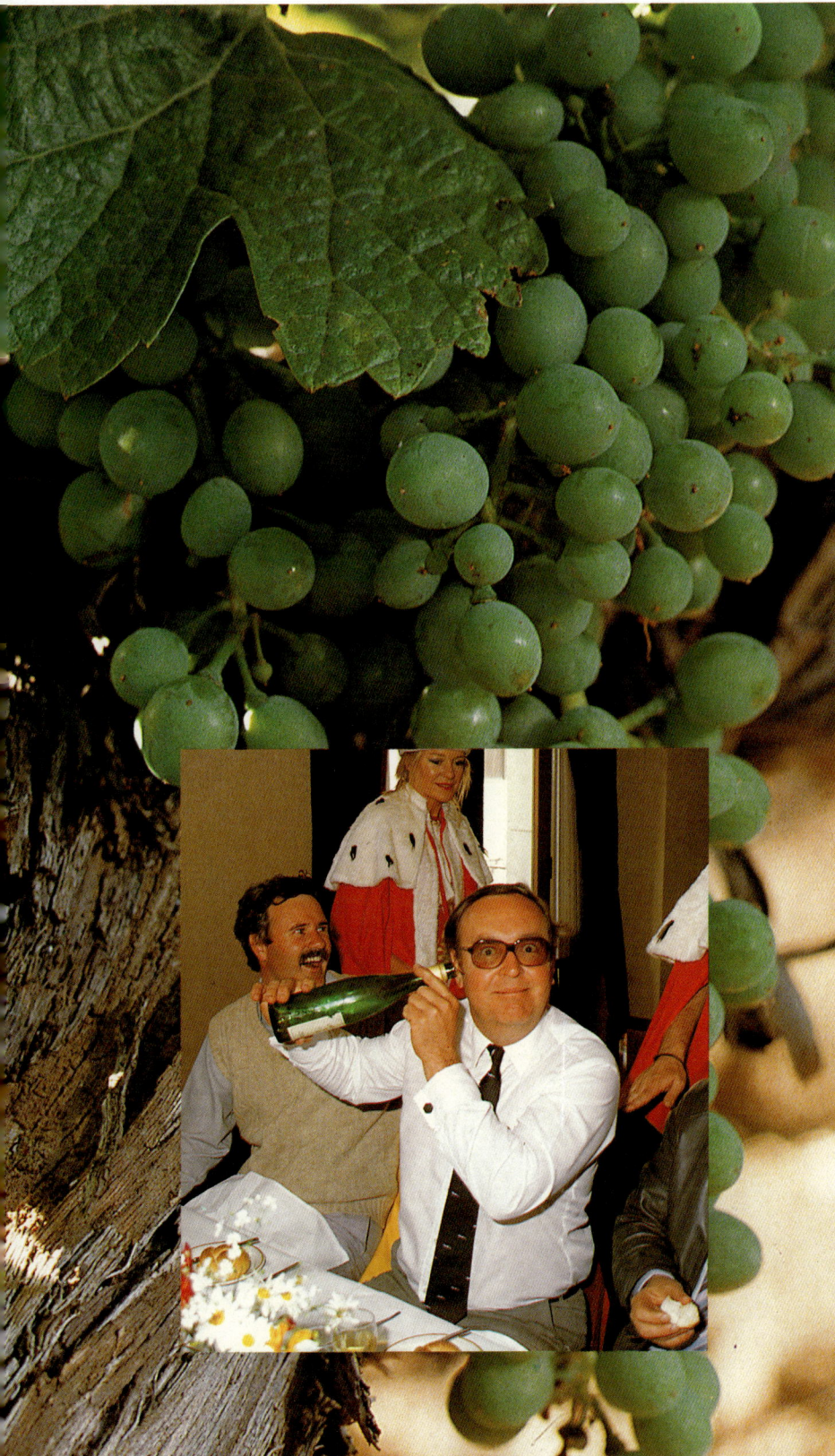

This is not a book about what the Ancients thought about wine, or how they made it (in spite of a little that follows).

It is, however, a rather sobering thought, pun intended, to consider how much wine history has gone before us: all those trillions of litres of juice that have laboriously climbed up the stems of billions of grape vines over recorded and unrecorded history, only to be turned into wine and poured down many a (grateful) gullet.

This is also not a book about the emotions or the science of wine or wine tasting — or about jaundiced views on the best wines and wineries of Australia.

It *is* meant to be a primer to help you learn how to enjoy Australian wines; to demystify them and to give you a feeling of confidence in choosing and ordering wine in most situations.

I see wine, as do many hundreds of thousands of Australians today, as an ordinary, everyday beverage. Certainly it can be a special drink. Most of the time for me, though, it's a drink that adds great pleasure to my meals, to the company I keep, the friends I have and make and the daily grind of working and living. Occasionally I drink too much. But, fortunately, wine is a forgiving friend.

Wine somehow seems to make the times around meals more gregarious, more enjoyable, more conversational and sometimes, if I know the wine-maker or the place the wine comes from, it adds a talking point or an anecdote to table talk. "Table culture" some Europeans call it, and it's all wrapped up with food and liking other people's company.

Indeed, wine possesses some powers that are akin to the magical. But while it has unusual properties and almost endless diversity, it *is*, at the bottom of the glass, just a drink.

What I have written here reflects my joy in wine, and my regard for it as an everyday beverage. I have stressed the many good things about it, and some of the bad. The opinions are mine; even the prejudices are mine, for which I make no apology except to say that you will make up your own mind when you taste the stuff, which is just the way it should be.

Robert Mayne

THE ETERNAL DRINK

Perhaps it all started in central Persia – I would like to think so, anyway. Maybe even near the site of what is now the city of Shiraz, which is some two hundred kilometres north of the Persian Gulf in modern-day Iran. To think that the first grapevines may have come from around there, where today it is strictly forbidden to sip the fermented juice of the grape!

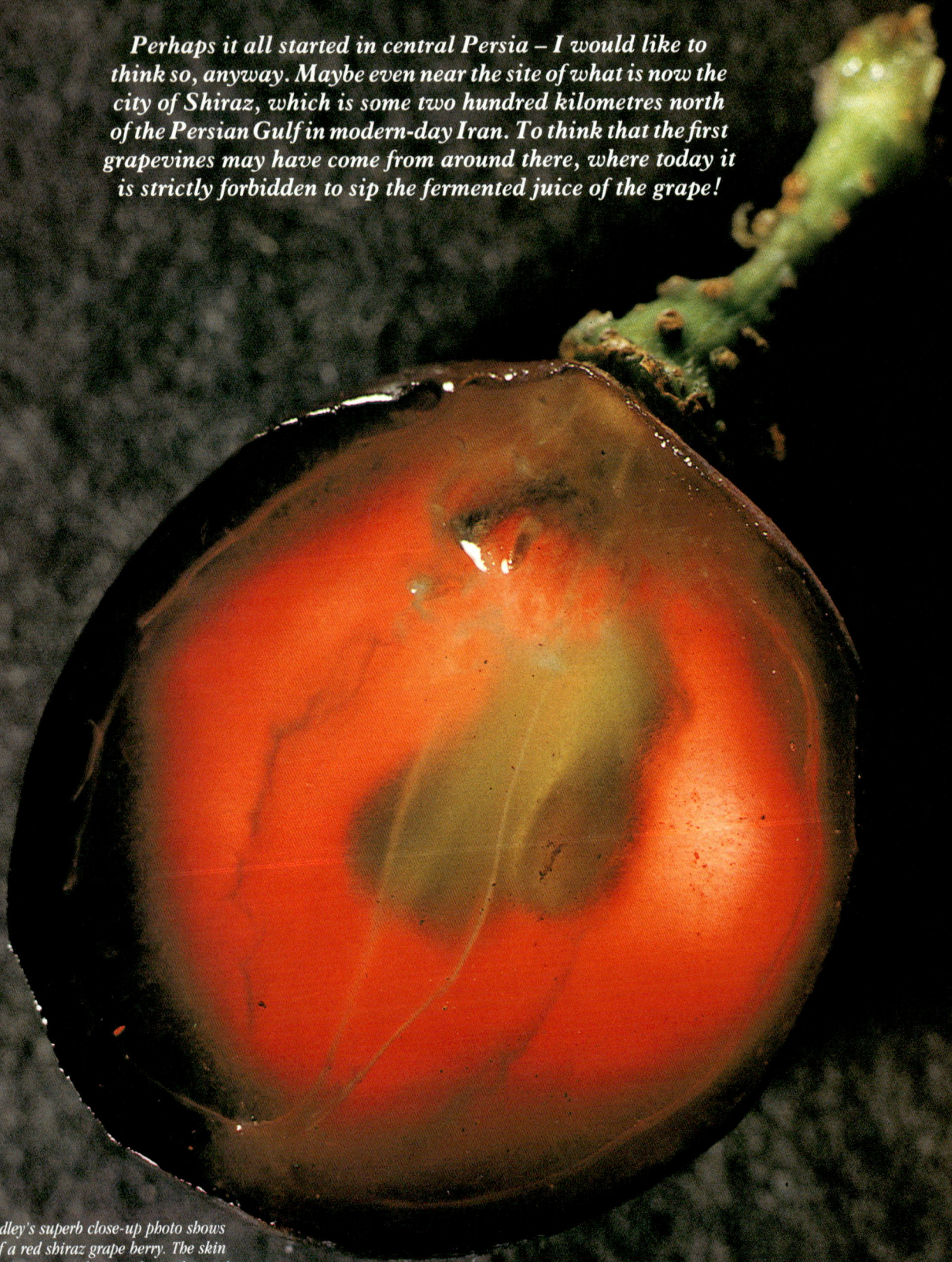

Milton Wordley's superb close-up photo shows the heart of a red shiraz grape berry. The skin helps give red wine its colour, and, together with the seed, its tannic flavours.

Wine goes way back into antiquity, perhaps 6,000 years. There are some signs that basic wines — rough reds, if you like — were made 10,000 years ago.

You can make wine, which is defined in all dictionaries as "the fermented juice of the grape", from all sorts of fruit. But in these past six millennia or so we have learnt that the fermented juice we most enjoy comes from one particular family of fruit. We know this family as *vitis,* and of course it comes from a fast-growing perennial vine of which undoubtedly the best branch for wine-making is *vitis vinifera* or the grape-bearing vine. "Vine" is defined in my dictionary as: "Any of a large and widely distributed group of plants having a slender flexible stem that may twine around a support or clasp it by means of tendrils".

The grape vine is indeed an attractive plant. Outside my back verandah four or five of them grow and, as I write this, it is early November and they are shooting wildly in all directions. Looking at them today at lunch time over the rim of a glass of shiraz red wine, it's easy to see what attraction they must have had five or six thousand years ago. In the summer heat around the fulcrum of civilisation, somewhere near the area joining Europe and Asia, the vines were green in the heat of summer; their abundant fruit was sweet, thirst-quenching, succulent and of course they provided shade in summer and allowed the sun through in winter when they shed their leaves. The leaves provided a base for the serving of food and a method of wrapping food for preservation and serving. (One I always enjoy is the Greek method of blanching the leaves and wrapping them around a mixture of rice and minced lamb and braising them in a little oil and lemon — dolmades!)

It is undeniable that those who walked the earth all those centuries ago enjoyed the fruit of this remarkable plant. What a joyful adjunct to find that this useful vine could, with a little help, produce a drink that made everyday life more bearable, even rewarding and enjoyable!

The earlier growers must have quickly stumbled on the secret: ripe grapes will ferment because the necessary trigger is found in the "bloom" you can see on the skins of the grapes. The bloom is the fine, powdery looking mist which is particularly obvious on the skins of ripe, red (or black) grapes.

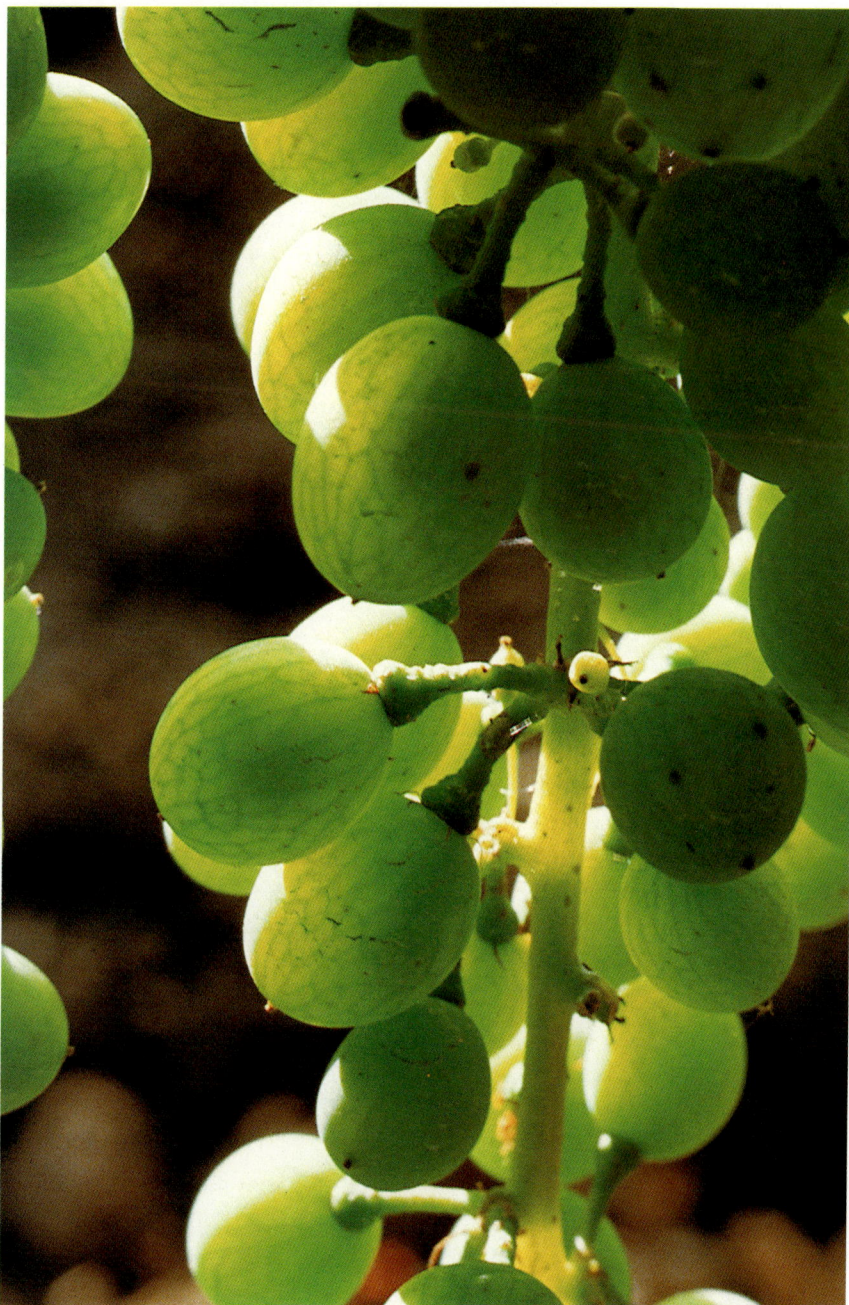

Unprompted by human hand, the yeasts in the bloom will eventually attack the ripe grape and start chewing up the sugar in the juice inside the berry. This is fermentation — the conversion of sugar to alcohol, with the by-products of CO_2 gas and heat. It did not take many accidental vintages, five or six thousand years or so ago, to persuade our forbears that fermented grape juice had many advantages over the unfermented juice.

The most obvious difference, of course, is that the plain juice of the grape berry is sweet if ripe. Throughout the growing season the grapes get more ripe as the sugar level increases. But fermenting the resultant juice changes the sugar content, in fact converts it into alcohol. Therefore, the finished product — wine — is normally drier in flavour, and along with the alcohol, makes wine as different from grape juice as a butterfly is from a caterpillar.

Alcohol is a volatile, flammable and colourless liquid with a penetrating odour and burning taste. There are two principal forms: ethyl alcohol (or ethanol) and methyl alcohol (or methanol, more readily recognised in the form of methylated spirits).

The one we enjoy drinking is a complex compound which answers to the name of C_2H_5OH, or ethanol. It is this chemical which turns plain old grape juice into a natural beverage of fascinating complexity: wine.

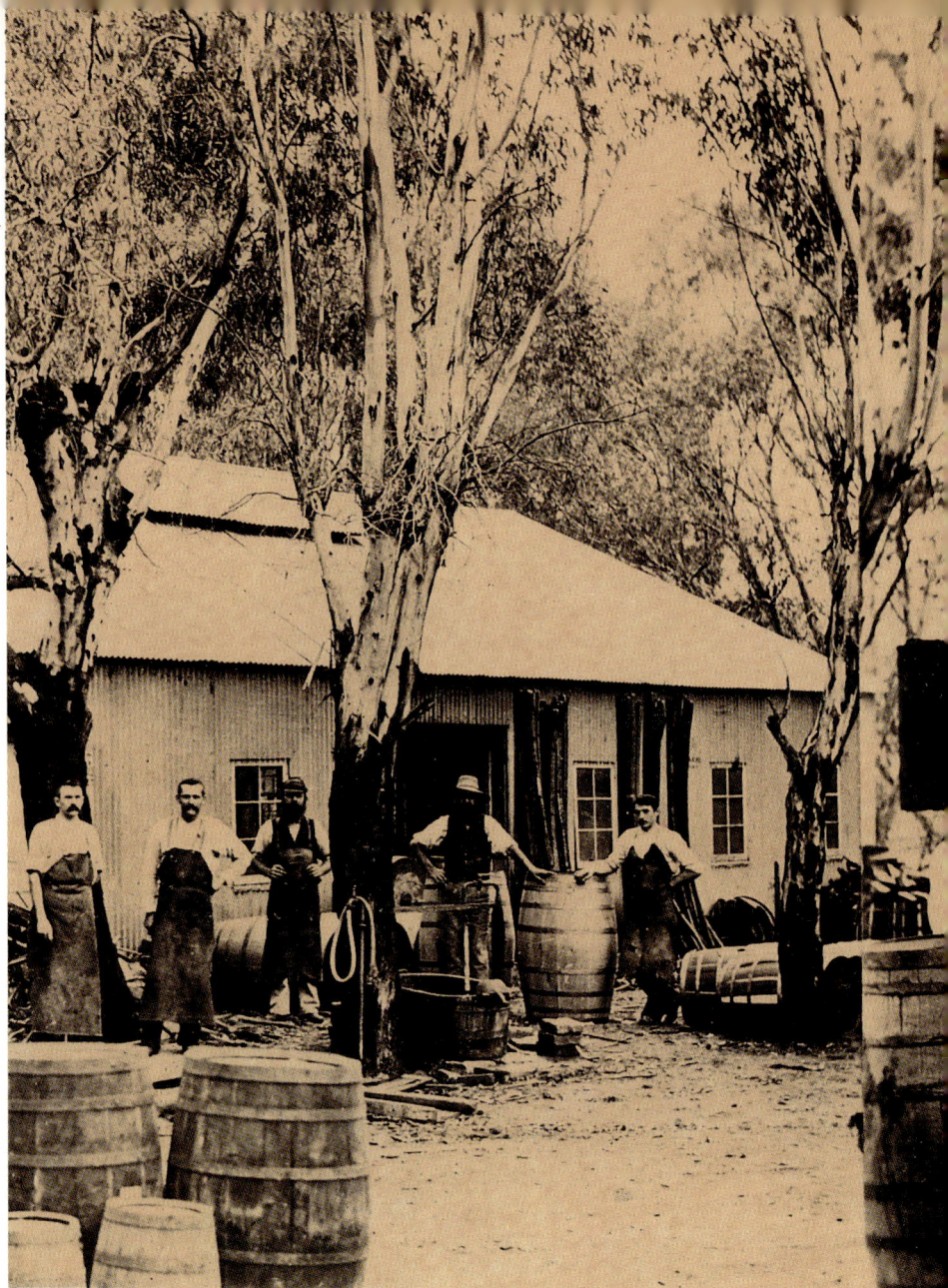

Making and repairing barrels at the cooperage at Seppeltsfield late last century. Coopering is a highly skilled trade, though coopers are hard to find today, when stainless steel is more commonly used for wine storage.

You can search far and wide in literature without finding a totally satisfactory explanation of why so many find the consumption of alcohol enjoyable and desirable. Clearly, the chemical compound of alcohol, in whatever form — wine, beer, spirits or pure — is absorbed into the system and has an effect on your body. The effects vary with the amount, with tolerance and so on.

The most appealing effects include, at least in moderate amounts, relaxed muscles, loosened tension and a general feeling of well-being. The social effects, of course, include a relaxation of inhibitions. Other benefits are a heightened appetite and aided digestion.

If all of these qualities were not clinically apparent to the ancient world, wine was certainly still worth the time and effort to grow and make. The vine spread north and east from Persia and found a firm home in and around ancient Egypt. We know they made red wines some 5,000 years ago, and that it was a drink of the relatively affluent. (Poorer Egyptians consumed a sort of beer made from a type of wheat.) Wine was mentioned in sacred texts: the God Osiris was known as "Lord of wine at the inundation" (the annual flooding of the River Nile). Red wine represented the right eye of the God Horus, white wine the left eye.

Wine has had a continuous place in religious history and, of course, today a number of the world's major religions use wine in services. It is no accident that men of God — monks for example — have played such a strong role in the development of alcoholic drinks. It offers some comfort in a life of self-imposed solitude and chastity, perhaps.

Wines, or to be more accurate, alcoholic beverages, have always inspired strong emotions. There are records of praise to the benefits and joys of wine from centuries ago, and if the articulate and noble felt this way about the stuff, "ordinary" people must have been just as grateful.

For Egyptians, the Nile Delta was a centre of cultivation for vineyards and vines in orchard gardens. The methods of crushing grapes were primitive but, in essence, not so different from the general principles employed in Australia and elsewhere in the world of wine today.

Wine drinking obviously had its own manners and etiquette. Wine was served from decanters and stone amphorae and probably from the storage jars in which it was fermented by its makers. They drank it, we know from many archaeological finds, from metal beakers; bowls baked from clay; a primitive form of glass; and from alabaster, among other vessels.

Wine was a widespread drink in the huge tract of what we now call the Middle East and Central and Southern Asia until religion entered the scene. Growing wine grapes in the Nile Basin and elsewhere in Egypt came to a sudden stop when the Muslims conquered the area in 624 A.D.

As a result, Egypt's vineyards were destroyed. Today, several thousand years later, the Islamic prohibition continues, though clearly, like the use of wine by wealthy Ancient Egyptians, some more affluent and aristocratic Muslims can ignore it or, at best, turn a blind eye to its use. Privileged Saudis, Muslim Iraqis, Egyptians and many other Arabs drink wine, Scotch or other forms of alcohol in the West and in the privacy of their homes.

This was, after all, the area of our world that gave birth to the grape vine and in its civilised sense, to alcohol. As with much of our culture, mythology, behaviour and folklore, religion had a lot to do with its birth.

Where would the civilised world of alcohol be without names such as the Monk Dom Perignon, the Benedictines, the American Christian Brothers, Australia's Sevenhill Jesuit Winery and France's Chateau Haut Brion, among others?

Timothy tells us in the Bible: "Take a

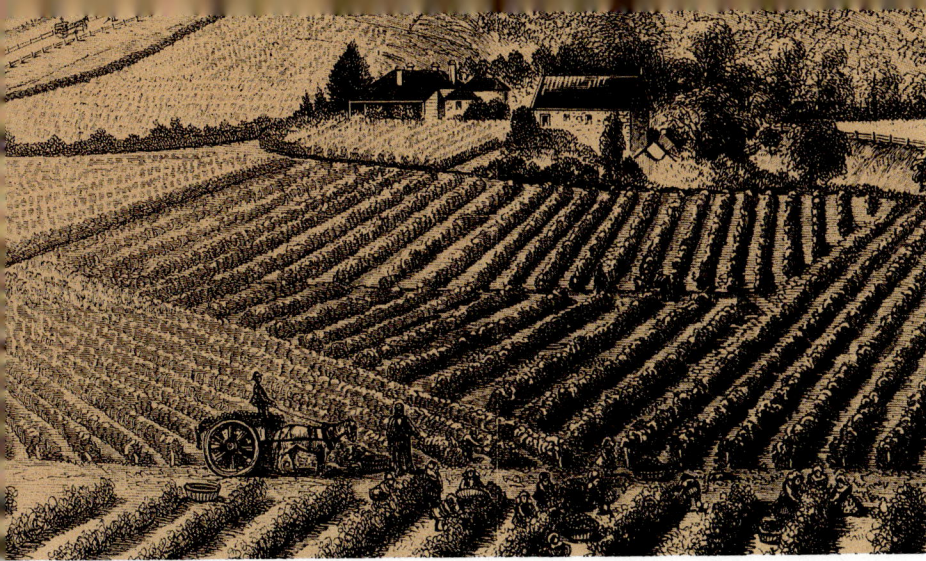

men, but the beauty of the stuff was once succinctly put by Winston Churchill, whose favourite tipples were Cognac and Pol Roger Champagne. He was berated over a dinner table by an irate matron: "Mr Churchill! You are drunk!" Churchill looked at her and said: "Madam, I may be drunk. And you are ugly. But in the morning, I shall be sober."

Today, people still rhapsodise about wine. Writers like Len Evans, James Halliday and many, many others fell thousands of trees annually with their words (and I've done my bit, too). But still the message tends to get confused and people forget that, when all's said and done, it's something you swallow to enjoy.

Listen to what South Australian wine enthusiast Remigio Galea — also a well known Adelaide restaurateur — had to say to wine writer Paul Lloyd in The Adelaide Advertiser on September 9, 1987: "A bottle is only as good as the company you drink it in. Together we can share the taste of the violins, the pepper, the soul of the wine maker. But maybe I'm too emotional."

Maybe he was. "Tired and emotional" was the phrase newspapers used to describe former Prime Minister Bob Hawke occasionally before he swore off hard drink. But even Australia's best known teetotaller still casts a wistful eye over a nice glass of wine and comments that, once, he would have enjoyed it.

What he really meant, I imagine, was summed up perfectly by a grand old man of Australian wine and one of our first and greatest wine writers, the late Walter James of Melbourne. He wrote: "Let wine be your joy, not your master."

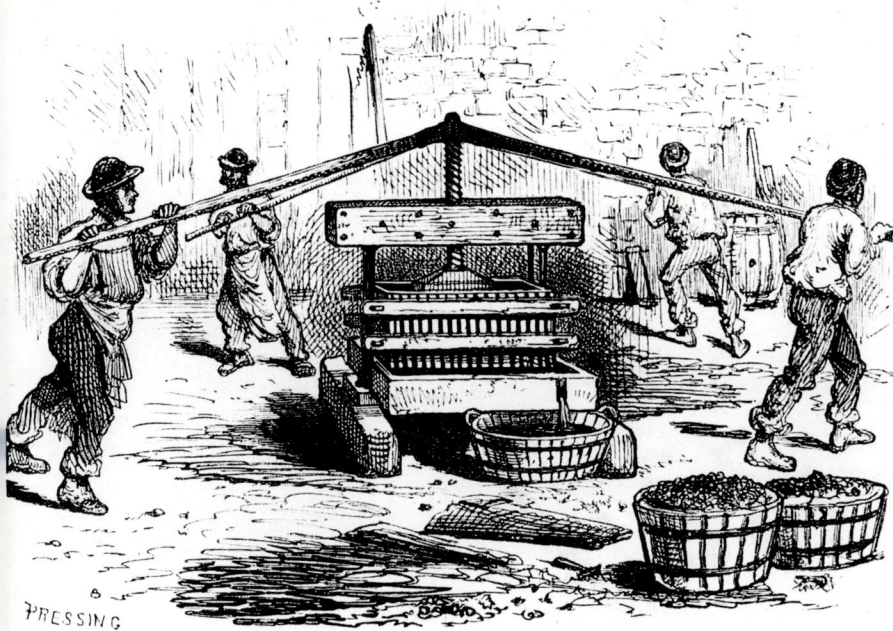

PRESSING

little wine for thy stomach's sake, and thine oft infirmities."

Even the religious orders which do not use wine as a sacrament — usually, by the way, "natural" wine rather than fortified wine — often prescribe grape juice instead. So ingrained is the fruit of the grape in cultures of the world.

The classics are full of references to wine, and it may help you visualise the Romans and Greeks as "real" people to think of Homer, Pliny, Julius Caesar or even England's Shakespeare — all of whom liked a drop — as regular guys with a glass of wine in hand.

In Egypt, Syria and Greece, wine was made, sung about, written about and obviously talked about just as it is today. To compare Dean Martin, Sammy Davis Jnr or Elton John — wine lovers all, by the way — to Plato may sound irreverent. But listen to

what the great philosopher had to say about it: "Nothing more excellent and valuable than wine was ever granted by God to mankind". The poet Homer obviously felt equally inspired when he wrote of "...a wine that was incorruptible and divine; it was so strong that never any filled a cup ... but 'twas before allayed with 20 parts of water; yet so swayed the spirit of that little, that the whole a sacred odour breathed about the bowl ..." (It sounds as though he may have been talking about a spirit, such as a brandy of some kind.)

Aristotle offered his view: "Wine was good for everybody except children and nurses." Another of the ancient philosophers, when asked if it were allowable for wise men to drink wine, replied: "Surely, you cannot think that nature made wine only for fools." He could have added, but didn't, that it has made fools of a few wise

HOW TO DRINK THE STUFF

Working out how to drink wine must be about as meaningful as Lauren Bacall's famous remark to Humphrey Bogart in the 1945 movie TO HAVE AND HAVE NOT: 'You know how to whistle, don't you? You just put your lips together and blow.'

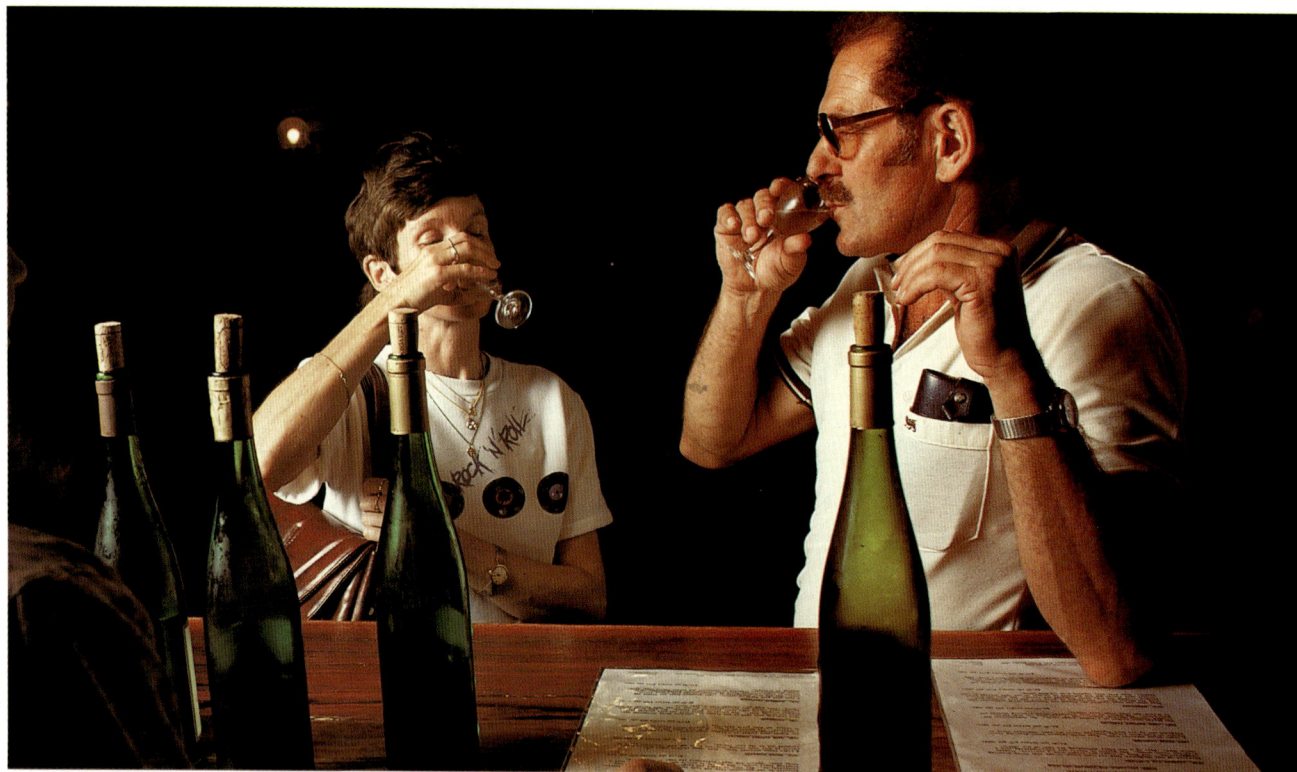

Swallowing wine is fairly easy. Actually drinking and enjoying it has a little more to it, particularly if you want to gain the maximum pleasure.

You don't drink wine because you're thirsty — if you do, you've got a problem. You drink it because you either like the taste, or you're trying to like the taste.

It's a fact of life that most who start drinking wine prefer to drink sweeter wines.

Most of us are brought up on sweet drinks — cordials, Coca-Cola, milk drinks, lemonade and so on. Australians consume some 50 kilograms of sugar a year, an amount which includes that used in the production of beer and wine. We also consume about a kilo of honey and three kilos of liquid glucose and syrups each year. We are high on the world list of sugar fanciers (number 10,

in fact). This helps account for the fact that we drink a lot more "sweet" wines than "dry" wines.

Don't be misled. There's nothing wrong with liking sweet, or sweetish, wines. I'm certainly not expressing any disapproval, as I happen to love sweet wines. But since I'm a bloke with catholic tastes, I also love dry wines. It's simply a matter of horses for courses. It is all part of the diversity of wine, just as it is with the immense cross-section of foods we can enjoy.

A vital point I want to make strongly — there is an important difference between sweet and fruity. They can be both fruity and sweet, or dry, yet fruity to your taste. You'll see what I mean, and hopefully taste it, a little lower in the glass. But remember: FRUITY and SWEET can be terms to describe one wine, but they can also be used separate-

ly to describe quite different wines. SUGAR flavours and FRUIT flavours can be present in the same bottle — or they can be separate.

So if you are starting on the road to wine enjoyment the chances are you'll like sweet wines. My children have been given the chance to have a small glass of wine since they were quite young. Though they seldom wanted it, the exception was when I opened a bottle of sweet (usually dessert) wine, and they jumped at the opportunity!

I believe, by the way, in the civilised European practice of educating children about the sensible use of alcohol, and making it available to them in moderate amounts at meal times, if they wish to drink it (they usually don't until they get to their late teens). People under the age of about 20 who drink wine, though, tend to be the exception rather than the

Tasting in the laboratory is vital to blending large volumes of wine for quality and consistency. Here Orlando's Robin Day and two colleagues discuss a range of the winery's flagship St Hugo Coonawwarra Cabernet Sauvignons.

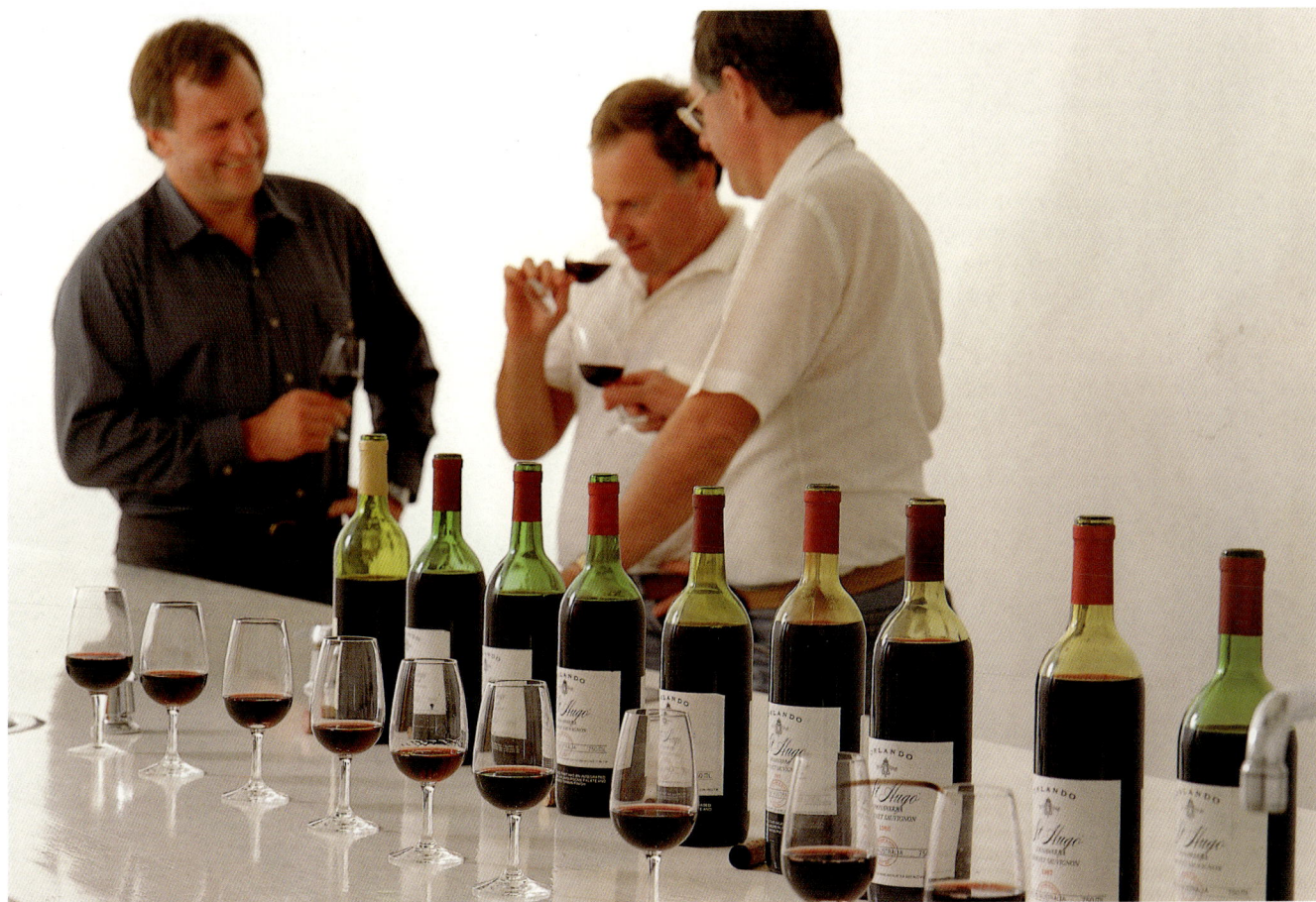

rule. Older people don't usually drink a lot of wine, which is partly a hangover from the days when spirits (such as whisky and gin) were more popular than they are today. But as today's wine drinkers get older, that situation will change and wine will have a more across-the-board appeal. At present, however, the majority users of wine are between the ages of 25 and 60.

We've gone through a wine boom in Australia in the past 15 years. The crucial time was the very middle of the 1970s, caused by tremendous popular growth in white wine. The reasons had a great deal to do with the vast improvements of technology for making white wines. Australian wine makers were making, at long last, very good whites in the German fashion — rieslings or fruitier whites — and an increasingly

affluent public started saying: "Hey, this stuff is okay. I like it!" Prices were low in a competitive market as makers tried to encourage wine consumption. Cask (bag-in-cardboard-box) wines were cheap, and quaffing wines remain excellent value today.

Our annual per-head wine consumption rose from about 11 litres to around 22 litres in just a decade, and then started falling back to the present level of just over 18 litres. Importantly, people were not drinking more alcohol, but less. The consumption of what is called "absolute alcohol" (that is, the amount of actual alcohol consumed per head, irrespective of whether it's in beer, wine, spirits or anything else) fell over a decade from 9.6 litres a person in 1976/77 to 8.7 litres in 1986/87.

The growth in wine sales has largely

been at the expense of beer. Beer consumption has fallen from a high of 143 litres a person to the present level of around 108 litres. Obviously other factors, such as random breath testing, played a part in this social change.

The most important factor was the widespread interest which developed in drinking wine and the improved wines that Australia's rapidly increasing number of wine makers were producing.

The development of the cardboard wine "cask", an Australian invention, boosted wine's popularity as a way of buying and consuming wine easily and cheaply. It became, in just a few years, an everyday drink instead of something extra special.

Perhaps, thanks to European immigration and overseas travel, the

Australian community at large started to realise that having a glass or two of wine with meals, whether at home or at a restaurant, was a fairly civilised and enjoyable thing to to. They started to realise, also, that there was a certain etiquette, rituals if you like, to accompany wine consumption. They just happen to make wine drinking a more enjoyable pastime.

By this I don't mean the sort of snobbish behaviour that wine people associate with those they call "cork sniffers". I simply mean a set of guidelines that enhances wine's pleasurable consumption.

An example may serve to highlight what I mean. A house guest we had at one time was a noted wine buff from Melbourne, which has always had a reputation for being a more wine-wise city than other Australian capitals. We got out the special glassware, which had been stored in a sideboard for months or longer, and opened a few special bottles of wine. I'd only been interested in wine for a year, as I recall it, and felt a bit intimidated by the expert about to grace our dinner table.

We poured the first glass of the expensive wine we'd bought, and waited for his views. "That's terrible!" he exclaimed, so I hastily removed the offending bottle and opened another, equally expensive, one. How's this? "Frightful!" he shouted, and after a bit more consternation he offered the opinion that there was something wrong with the glasses.

We examined some clean glasses and it soon became evident that storage in our timber sideboard had permeated all of our wine glasses with the woody odour of furniture polish!

So, be careful about storing wine glasses in oaky or camphorwood places. Wash the glasses first, if in doubt. And, in other cupboards, stand the glasses right way up for storage, rather than rims down where they can pick up timber, plastic or other odours.

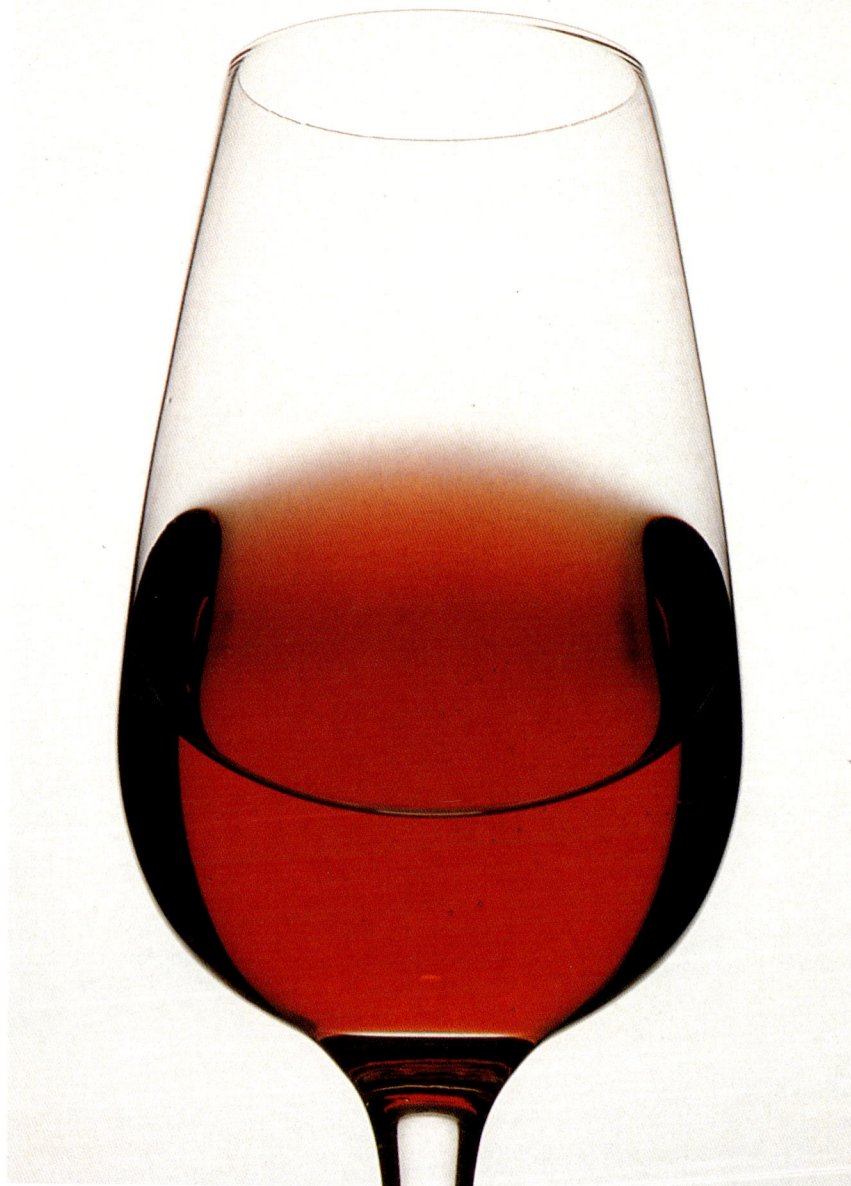

There are certain practices that make drinking wine more enjoyable, but they don't have to be followed. The bottom line, I have always believed, is that you have to like the drink. For the most part there aren't many hard and fast rules about how to drink it.

Drinking out of glass seems to make it a more enjoyable experience. That's because glass (if it is clean, anyway) does not affect the delicate flavours of the wine, and it also lets you see the colour of the wine.

Colour is a very important part of the appreciation of wine's quality. It also has a lot to do with the wine's appeal, as it does with food. How boring food would be if it was all the same colour. I was looking at some dog food pellets the other day; they were coloured red and green. Dogs can't possibly appreciate this subtle piece of marketing, as they're colour blind. Obviously the colour is aimed at the owners, who buy the stuff.

Wine colours vary greatly, with the two basics (red wine and white wine) having almost endless permutations. When I compiled "The Great Australian Wine Book" several years ago, we devoted a photographic section to the colours of wine. It was a fascinating exercise, both looking at the variety and coping with the technical problems of photography. If you're interested in photography, one of the problems faced

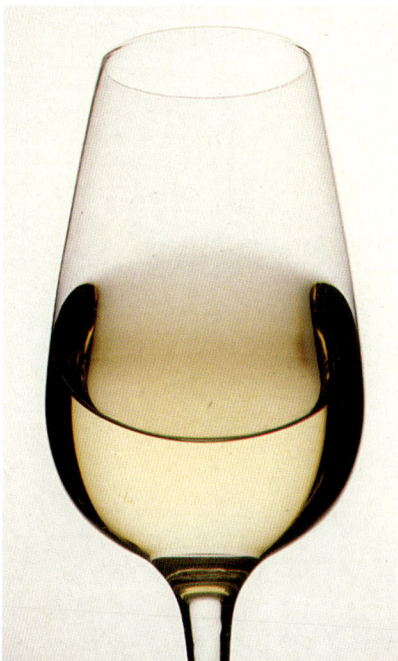
This young chardonnay wine is pale at one year of age.

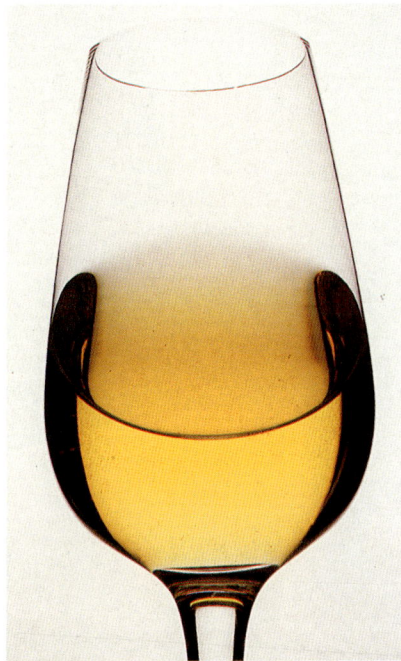
Chardonnay picks up colour after six years in the bottle.

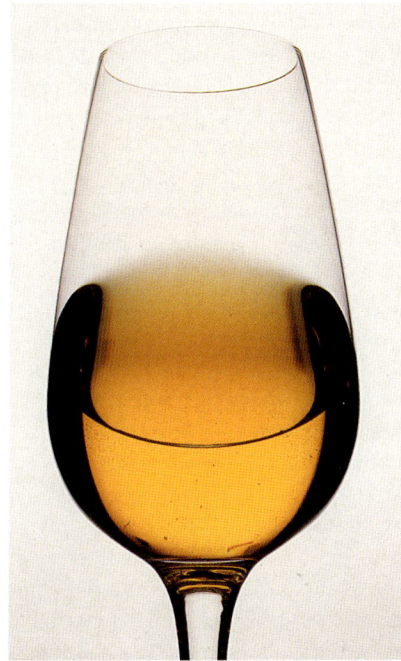
A botrytis-affected sweet white at just three years of age.

by photographer Milton Wordley, (who took many of the photos in this book) with that project was that the wine was held in a glass with a clamp and then back-lit ... the toughest problem to solve was that the wine in the glass acted as a natural lens, showing all sorts of things nearby, including the Kodak colour correction card!

I always enjoy looking at the rich colours of a good, aged white wine, or the brilliant hues of a good young red. The colours I consider to be the most visually appealing, though, are the brilliant (using the word in its colour sense) shades of a really well-made rosé wine. Outstanding examples of the sort of colours I mean can be found in the rosés of Geoff Merrill, Houghton and Rockford Alicante Bouchet, but they must be young wines as they lose colour with age. They are a vibrant red/cherry/pink, often with shafts of blue running through as you hold a glass up to the light. Try a good rosé to see.

Wine glasses can be any shape or appearance, but experience has proven that the best ones have flute-like or tulip shapes. There is now an International

Standard for wine tasting (or judging) glasses and the International Standards Organisation's (ISO) specification for this glass give us a shape known commercially as the XL6 glass. I find this glass, if well made, suitable for use just about anywhere and in fact I use them on my dinner table for reds and whites when we have dinner parties, and sometimes even for sparkling and dessert wines.

But just about any kind of plain, stemmed glass will do. Avoid coloured glass as it doesn't allow you to properly assess the colour of the wine. Also avoid pewter, steel, wood or other gimmick containers as they can taint the wine.

Most plastic glasses are fine for casual drinking — picnics and, especially, poolside drinking. You can now buy some plastic glasses that look very much like actual wine glasses (though without that nice feeling of glass itself). Paper cups are okay when there's nothing better available or if you really want to be mobile!

All you really need to enjoy drinking wine is the wine itself, a glass and a bottle opener.

In novelty or gift shops you'll notice openers of an incredible range of shapes and sizes. Many of them are gimmicky and next to useless.

The best all-round and reasonably priced opener is one simply called "The waiter's friend". That's because it's compact and a wine waiter can carry it in the way you've often seen them doing it in restaurants: stuck into belt or cummerbund, or in the apron pocket.

It has a fold-out blade for cutting the neck capsule away. And it has a fold-out screw to insert into the cork, plus a little lever to help you remove the cork. Some combine the lever with a crown seal (beer bottle top) remover. The waiter's friend is a simple and effective opener, but some are better than others. The best ones seem to be French. (One very good brand name is SCOF.)

What makes the SCOF opener better than others is a two-fold design advantage. One is the way the thread of the corkscrew itself is designed. It is cleverly shaped so that the thread can quickly gain a purchase on the top of the cork, and a small groove around the outside of the thread helps it both enter the cork and hold it tightly when you start pulling it out. The second is that the lever sits comfortably on the neck of the bottle and does not slip away when you apply the upward pressure.

The trick in pulling the cork out of a wine bottle is a simple one. But until you recognise it, you'll have trouble.

Here's how to do it: Cut the top of the neck capsule with the knife and flick it away. Wipe the neck if you need to remove any deposits or dust. Holding the bottle by the neck, insert the corkscrew and rotate it. (Another way is to rotate the bottle.) When it's in deeply, put the shoulder of the lever on the neck and pull it up *but* in such a way that the corkscrew itself remains vertical. You need to pull the corkscrew body off to an angle — about 20 or 30 degrees — to pull the wine cork deftly like the professionals do.

Notice that I've been talking about bottled wine — there's no secret to opening casks or flagons. More importantly, good wines come in glass bottles. For the most part, that's what we'll be talking about here. For while there are some "quality" wines put into casks — Yalumba started it with a range of good two-litre wine casks — most quality wine is packaged and sold in 750 ml glass bottles.

Sometimes bits of cork may fall into the wine — mainly from old corks. This can happen if the corkscrew goes right through the bottom of the cork, which you can usually avoid. The way to get rid of the cork crumbs is to either strain the wine (tedious) or more simply, flick the neck over the sink, getting rid of the top couple of spoonfulls of the wine bearing the cork pieces.

The only other thing you need to worry about is actually pouring the wine. Do it slowly to prevent slopping and dripping.

You can do what some wine waiters do, and twist the bottle as you raise it

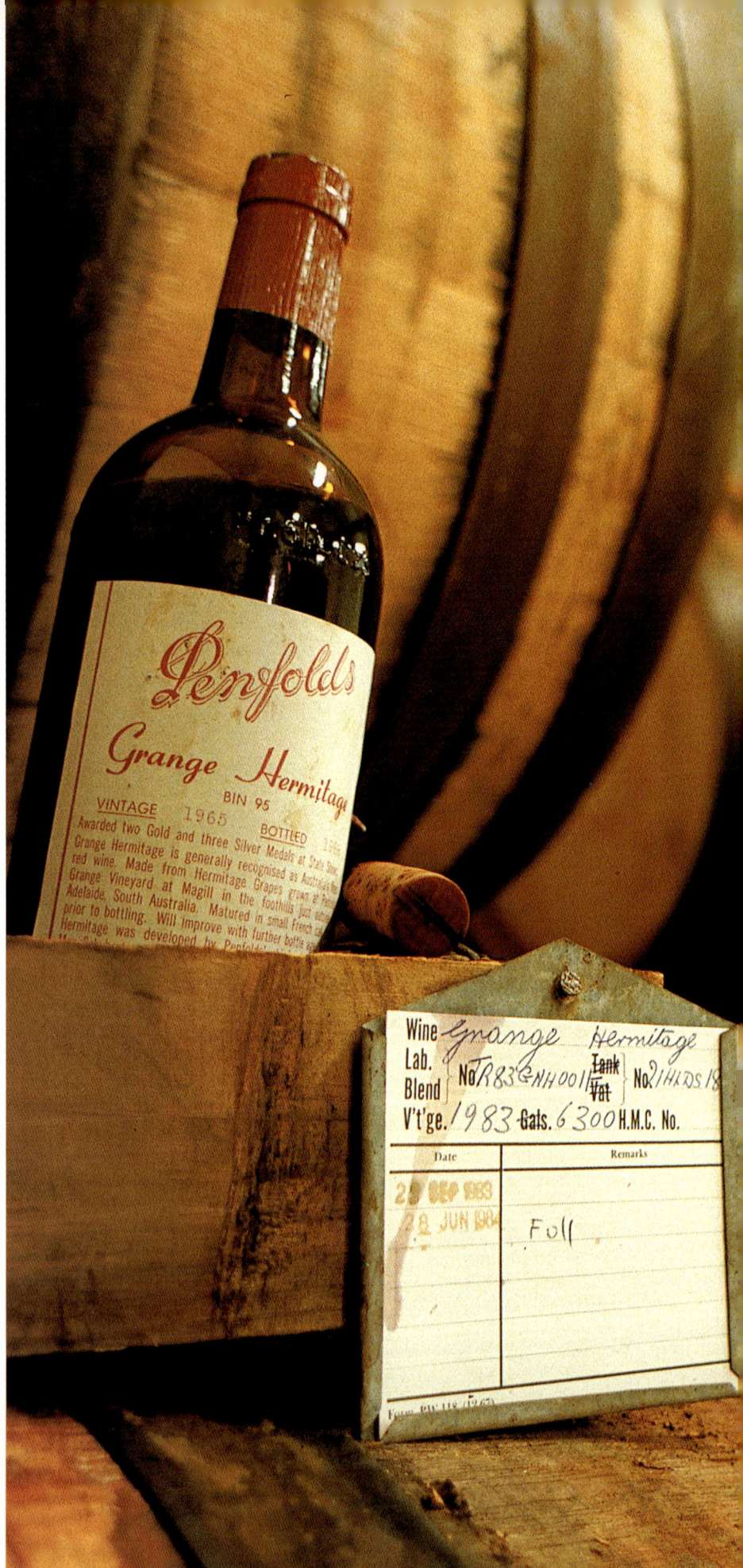

Wood is the magic wand that turns fermented red grape juice into the wonderful substance, dry red wine. The oak may come from France, Germany or perhaps America, and most reds will spend a few months to a few years lying in casks like this before they are ready for bottling – and later for enjoyment.

after pouring. It looks pretentious, but it works if done properly. Careful, measured pouring will do the same thing. There's also a range of gadgets you can buy to do the same job. But who wants to mess about sticking a pourer into the neck of every bottle of wine you drink?

The amount you pour into a glass is important. Among my pet hates are wine waiters who overfill glasses, or who fill your wine glass every three minutes, usually when you aren't looking. That way you lose track of how much you've consumed — and they make more profit, of course.

Wine glasses should never be filled more than about two thirds of the way to the top.

Temperature is also important — even vital — for enjoying wine. In our country temperatures are usually a good deal higher than they are in Europe. That's why the buzz words "room temperature" became such a part of the wine catechism.

Nevertheless, Australians tend to serve our wines at less-than-ideal temperatures. In general, we serve our white wines too cold and our red wines too warm.

The ice buckets so beloved by most restaurants are often quite unnecessary. A bottle of wine which comes from the chiller or the refrigerator is quite cold enough for enjoyable consumption on a hot day without being immersed in icy water and reduced to almost zero. By the way, the alcohol in wine prevents it from freezing until it gets to minus 4°C.

Don't hesitate to tell waiters not to put your bottle of white wine in the ice bucket, but to leave it sitting on the table, if you think it will become too cold — one of the reasons they're reluctant to do this is that their boss tends to chastise them for not supplying an ice bucket, and you often have to make your point very firmly as the wine arrives.

The reason why wine should seldom be placed in ice buckets is a simple one. Most whites taste better, and less like (expensive) iced water if they are served at between about 5°C and 10°C. Put your white wines in the bottom of the refrigerator for about 40-60 minutes or, if the need is more urgent, slip them into the freezer for 10-15 minutes to get the right temperature.

If your need is really urgent, wrap the bottle in a piece of moistened cloth such as a tea towel. It doesn't have to be wringing wet, just quite damp. Then put the bottle in the freezing cabinet for 10 minutes. The cold transfer takes place very quickly.

Don't hesitate to pop an iceblock into a glass of wine, either. It will water the wine down somewhat, but with most inexpensive commercial wines that won't matter much. It may even help, as it will reduce the alcohol you consume per glass.

Red wines should be served at between 12 and 18 degrees, preferably at about 15 degrees. The reason we tend to consume reds too warm is that our summer room temperatures are usually somewhere in the 20s, even the 30s or higher. Up to half an hour in the refrigerator door fixes the problem.

You can buy those temperature bands that wrap around a wine bottle to indicate whether it's at the correct serving temperature.

Champagne needs to be a little colder than white wine, say 4-10 °C. Fortified wines, similar to reds, may be a smidgeon warmer. Rosé (pink) wines should be treated as whites.

But commonsense is the best guide. Drink wines the way *you* enjoy them.

RECOMMENDED READING : The main wine consumer magazine in Australia is *Winestate*, available from newsagents nationally, bi-monthly. This magazine reviews new Australian and some imported wine releases and conducts regular area and style tastings, and is a good source of advice about wines and wine-related activities.

WINE RECOMMENDATION : Try a bottle of Seaview Cabernet Sauvignon and serve it at room temperature if it's cold, or chill it a little if it's summer and hot. A well made and priced red from the Penfold/Wynn wine group, Australia's biggest wine-maker.

WHY WINE TASTES LIKE, WELL... WINE!

Every season, at the end of winter, a million grapevines show the first signs of life. They've been dormant over the cold months, changing the face of the vineyard landscape quite dramatically. Where I live, outside the town of McLaren Vale, South Australia, the vines are brown in winter and the Southern Mount Lofty Ranges, in the background, are green. Then, as spring approaches, the rains slowly retreat and the hills turn brown. As summer comes, the vines bloom into a sea of green leaves.

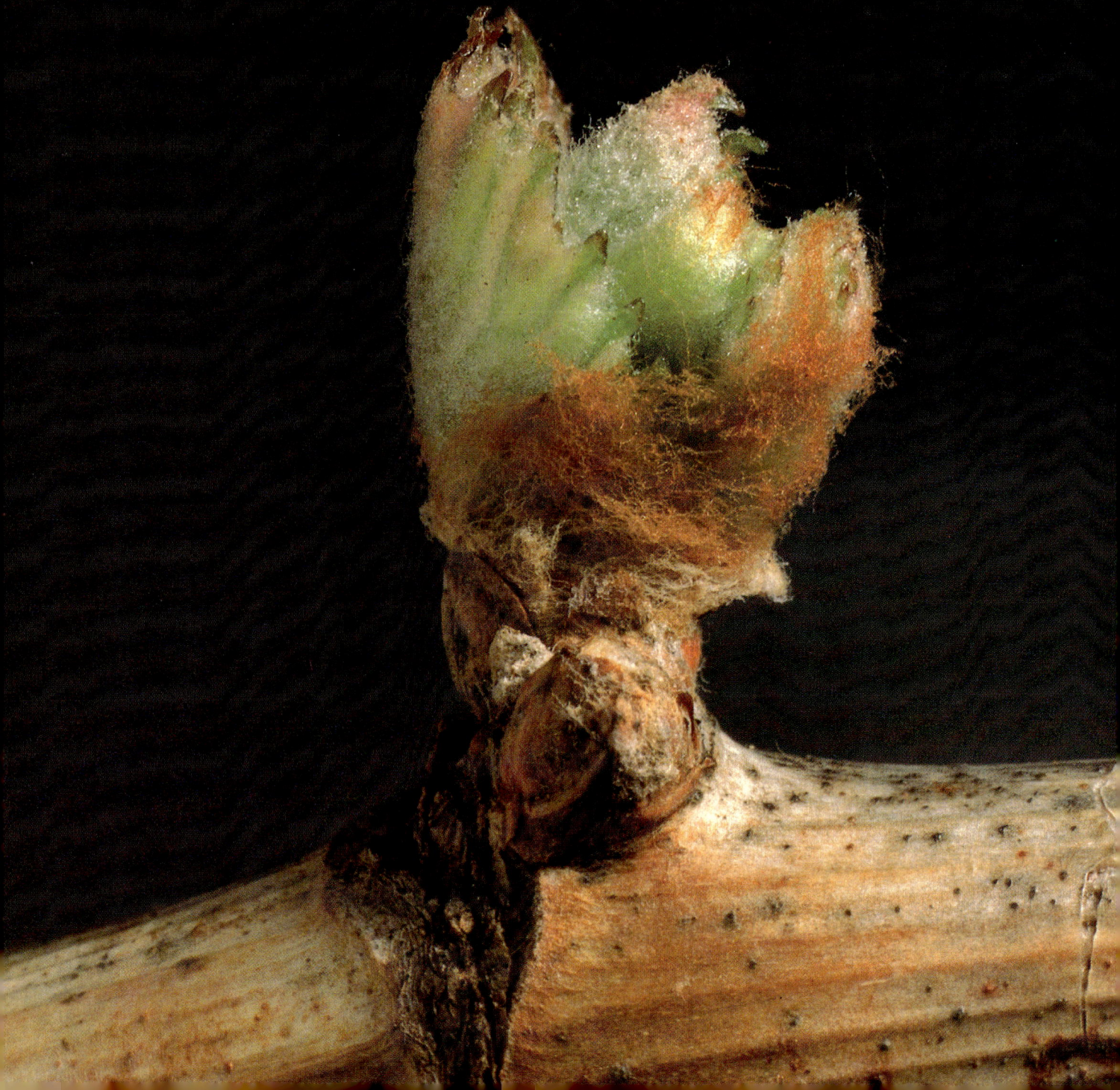

Right: *A little later, the first embryonic bunches of grapes follow the flowering.*

Left and below: *The magic of budburst in late winter or early spring, as dormant vines shoot their young leaves out to greet the warmer sun, and the annual cycle begins again.*

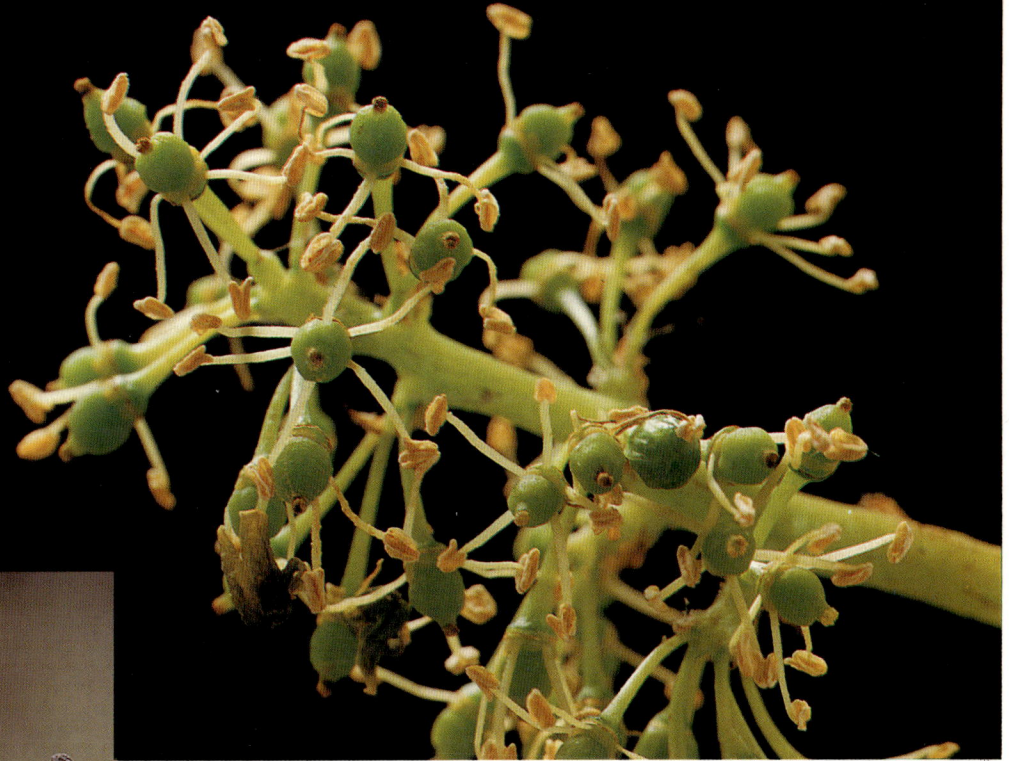

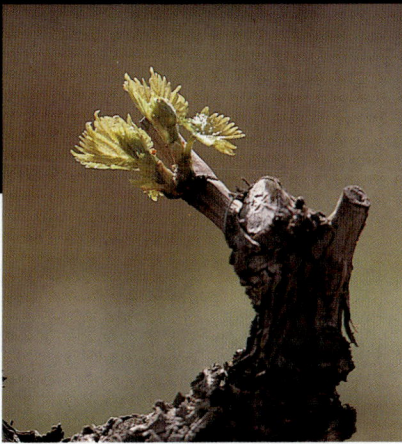

Below the surface, the roots gather nutrition and moisture for the growth above. The taproot of a grape vine can go surprisingly deep, sometimes as far as ten metres, to locate moisture.

First come the buds, usually in late September, early October. From the buds come vivid green shoots which turn into leaves, a magical sight which never fails to delight me. The leaves unfold as the canes start to grow rapidly. Grape vines are usually pruned in the winter months, and no matter how hard you prune them, they find the vigour to burst into life and put out canes for metres; a vigorous vine in good conditions can grow up to five centimetres a day, and continue growing almost to harvest time.

Anyone who has seen the vigour of vines growing out of a bitumen street pavement and spreading over an overhead canopy each year can appreciate

their tremendous vitality. Most of the vines which grow over verandahs, pergolas, patios and shop fronts are the so-called Glory Vine (which goes by the unlikely scientific name of *Aramon x Rupestris Ganzin Number 9*). They are very decorative, turning to gold/red/crimson colours in autumn, but they bear no fruit; the colour, incidentally, is often exaggerated by a virus infection.

The grape-bearing vine *Vitis vinifera* is different in that it puts quite a lot of energy into bearing fruit. The fruit is used for a number of purposes: eating fresh; as dried fruit (raisins); as a refreshing drink (grape juice); and, of course, in its fermented form as wine.

Vitis vinifera plants are an extraordinarily diverse group among an even wider-spread family. There are many other forms of grape vine (North America has one called *Vitis labrusca*). Centuries of experience have told us that *vinifera* is the one which produces the most palatable wines. There is more to viticulture (the skill of growing grape vines) than just the physiology of the plant itself, and the surrounding terrain, soils, climate, rainfall and so on. The hoary old description ("It comes from the southern slopes of the hill"), while having some importance in sun-starved

parts of Europe, indicates the importance of the whole range of things which produce the type of fruit which is the raw material for the end product — wine.

It is popular among the wine knowledgeable to use the French word *terroir* to describe this whole "coming together" of factors which influence the final, ready-for-harvest grapes.

Understanding all the processes and goings on in the vineyard are not vital to enjoying a glass of wine. Grape growing and wine making is, though, a very skilful business and Australians, even with over 200 years' wine making behind us, are still groping around, knowing that some places grow better grapes than others, but suspecting that we have not yet identified many of the places throughout this vast continent where it will be possible to grow not just wine grapes, but wine grapes which yield wines of quality.

For a century and a half tolerably good to exceptional grapes have come from many parts of South Australia, New South Wales and Victoria. Now, very good wine grapes indeed can be grown in many other parts of Victoria (particularly), in the higher and in some cases cooler parts of South Australia such as the Adelaide Hills, in cooler parts of Queensland, in Tasmania and parts of

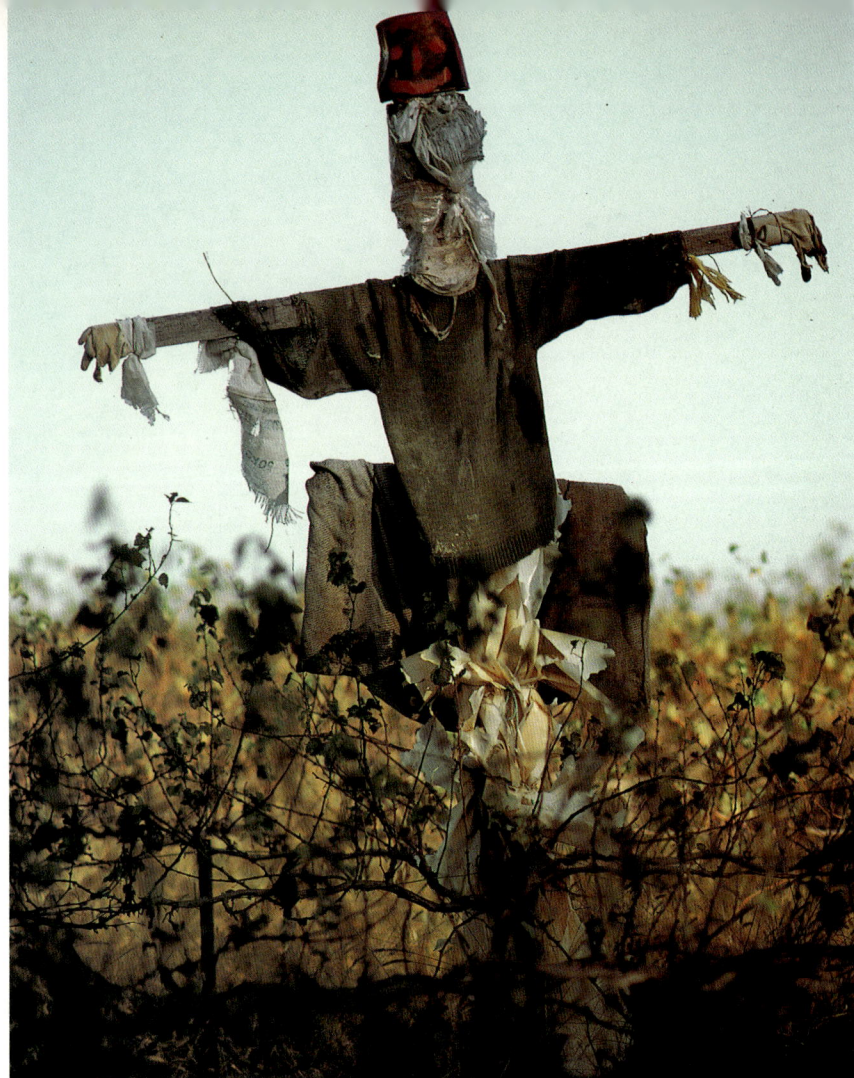

A mute but vivid guard against predators in the vineyard. Vignerons use guns, hooters, ultrasound, scares and even shouting and screaming to keep birds away from their sweet, ripe grapes.

south western Western Australia.

It is, like many other agricultural pursuits, often a frustrating business of tedious and costly trial and error. In the lovely Margaret River area of Western Australia, now producing some excellent wines, flocks of silver-eye birds, thousands of them, have regularly descended on the ripe grapes and eaten most of the crop. In the Hunter Valley of New South Wales it often rains, nay, buckets down, at the crucial harvest (vintage) time. In 1983, to pick a notable example, the vines of South Australia had struggled through two years of harsh drought; then came the Ash Wednesday bushfires, taking scores of lives; finally, as disillusioned wine makers prepared to pick the fruit they still had on their vines, near-torrential rains spoilt crops, flooded parts of the Barossa Valley, bogged tractors at Coonawarra and Padthaway and generally made life miserable.

That vintage was one of the harvests that could be described as an exception that proves the more general rule that Australia has, most years, very good and very reliable grape crops. There's plenty of sunshine — sometimes too much — and in the huge, irrigated vineyards along some of the major river systems in the south-eastern corner of the country there are abundant crops to be picked and transformed into good, reasonably priced wine.

Obviously, our Southern Hemisphere vintage happens at the other end of the year to the European and North American harvests. While the grape vines of France, Germany, Portugal and Spain are picked in August, September or October, Australia's vines are dormant. By Christmas time, our vines are heavy with abundant leaves and small bunches of fruit.

The ripening process is fascinating. The grape berries swell as moisture is pumped up the stems. The grape berry contains mainly water, at least by volume, but there

are small yet significant amounts of sugar and its level increases as the summer progresses. The increase in the natural grape sugar content is what interests the winemaker, sitting on the sidelines ready for the annual harvest, called the "vintage".

As the sugar level increases other significant, and subtle, changes occur in the chemistry inside the juice held by the grape berry's skin.

The most important change is the decrease in the acids. Acid is an important flavour constituent of wine and the wine-maker is determined to pick his fruit when the "balance" is at its most desirable. Think of it as a pair of scales — sugar goes up, acid goes down. When they are somewhere near level, the wine-maker rings his staff, or the grape grower, and says: "Go for your life!"

So the harvest begins. Fortunately for most winemakers, especially the bigger ones, different types of grapes ripen at different times and in different places. Otherwise the vintage, which in recent

years has yielded over half a million tonnes of wine grapes, would be impossible to manage.

Picked by hand and increasingly by big, tractor-like mechanical harvesters, the fruit comes pouring in. If mechanical harvesting machines are used, the picking can go on at night as well as during the heat of the day. The cool fruit so obtained is generally considered to give wine makers better quality. Growing grapes in cool climates is all the rage in Australia these days, and that's one of the reasons why Victoria, the Adelaide Hills, high parts of New South Wales and to a lesser extent Tasmania seem to be the wine making "flavour of the decade".

A lot of planning has gone on before the vintage begins. Machinery is made ready, and estimates are prepared of how much fruit is likely — and revised as the season wears on. Marketers work out how much they are likely to need of each wine style and vineyard workers keep the weeds and pests under control,

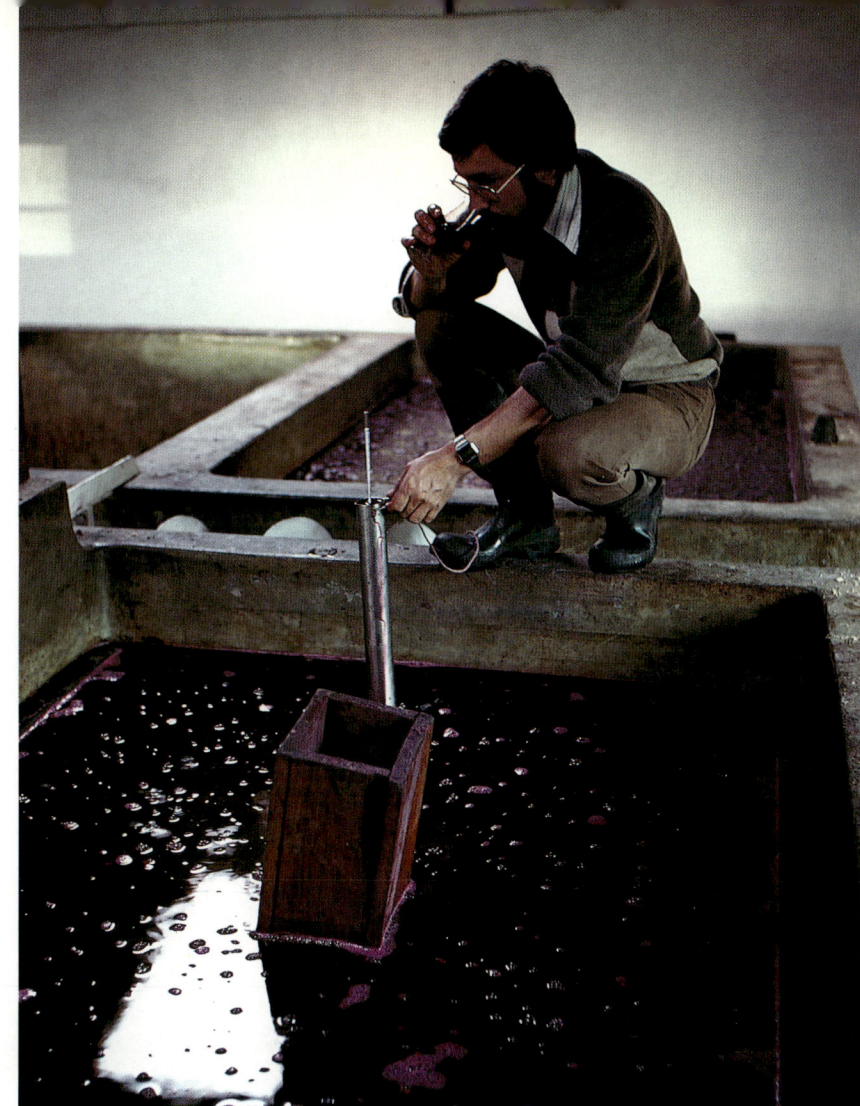

Barossa Valley winemaker Stephen Henschke samples his fermenting red wine. Some makers believe that older open concrete tanks, like these, produce wines with more flavour than modern stainless steel tanks.

if they can. Grape vines can be hit by parasites and diseases, and spraying is used to control problems like Downy Mildew. They go light on sprays, if they can, as the harvest approaches.

The world of wine does not take kindly to finding chemicals in wine, especially in export markets. Detailed analyses on wine imports make sure there are not more than absolutely minute concentrations of leftovers from pesticides and fungicides, measurable only in Parts Per Million (PPM).

Here is where Australia has a natural advantage over its overseas competitors, and why our exports have been rocketing up so dramatically in recent years. As I write this, for example, the United Kingdom market for Australian wines, already our largest export market, is zooming up at an incredible 80 per cent a year.

The natural advantage is partly Australia's benevolent climate, partly our long experience in winemaking, partly good management and, most notably, reflects the purity and antiquity of our soils and our clean skies. The grapes we harvest the first few months of each year should be as pure as we can make them, and the wine-maker's aim is to interfere with them as little as possible.

The ripe grapes first go to the crusher, usually a stainless steel or concrete pit with a worm-like screw at the bottom. Here the first juice extraction is performed. The resulting pulp, usually minus the stalks and pips, goes on for further pressing with a mechanical press. Modern technology has stepped in again and many wine makers now use rotating steel mesh presses into which they pour the grapes, which are crushed by an air bag which expands inside the cage, gently pressing the juice from the berries.

It's surprising how much more juice can still be extracted. This juice is more heavily flavoured by the contents of the skins, coarser if you like, but it has uses in flavouring the rest of the grape juice,

particularly for red wines where tannins (from the skins) are important.

Grapes come in two basic colours (which is at least one more than Henry Ford's famous Model T car): white and black, sometimes described as red. Around these two basic colours, though, are subtle variations: some are pink, some green, some deep purple, some black and some shades of red. But inside the skins, which provide the colour, most of the flesh of the ripe *vinifera* berry is green, and so is the juice. In red wines and rosé wines, the colour is extracted from the skins. The more contact the wine-maker gives the wine on the crushed skins, the deeper the colour in the finished wine.

Making good wines is a complex skill and a demanding occupation. Some people learn by going to winemaking school. They usually spend three years full-time, or more part-time, studying the science of wine making — œnology, pronounced "EN-OLO-GY". Others

learn on the job, and some of Australia's best winemakers gained their skills this way. Some obtain other professional qualifications, usually science related. One popular background is a university degree in agricultural science, stressing wine's strong roots in the land.

The wine-maker's handling of the juice, starting in the vineyard and finishing later (maybe months later, in some cases years later), powerfully influences the quality of the finished wine. To make a good wine, you must start with quality fruit; a great wine-maker can't make a great wine from bad fruit, though the reverse can (and does) happen.

Here's how wine-maker Wolf Blass describes it: "Wine quality can only be achieved by continual, exhaustive and close supervision at all stages of production. This starts at the vineyard and continues at the crusher. Anything which is neglected at these stages can cause the race to be lost before it

The rigours of winemaking last century are graphically illustrated by this shot of a huge jarrah wine vat being unloaded from a dray at Chateau Reynella in South Australia. Things are easier today...

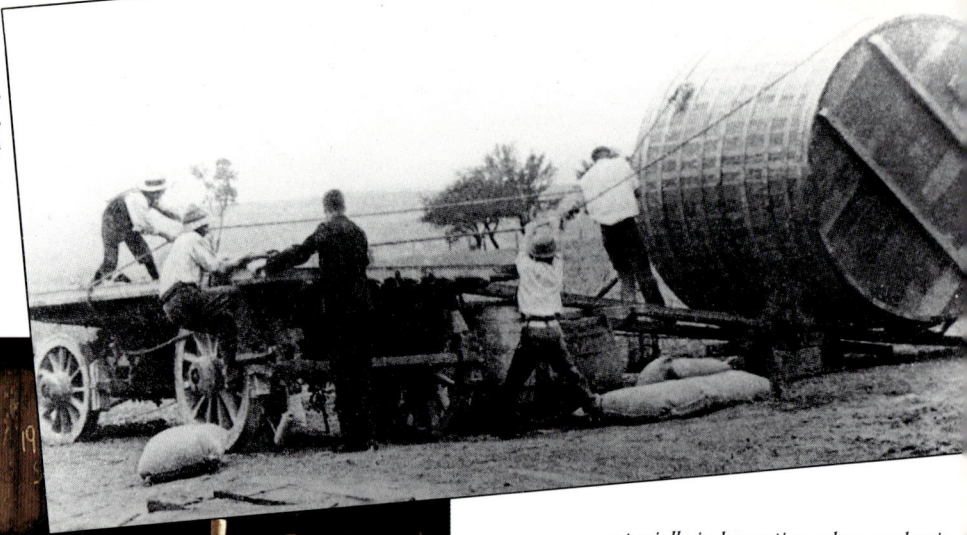

*... especially in harvesting, when mechanical harvesters, **right**, can work in the cool of the night to bring in the grapes under floodlights.*

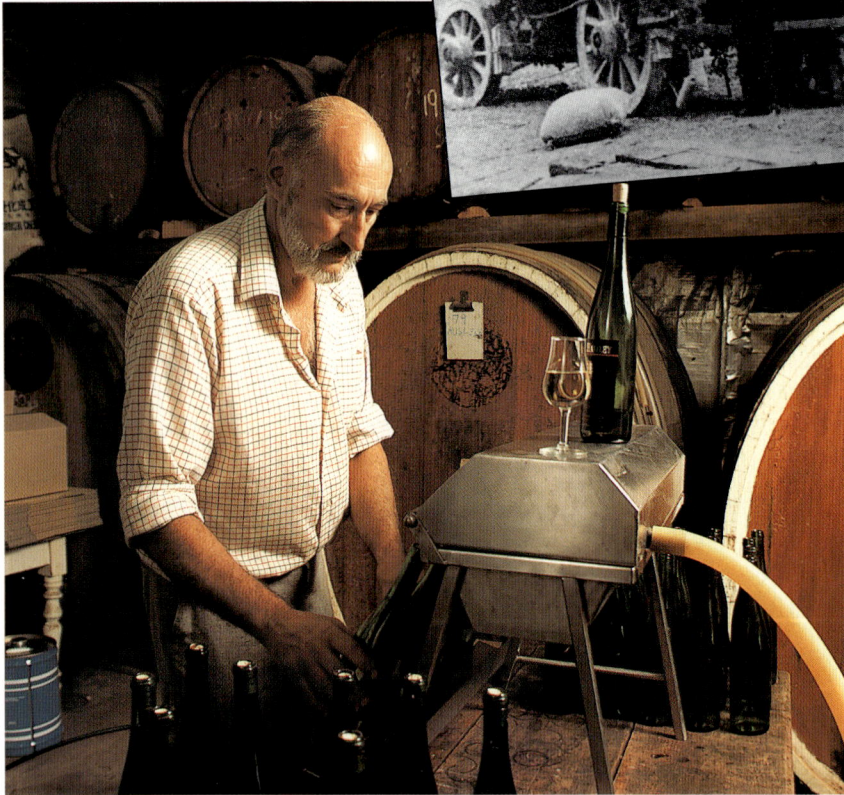

Left: *Small winemakers have to do it all themselves, including grapegrowing, wine-making and finally bottling – which is probably part of the pleasure of the business.*

begins."

As the juice moves from vineyard to crusher and through the winery, the transformation or fermentation takes place. This can happen in just about any container, though one which will not taint the wine is obviously desirable. In the early days stone vats and wooden casks, preferably made of a very hard wood such as jarrah, were used. Then came slate and later concrete vats, some of which are still in use in some wineries (and which have to be lined with wax before every vintage). Finally stainless steel provided what is probably the most hygienic, most efficient and easy-to - clean and relatively inexpensive fermentation and storage vessels. With the stainless steel winery technology came some of the great wines we take for granted today.

Inside each of these tanks, often

holding 20,000 litres of grape juice, the miracle of fermentation takes place. Today it's also something of a techno-logical miracle. The fermentation that has happened since grapes first grew still occurs. But now it is carefully controlled by man (and women, as there are an in-creasing number of female winemakers).

Yeasts eat up grape sugar and turn it into alcohol and CO_2.

The by-product of this fermentation is heat. But winemakers today know that fast fermentations, running out of con-trol like a berserk nuclear reactor, develop all sorts of "off flavours", pro-ducing wines that the ancients must have often consumed, but not the sort of thing you'd enjoy today. Unpleasant by-products of such fermentations include chemicals such as hydrogen sulphide (H_2S or "rotten egg gas"). You can still find them in poorly made wines, and

this, among other things, is what wine judges are looking for, even in minute amounts, as wine faults. These are con-sidered very bad form and will result in a wine being dismissed out of hand at any serious wine competition in Australia.

The secret to good, modern wine making therefore is temperature control. Some wise old wine makers, even in the last century, managed a primitive form of temperature control by throwing ice blocks into fermenting wine. Another way is to go underground, or insulate your winery.

But refrigeration, combined with stainless steel tanks, has given wine mak-ers the tool they need. Coils inside the tanks pump brine from refrigeration equipment through the juice or the fer-menting wine, holding the juice as juice for as long as the wine-maker needs to, during or after vintage, to work out

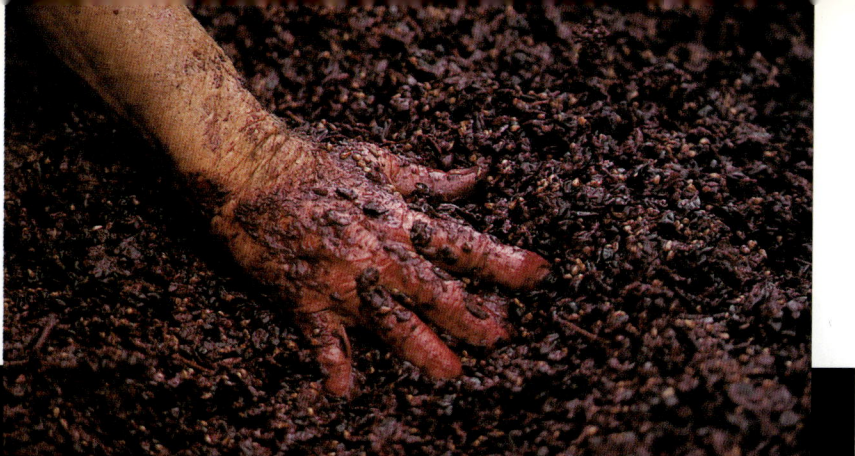

The crushed grapes, including skins, juice and seeds, are known as 'must'. And there's more in it than you realise.

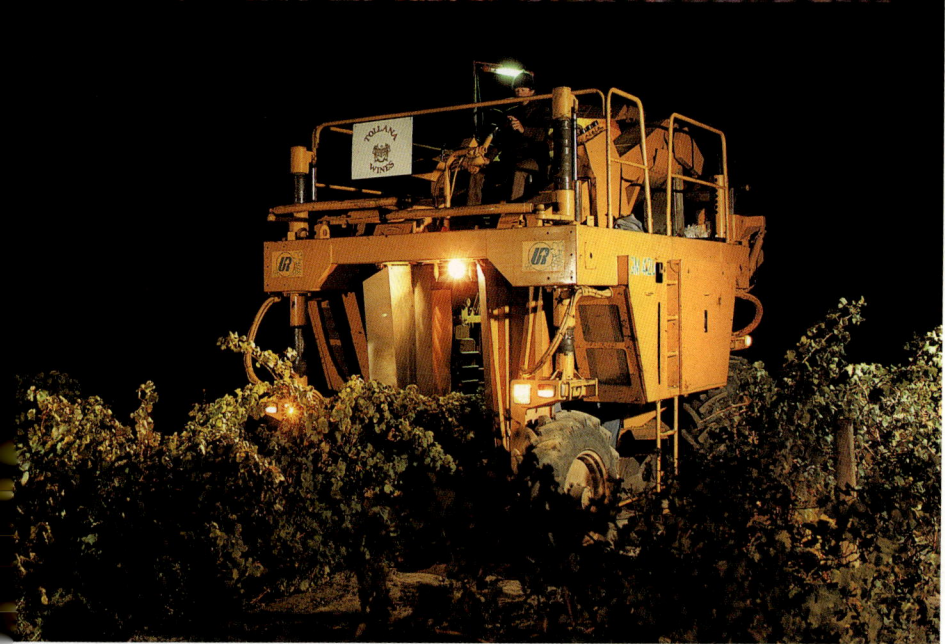

around your tongue.

The fruitier whites (perhaps described as moselles) are usually in the 15-30 g/l range. But don't forget: it's often easy to confuse fruit flavours with sugar.

There is an incredible range of flavour components for wine makers to play with, depending on grape variety, the growing area, the season, the wine making technique and whether or not he wants to add acid to the wine (sugar addition is illegal in Australia, though not in Europe).

Wine contains some 300-400 chemical compounds, making the flavour permutations almost endless. And of course they can change with age, sometimes for the better, sometimes not.

All this is what makes wine the endlessly interesting drink it is.

what should happen next

Then, when ready to kick things off, the wine-maker gets some laboratory-bred yeasts, known to do the job the way he wants, and he injects them into the tank, and raises the temperature to around 12-18°C. That's warm enough to allow the fermentation to start and proceed, but low enough to retain all of the desirable, and delicate, grape flavours.

Such fermentations may take weeks, even months, but the result (especially with modern white wines) is wine of flavour, finesse and great drinkability. Furthermore, the wine-maker can make a wine to the specifications desired by not allowing the fermentation to go on gobbling up grape sugar until it's just about all gone, and a "dry" wine remains. There is evidence that the public palate, if there is such a thing, is "drying out" as consumers go to wines like chardonnay. But there is still big demand for fruity and slightly

sweet wines. The technology our wine-makers now have allows them to stop the fermentation before the yeasts, behaving like little Pac Men, if you like, have gobbled up all of the natural grape sugar.

Our wine-maker uses refrigeration equipment to drop the temperature of the fermenting wine to somewhere approaching zero, and the fermentation grinds rapidly to a halt. But this leaves a little natural grape sugar in the wine, if that is what the wine-maker wants. That touch of leftover sugar is called "residual" sugar, and that's one of the things that makes white wines so popular today. In most "commercial" whites (say wines such as Wolf Blass Rhine Riesling, Seaview Rhine Riesling, Hardy's Siegersdorf or Orlando RF Rhine Riesling) the residual sugar level is around 7 to 15 grams per litre of wine. A level of around 7 g/l is considered quite dry, but you can still taste it, pleasantly, as you roll the first mouthful

RECOMMENDED READING : Most major newspapers and some magazines publish wine columns and they vary greatly in expertise and quality. Huon Hooke in *The Sydney Morning Herald* and Ian Mackay in *The Age* in Melbourne both know what they're all about, as does Tim White in *The Australian Financial Review* and David Bray in *The Courier Mail* in Brisbane. I also enjoy the down-to-earth words of John Lewis in the *Newcastle Herald*. You can learn a lot from columnists such as these and others and, of course, the more learned .James Halliday in *The Weekend Australian* each Saturday.

WINE RECOMMENDATION: Try a bottle of Wyndham Estate Traminer/Riesling and you'll taste what residual sugar brings to white wine.

WINE & YOUR HEALTH

Too much alcohol is bad for you. That we know from social experience and medical evidence. In excess it can harm the heart, the brain, the liver and other organs, and its potential to cause social disruption is also obvious.

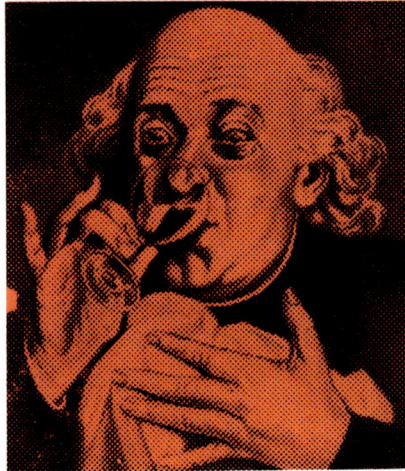

'Bonne Bouche' – *the jolly prelate imbibing. This image of Bleasdale remained familiar to generations of Australians long after his death, as an advertisement for Atkin's Quinine Wine.*
(State Library of Victoria)

But there is good news. Increasing evidence shows that moderate consumption of alcohol is actually good for you and is likely to prolong your life. As drinking alcohol is usually a pleasurable social experience, doing what you enjoy and knowing that it is actually good for you is both reassuring and rewarding.

Moderation is, of course, the key to sensible drinking. The problem is that authorities, and others, disagree about what is "moderate" drinking. Influential lobby groups are very vocal about alcohol use and abuse. Many among them argue that all alcohol consumption is bad — the sort of social voice that inflicted the disaster of total alcohol Prohibition on the United States in the l920s. As Americans and others have discovered, prohibition of alcohol (or drugs, or gambling, or just about anything) seldom works and creates its own underworld of avoidance, crime and contempt for the law.

Those who argue against alcohol seldom do so for utterly wrong motives. A lot of damage is done in our community and to our community by alcohol abuse. The answers, however, lie not with what we might call neo-prohibitionism, but with sensible regulations, proper education and a respect for alcohol as a social drug when properly approached.

I believe that it is important to differentiate between wine and other forms of alcohol. For while alcohol is good for you in moderation, wine occupies a special place among all the various forms of liquor.

How we deal with alcohol varies from country to country, culture to culture, family to family and individual to individual.

Many Europeans regard it is a part of everyday life, hardly worth commenting on; people in other countries think of it only as a drink for special occasions, a mystery substance to be removed from the bottle like a genie.

Australia is having a love affair with wine, though not all are sharing in it. As we continue to enjoy high quality and moderately priced wine, so its acceptance grows.

So there is a growing body of medical and research opinion that shows reasonable consumption is not harmful and can, indeed, be beneficial to your health.

But what is moderate consumption? The answer has to be a general one. Generally speaking a standard (about 125 ml) glass of wine is equivalent in alcohol content to a "standard" (about 285 ml) glass of beer or a nip of spirits. Remember that an ordinary bottle of wine (750 ml) holds six glasses of wine. The arithmetic is obvious: consume a bottle of wine between four people at a restaurant over dinner and (assuming you've all shared the wine equally) you've had one and a half glasses each.

This is about 190 ml of wine; drink two bottles between four people and you've consumed about 375 ml of wine each, which is three glasses, or half a bottle. Or, in another way, if the wine has an alcohol-by-volume content of 10 per cent (just a little lower than average) you've consumed 375 ml of wine, including 37.5 ml of actual alcohol.

The most generally accepted figure for "moderate" consumption these days is around four standard glasses of wine (or the equivalent in beer or spirits) for an adult male, two glasses for an adult female. This is encapsulated in the advertising campaign which has been run for several years by the alcoholic beverage industry with the slogan "Four men, women two ".

A recent development in the wine industry is of relevance here. For years wine makers experimented with reduced alcohol wines, just as the brewers played around with "Light" beers. The early Light beers were pretty crook, mainly because reducing the alcohol took out some of the flavour components, both as alcohol itself and because the process also removed some of the flavour esters.

The processes initially used to lower alcohol involved heating the beverage under a vacuum and distilling off some of the alcohol.

Now two major wine makers seem to have found better ways of doing the job and the resulting Light wines are quite good. In late 1992 Orlando and Seppelt, presumably to be followed by others, released chardonnays and a cabernet sauvignon which had about half the normal alcohol content, or just over 6 per cent alcohol by volume. One of the techniques used is centrifuging. One can drink twice as much of these wines as of "standard" wines of 11-13 per cent alcohol.

Those with illnesses should obviously consult a doctor before drinking. Pregnant women should seek medical advice about drinking, and should certainly drink in strict moderation, if they drink at all. Be aware that even small amounts of alcohol **may** have an effect on an unborn child.

As a rule of thumb, half a bottle of wine a day, consumed at or around meal times, is moderate consumption for normal, fit adults. These levels may err on the conservative side, and some people can drink somewhat more than this and still be within the "moderate" band of drinkers. At least these levels give an idea of what most medical researchers think is reasonable.

Alcoholism, problem drinking which cannot be controlled, is generally recognised as a disease, one which requires treatment of one kind or another, and one which most alcoholics cannot cope with by themselves.

Clearly, encouraging anyone with an alcohol problem to drink is foolish. They can't cope with even moderate drinking, failing to stop when that level of alcohol intake is reached. And, of course, people taking drugs or medication are discouraged from drinking alcohol too. Many forms of medication, such as decongestants and cold or 'flu medicines, promote drowsiness and other side effects which can be a considerable problem, particularly if you're driving.

Moderate drinking is good for you, all other things being equal. Since the early 1900s, scientists have studied the relationship of alcohol consumption to longevity. It became apparent that heavy drinkers (more than nine drinks or the equivalent of one and a half bottles of wine a day) had a death rate almost twice as high as that of moderate drinkers and abstainers.

More recently, researchers have examined the effects of abstention and moderate drinking on the overall death rate. The results were intriguing. For example, the Honolulu Heart Study (published in the *American Journal of Medicine* in 1980) concluded that the rate of coronary heart disease decreased by about 50 per cent with moderate drinking (two to three glasses a day).

In a more graphic example, an American, Dr La Porte, wrote in *Recent Developments in Alcoholism* that "alcohol consumption is related to total mortality in a U-shaped manner where moderate consumers have a reduced total mortality compared with total non consumers. Clearly, the results imply that moderate consumption ... is not detrimental and may in fact be beneficial for longevity." (By definition, those on the other side of the "U" are at considerable risk.)

Much research on alcohol's effects on human health has been done in the United States over the years. One of the largest was

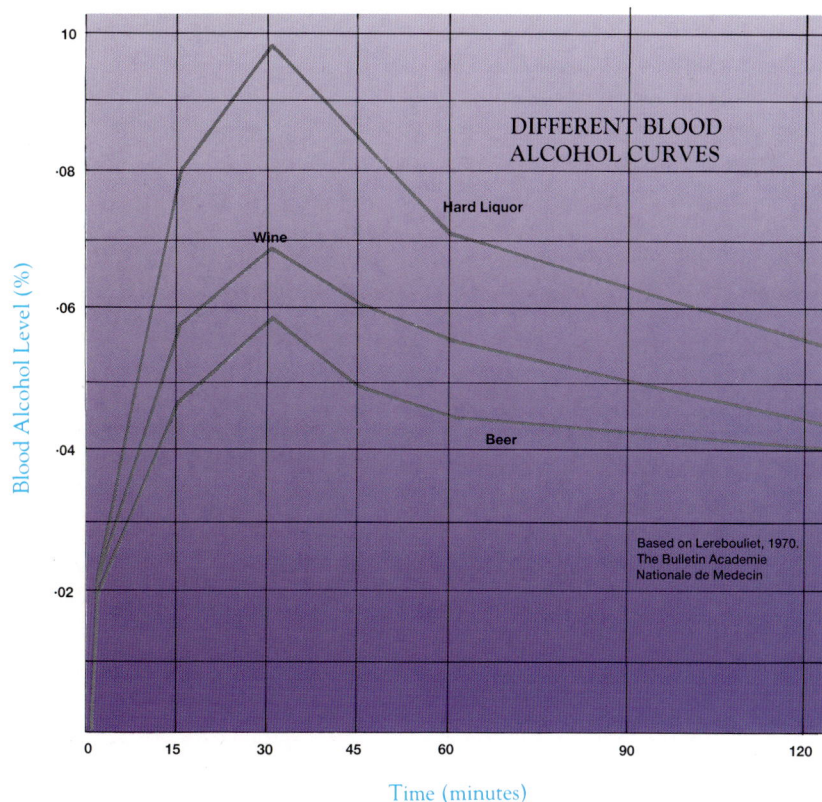

conducted by the Kaiser Permanente Hospital Health Plan, published in the American *Annals of Internal Medicine* in 1981. Some 87,000 people were interviewed as a part of the study. Over 8,000 people were carefully matched and divided into four equal groups:

- •Those who did not drink at all;
- •Those consuming up to two drinks daily;
- •Three to five drinks daily;
- •And six drinks and over a day.

The scientists monitored the subjects for 10 years. The results showed that the moderate drinkers (up to two drinks daily) live longer and are about 27 per cent less likely to die from all causes than either abstainers or heavy drinkers. The reason for this increase in longevity for the moderate drinker appears to be lower rates of heart disease. This has yet to be fully proven, though there are theories about it.

Moderate drinking appears to yield some cardiovascular protection. Higher than normal levels of high density lipoprotein (HDL) were noted in moderate drinkers. High levels of HDL reduced coronary heart disease and the theory is that HDL has this effect by clearing cholesterol from the arterial walls and then shifting and removing the cholesterol. Experiments have shown increases in HDL levels immediately

after consuming alcohol.

In 1985 *The Journal of the American Medical Association* published the results of research at the Stanford Center for Research in Disease Prevention which showed that moderate alcohol intake (they defined this as one to four drinks a day) increased the concentration of HDL in the blood. Further research indicated that some elements of HDL itself were increased by drinking, and these fractions (apo A 1 and apo A 11, if you're interested) are thought to be the most protective.

Further research, in various parts of the world, shows that wine, or something in it, offers more specific protection against heart disease than other forms of alcohol. The British medical publication *The Lancet* reported in 1979 that high rates of wine consumption had the strongest association with low rates of mortality from heart disease. Another piece of research in 27 countries showed that there is a firm association between low rates of human mortality due to heart disease and a high level of wine consumption relative to total consumption.

Perhaps the most sensible overall advice about drinking and health appeared as an editorial in *The New England Journal of Medicine* on March 29, 1984. While warning against heavy drinking and advising caution to abstainers, it commented: "... for a moderate drinker who has demonstrated the capacity to maintain intake at acceptable levels, there is no compelling reason to change that lifestyle and eliminate a pleasurable and possibly beneficial habit".

The arguments for sensible wine consumption over hard liquor appear compelling. For example, distilled spirits consumed on an empty stomach result in a 33 per cent to 130 per cent higher peak blood level than the equivalent amount consumed through drinking wine or beer.

Since wine is more likely to be consumed around meal times, it is important to note that peak alcohol levels for wine and beer are lower than distilled spirits consumed at or after a meal. Distilled spirits (whisky, for example) cause higher peak blood alcohol levels even when diluted to the same alcohol concentration as beer.

And when equivalent amounts of alcohol are consumed, the impairment of physiological and psychological parameters is greater with spirits than with wine or beer.

In plain language, you get drunk quicker on spirits. Probably on beer too, since it is more often consumed on an empty stomach and the gas seems to speed alcohol absorption.

Wine also contributes energy and nutrients to our bodies. The calories we don't always want, of course; a standard glass of dry white or dry red table wine at 12 per cent alcohol by volume contains around 100 calories, and less than 1 per cent sugar. Wine is a complex liquid — as we saw earlier — it has well over 300 known components, and it's likely that some of these (other than alcohol) may be responsible for wine's "good" effects.

Wine contains vitamins, too — not in large amounts, but they are there. There is riboflavin, niacin, pyridoxine, folate, biotin and traces of thiamine and Vitamin B_{12}. Wine has virtually no fat-soluble vitamins or Vitamin C. In general, reds contain more vitamins than whites (though marginally so), possibly because the extra pigments in red wines protect the vitamins from light.

The complexity of wine can also be grasped by analysing the minerals in it. These minerals vary, due to what goes into the grapes from the soil and elsewhere. But there is calcium, copper, iron, iodine, magnesium, phosphorus and zinc (all in minute amounts), *plus* many trace elements such as chromium and silicon. Speculation in medical journals has linked low dietary levels of these minerals to increased coronary deaths.

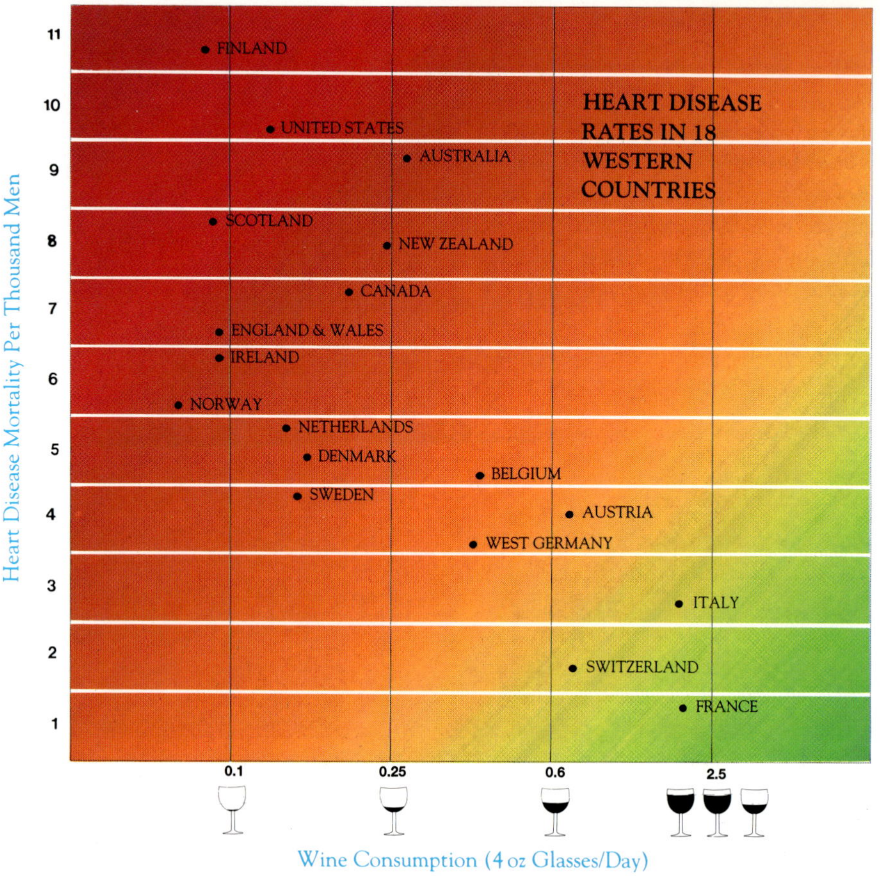

HEART DISEASE RATES IN 18 WESTERN COUNTRIES
Heart Disease Mortality Per Thousand Men
Wine Consumption (4 oz Glasses/Day)
11
10
9
8
7
6
5
4
3
2
1
0.1
0.25
0.6
2.5
FINLAND
UNITED STATES
AUSTRALIA
SCOTLAND
NEW ZEALAND
CANADA
ENGLAND & WALES
IRELAND
NORWAY
NETHERLANDS
DENMARK
BELGIUM
SWEDEN
AUSTRIA
WEST GERMANY
ITALY
SWITZERLAND
FRANCE

There are other ways in which wine is good for you. It has historically been recommended for the treatment of iron deficiency anaemia and to help vegetarians increase their mineral absorption. A Scandinavian study showed that four times more iron was absorbed from white wine than from the same amount of iron dissolved in a 12 per cent alcohol solution.

It also aids the digestive process. Wine is known to increase the secretion of the hormone gastrin, and increases in gastrin help stimulate the digestive process.

From all this we know:

- Wine consumption yields lower blood alcohol levels than does consumption of other forms of alcohol;
- It helps with the absorption of important nutrients;
- It has nutrients and minerals of its own;
- And it stimulates the digestive process.

Less scientific is wine's role in relieving tension and stress and promoting better sleep. One study, in 1963, showed a great difference in the action of wine (compared to a control solution of 12 per cent ethanol in water) in the reduction of tension. This may be due to the slower absorption of alcohol from the digestive tract. Scientists have found trace components which are known to possess tranquillising properties, including gamma hydroxybutric acid, ellagic acid and phenethyl alcohol, which may contribute an additional relaxing effect on the brain.

Of course, wine also promotes your appetite — try a glass of dry sherry just before a meal — which can be a problem for dieters. Many enlightened hospitals and old age homes use wine, especially sherry, for this purpose.

Used sensibly, wine can be very good in many ways. What it is in wine (if indeed it is one thing, which is unlikely) we don't exactly know. The medical research done some years ago at the University of Cardiff, Wales, demonstrated the sorts of effects on heart health that I described above. They did not know what property it was in wine that did the job, but, they added, "Why bother to find out, when the medicine already comes in a most palatable form?"

I'll drink to that prescription, doctor. Moderately, of course.

RECOMMENDED DRINKING : A bottle of Wilson Cabernet Sauvignon, or if you can't locate that, try.one of the "Pierro" wines from WA's Margaret River, founded in 1980 by local doc Michael Peterkin. Beats anaesthetic any day, and is also cheaper than seeing a doctor.

T R I L O G Y ®

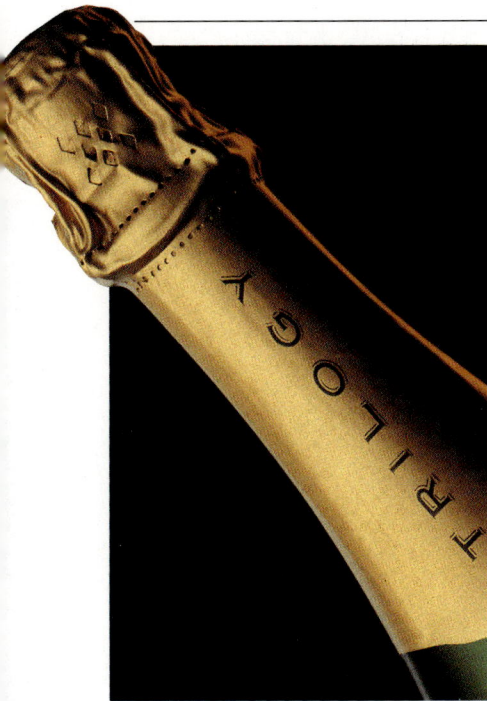

A celebration of
the three classic...

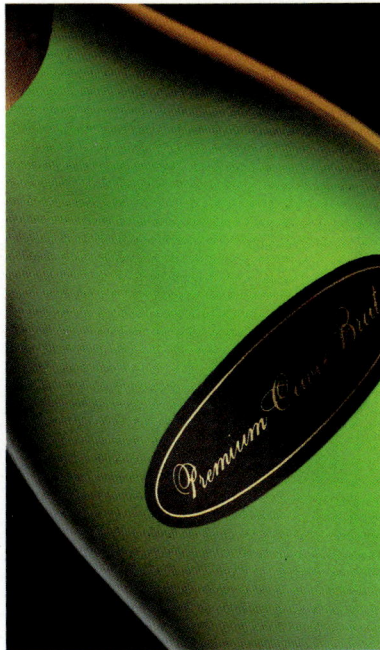

champagne
grape varieties...

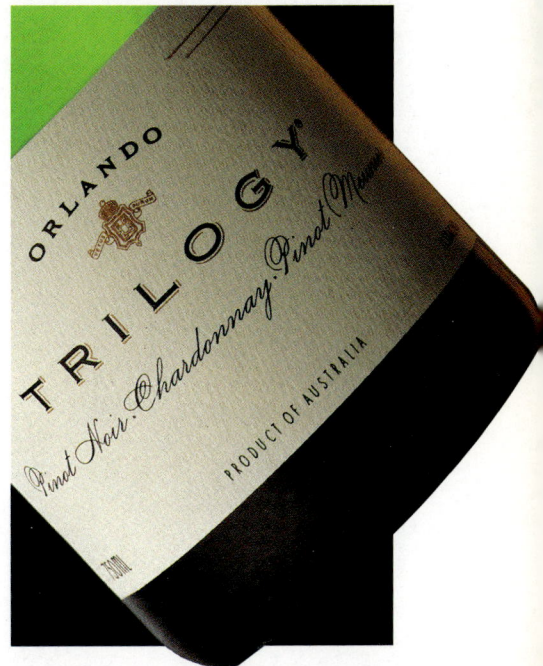

Trilogy from Orlando is a celebration of the three classic champagne grape varieties in a singularly stylish new Cuvée Brut. Trilogy is composed of Pinot Noir – adding depth and intensity of flavour, Chardonnay – providing crisp delicacy and elegant fruit characters and Pinot Meunier – adding finesse and balance to complete the Trilogy. New Orlando Trilogy is a blend of tradition and artistry combined to produce the subtle flavour and personality of a classic Cuvée Brut.

T R I L O G Y ®
from Orlando

ALL ABOUT WHITE WINES

They put wine on the agenda for most of us

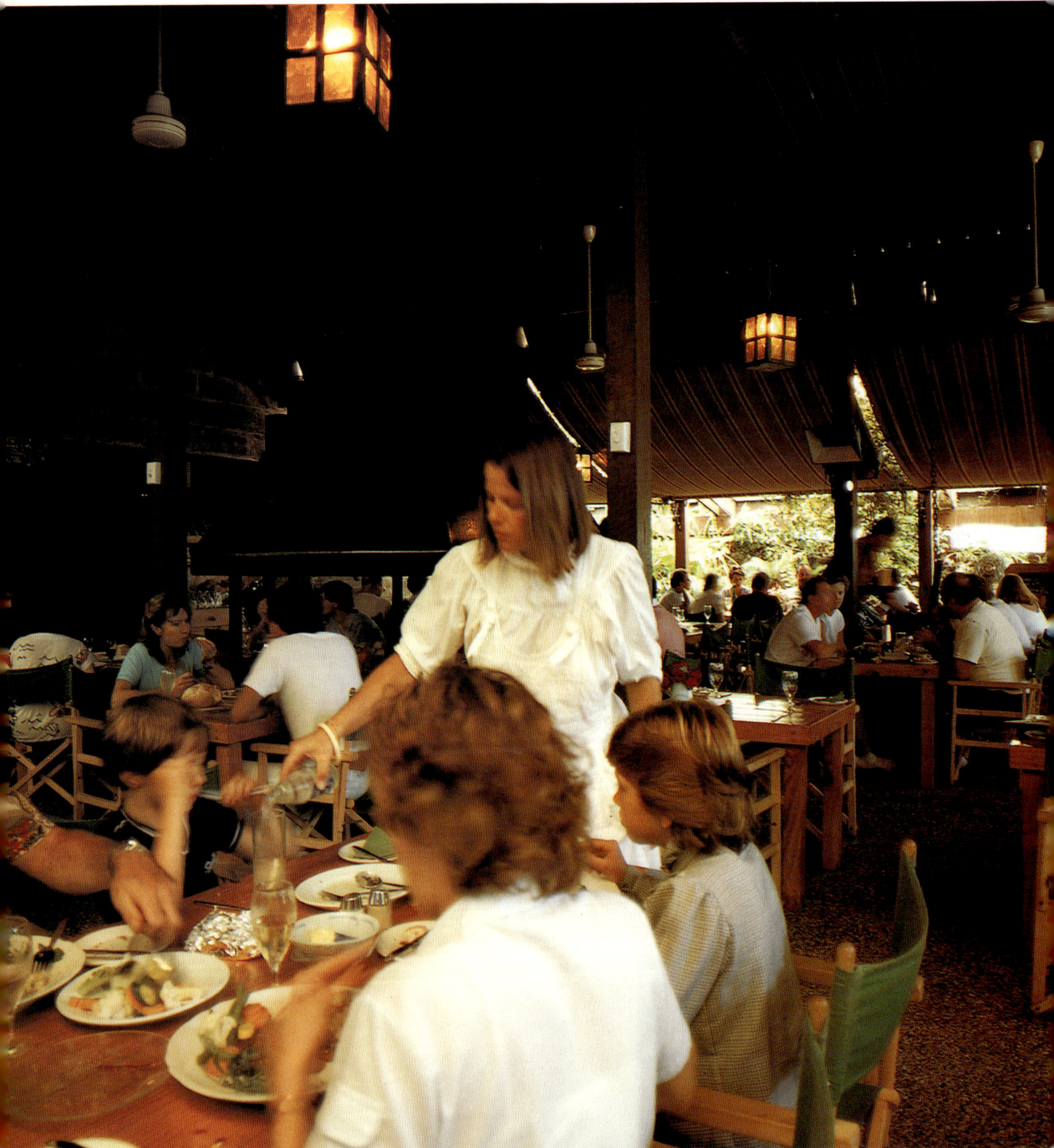

To many people, white wine is wine. They start drinking white wine (maybe bubbly white) and stay with it for a very long time, if not for all of their drinking lives.

Many will protest that they don't like red wine (or red wine doesn't like them). Fair enough. There is enough variety in whites to enable you to drink a different wine every day of your life and not repeat one.

Cool white wine is a drink admirably suited to much of our Australian lifestyle. As with most other forms of wine, an understanding and appreciation of white wine, and more enjoyment from it, can best be gained by realising the difference between the two broad "styles" of wine. They are at the core of what wine is all about:

GENERIC WINES

are labelled after the old European wine types and areas. Generic wines include White Burgundy, Chablis, Hock (a name seldom used these days for whites), Claret, Burgundy and so on. While there are plenty of good branded wines of this type around (e.g., Jacob's Creek Chablis, Houghton White Burgundy, de Bortoli Sauternes, and so on), and most are excellent everyday drinking, they generally tend to be made to a formula. With big branded products such as these, consistency is a paramount requirement from the wine-maker, and an expectation by the consumer.

These wines are usually of extremely high quality. They are generally reasonably priced, because economies of scale mean that costs can be kept down. To make these wines, you need high technology; high levels of quality control; wine making and production skills of a very high order; and skilful marketing support.

Often these wines have launched many a wine drinker. Millions of litres of generic wines are sold and quaffed annually from cardboard casks (the wine industry knows them as "bag-in-box") under generic labels: Stanley Moselle; Lindeman's White Burgundy; Orlando

Our tastes in wine have been getting drier. More Australians are eating out and enjoying bottled wines with their restaurant meals. A little knowledge will help your enjoyment and cut costs.

Coolabah Claret and so on. Generic wines often not usually reveal their grape origins. Instead, a blend of different grape varieties is usually used to obtain the desired flavour/sweetness/dryness, or whatever. Some of the big selling moselles may contain half a dozen or more white grape varieties, with a heavy dependence on the aromatic and pungently flavoured white grapes such as muscat. These grapes are known as multi-purpose grapes. They can be used for wine making, for grape juice, for fresh grapes or for drying. They usually bear fruit heavily, especially in the irrigated river regions of Australia, and are comparatively easy to grow. They are also cheaper than the varieties used exclusively for making varietal wines.

People's tastes in white wine constantly change. While there is clearly no such thing as an average wine drinker — tastes vary according to age, experience, income and so on — there is an obvious switch in preferences for drier (less residual grape sugar and more dominant wood flavours) among the top selling wines in Australia.

It is interesting to see what Australians choose to drink in the wine market today. In late 1992, of the top 10 selling white wines, four were generic and one (Traminer Riesling) "sort of" generic. Here's that cobbled-together list (with the generic style wines in **bold type**): See above right.

Some of these wines vary in grape content, for example, the Queen Adelaide Riesling. But there is a clear trend, with wines like Ben Ean continuing to fall and the chardonnays growing in sales. The so-called Traminer/Riesling wines also pose a problem with identification. Traminer and Riesling are two different grape varieties, though names on wine bottles often indicate a style of taste (a generic wine), rather than a guide to the actual varieties. Expect a wine which is probably

TOP SELLING BOTTLED WHITE WINES

1. Woodley Queen Adelaide Chardonnay
2. **Houghton White Burgundy**
3. Wyndham Estate TR 2 Traminer/Riesling
4. Woodley Queen Adelaide Riesling
5. Orlando Jacob's Creek Chardonnay
6. Wolf Blass Rhine Riesling
7. Hardy's Siegersdorf Rhine Riesling
8. **Orlando Jacob's Creek Chablis**
9. **Tyrrell's Long Flat White**
10. **Brown Brothers Moselle**

fairly fruity and fairly sweet when you see traminer/riesling on a label, though not necessarily made from the two varieties.

Generic wines are also beginning to identify their origins: Jacob's Creek Claret, for example, has for some years stated that it is made from a blend of three red grapes — shiraz, malbec and cabernet sauvignon.

And late in 1992 the Australian wine industry reached agreement with the Europeans that we would phase out the main generic names, and instead rely on other descriptions, particulary descriptions relating to the grape varieties used to make the wines.

The road to wine appreciation and enjoyment is much smoother if you take just a little time to acquire some knowledge about, and understanding of, a

It's good to drink but some wines are better than others.

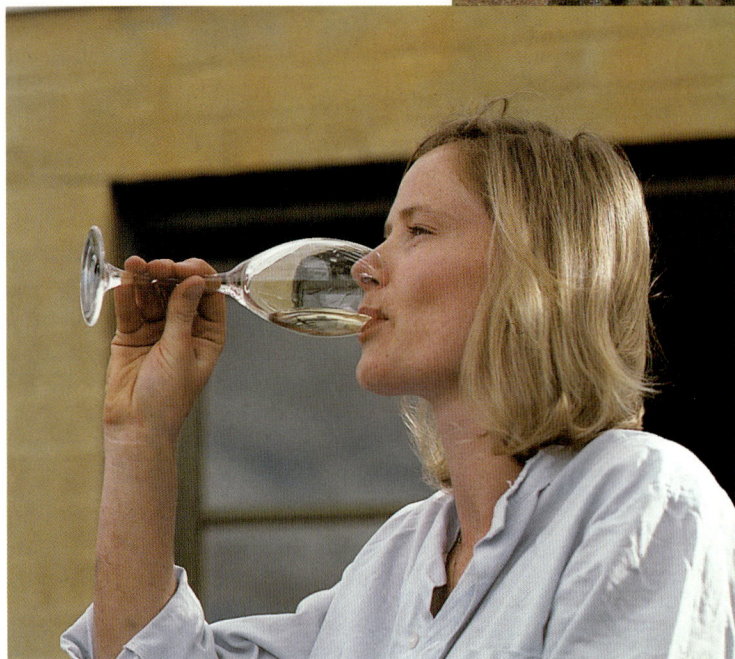

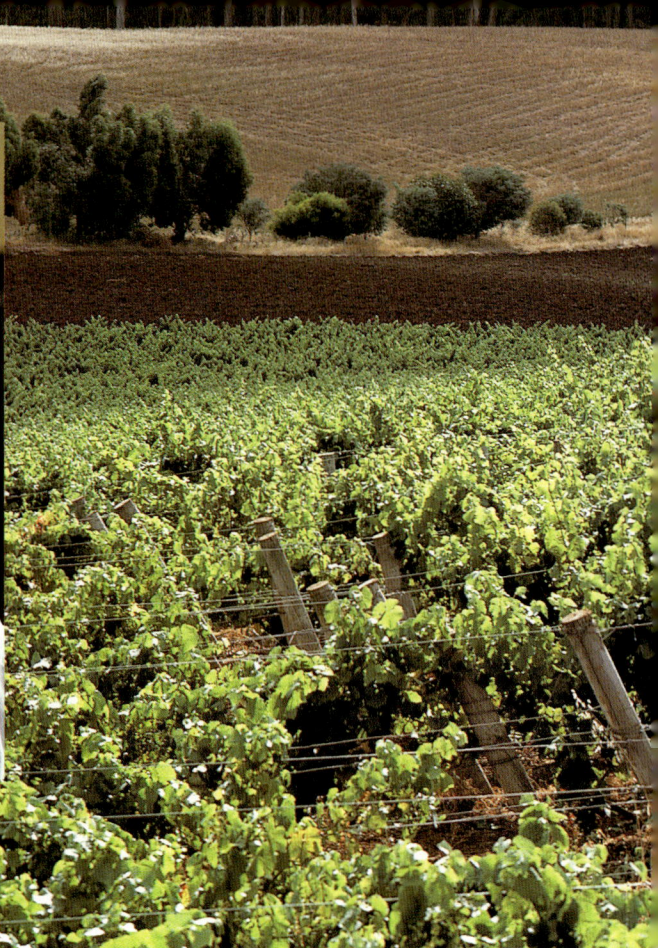

Riesling is one of the great flavours of the world of wines, and Australia's sunny vineyards produce some magnificent — and underestimated — examples of this grape variety which makes wines right through from dry to sweet.

number of grape varieties that go to make:

VARIETAL WINES

The label will indicate which grape varieties went into the making of the wine. Under Australian law, a wine-maker describing a wine by a varietal name must put at least 80 percent of the nominated variety into the bottle. In practice, a wine described as a Rhine riesling will usually have 100 per cent of that grape variety.

I have no doubt that with the continuing boom in the white variety chardonnay, many makers of big-selling brands are taking advantage of the law's letter, using 80 per cent chardonnay and 20 per cent of blander and cheaper varieties, perhaps semillon or palomino, to top up and maximise profits by minimising costs.

If two varieties are listed on a label, the dominant variety should come first, unless they are equal, in which case either can go first: for example, chardonnay/semillon, which is legal and has the desirable advantage, from the marketing viewpoint, of putting the trendy word

"chardonnay" first.

Here are the main white varietals, with a few comments and a few nominations of generally good examples of the style.

RHINE RIESLING

Riesling (as I prefer to call it, without the name of the German river whence the variety originates) still produces some of the best white wines in Australia. Australian wine makers have had a great deal of experience with riesling, and while we make different rieslings from the Germans, Austrians and Americans (whose Johannisberg rieslings I find unpleasant), the Australian style is generally a very enjoyable drink, particularly pre-meal or with light foods such as fish.

Riesling, when well grown and made, produces wine which has what is called an "aromatic" character. It is pleasantly perfumed and a sniff of a fresh riesling is often reminiscent of passionfruit, peaches, apples or tropical fruits. The wine can vary from sweet to dry, but the fruit flavours should be quite dominant. The wines are usually most drinkable when young (less than two years old) and many

will gracefully acquire bottle age. With this maturity the characters will change, the colour darken, but a year or two of cellaring, even for a commercial wine, will provide a very rewarding drink.

Among the outstanding Australian rieslings are Yalumba Pewsey Vale and Heggies; the better (i.e. more expensive) wines of Lindeman and partner Leo Buring; Orlando with St Helga and RF rieslings, among others; Hardy's with Siegersdorf, Mitchelton, Petaluma, Seppelt Black Label, Woodstock and Wirra Wirra from McLaren Vale, Mitchell and Tim Knappstein and Eaglehawk from the Clare Valley.

It's interesting to note the dominance of South Australia in the above recommendations. While there are some good rieslings grown elsewhere (Piper's Brook in Tasmania; Houghton in WA — and a few from the Upper Hunter Valley, among others) South Australia indisputably produces the finest rieslings of Australia.

Riesling also makes some excellent sweet white wines. In the right circumstances, a glass of a really good, complex sweet white can complement an appropri-

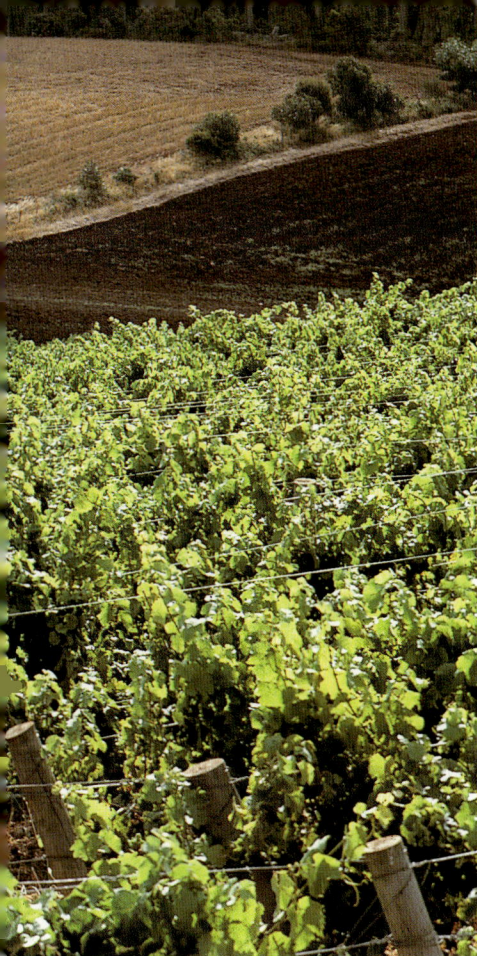

ate dish beautifully. Desserts are the obvious benefactor for such a sweet wine, but a good one can also usefully accompany many cheeses, and some fruits.

Every now and again, ripe riesling grapes are attacked by an unusual mould, called *Botrytis cinerea*. Warm and wet conditions in vineyards promote the movement of the spore of Botrytis. When they land on the sugar-ripe grape berries they start sucking the water from them through the skins. This has the effect of concentrating the flavour substances inside the berry, and also concentrating the sugar. As the grape bunches turn a disgusting looking grey/green colour, and shrivel up, the Botrytis keeps attacking, and at the right stage a smart wine-maker can pick and crush them. The very sweet juice can then be fermented into wine and the results, when properly done from thoroughly Botrytis-infected vineyards, are wines of amazing richness, sweetness and complexity of flavours.

These wines are therefore sometimes called "Noble Rot" wines, and they produce some of the great sweet dessert wines of France and Germany, wines much sought after. The most famous is proba-

bly France's Chateau d'Yquem, and these wines can cost hundreds of dollars for a single bottle.

In certain, though unpredictable, conditions, the same sort of thing can happen in Australia, and fine examples have been made by wine makers including Len Evans's Family, Petaluma, Brown Brothers, Hardy's (notably in 1985 and 1987), de Bortoli, McWilliam's, Woodstock, Rosemount and Yalumba.

The spectrum of sweetness ends with Botrytis affected wines. They are the Rolls-Royces of sweet whites, or "stickies" as some call them. And while riesling is the base for many, some of the other white grape varieties also make good sweet whites — semillon, muscat and sauvignon blanc among them.

Australians owe a real legacy to the German rieslings, the wines that come from the areas such as the Rhine and Mosel Valleys. From Germany we have also acquired the hierarchy of sweetness in riesling wines. The longer you leave the grapes hanging, of course, the higher the sugar levels and the more sweetness (or higher alcohol, which ever the wine maker chooses) you get in the finished wine.

In Germany, with a generally cool to cold finish to the vintage, fully ripening the grapes can be a real challenge, as it can be in France. As a result, wine makers and grape growers tend to opt for grape vine clones that yield ripe grapes fairly early, before the frosts can destroy the crop. The alternative to fully ripe grapes is to add sugar to the fermenting grape juice — cane sugar or beet sugar, for example — which takes the place of grape sugar and translates, of course, into alcohol. This practice, called "chaptalisation", is legal in Europe though it is, in theory though not always in practice, strictly controlled. In Australia, with high sunlight levels throughout much of the country, the practice of chaptalisation is illegal.

Australia has widely adopted the German system of sweetness levels in wine, but these are not always clearly defined here. Their use is more a compliment than anything else, and a reflection of the strong Germanic influence in the Australian wine industry. Orlando, with its origins in the Gramp family of immi-

grants, is a good example. Some of its wonderful whites, in particular their Steingarten rieslings, are quite German in style.

Here's how rieslings should rate on the scale of rising sweetness, then:

Spätlese is a wine made from riper-than-normal grapes; if you believe that sweet wines are not your bag, some of the better made spatlese wines may surprise you. Orlando has been a notable maker of such wines.

Auslese is the next up the sweetness scale, and will also be pretty fruity. Good fresh fruit wines.

Beerenauslese. Sweeter again, and should be full of fruit. High sugar levels are pretty easy to get in Australia (but not in Germany), but do not necessarily have that extra complexity one is looking for in wines of this description.

Trockenbeerenauslese. Very sweet indeed, usually rare and expensive. A term not often used in Australia.

Riesling is a versatile wine grape variety which gives quite different tasting wines, although generally recognised as part of the riesling family, varying from one part of Australia to another.

There is an area of confusion. The word "riesling" by itself can describe a blended (generic) wine style, though this use of it is fading. In general, Australian wine makers denote pure riesling by using the words "Rhine riesling".

The other strange aberration, now largely gone, was the use of "Hunter River Riesling" to denote a drier style which, many years ago, was actually identified as the white variety semillon. Few makers hold on to this curious anomaly, though one that did for a long time was McWilliam's with the Elizabeth "Riesling" from their Mount Pleasant Hunter winery. (The wine is now accurately identified on the label as "Elizabeth Semillon".)

CHARDONNAY

Chardonnay is to dry whites what riesling is to the fruitier, more aromatic styles.

Like riesling, it can produce some exceptional wines. Whether you like it or not depends on personal preference. If you have a typical palate, you'll probably prefer a riesling-style wine first, then maybe move on to a drier white wine, such as chardonnay, later in your drinking career.

It is a more difficult grape to grow and turn into wines. Yet it can produce some outstanding dry, yet full-flavoured, whites. And, handled properly, it takes to wood ageing (in oak barrels), like a duck to water. Like most red wines, chardonnay gains an extra complexity when it is given good wood treatment.

The problem is, and it has been clearly noted by many wine judges, that many Australian wine makers, in their haste to make a buck out of the trendy new drink called chardonnay, have been overdoing the wood and forgetting about the fruit flavours. I have heard Len Evans say many times, in his summation of the judging at the Sydney Wine Show, that the chardonnay classes lacked fruit and had poor wood treatment. (This means old wood, sour wood, off flavours coming from the barrels, or use of oak chips, which is quicker and cheaper.)

The chardonnays which usually win gold medals at most of the wine shows show strong fruit flavours and light but deft wood treatment. In itself oak adds extra, almost spicy "sweetness" to wines, but they should all, including reds, be redolent of fruit. The different components of wood, fruit, alcohol, acid and so on should all marry together — the wine should taste good, and the flavours should linger pleasantly in your mouth. If not, ask yourself whether you really like the wine.

Several makers of the more affordable chardonnays can demonstrate to you what I mean. Chardonnays rocketed in price when the chardonnay grapes were scarce, but now there's more around prices are generally reasonable. Some of the wines from Lindemans, Seppelt, Hardy's and Wynns (all from the southeast of South Australia, mainly Padthaway), the better Rosemount Chardonnays, Rothbury's Cowra Chardonnay, Peter Lehmann from the Barossa, and Orlando's fine value-for-money RF and Jacob's Creek Chardonnays, are good examples and fairly priced.

Chardonnay is the great white variety of the Burgundy and Chablis areas of France, and has assumed trendiness in California, where very ripe grapes and plenty of wood treatment have given rise to some very good, but very expensive, wines. They tend to the "buttery" and high alcohol end of the spectrum; you sometimes feel you are drinking them for interest rather than enjoyment. That's fine if you like that, but the Australian styles of chardonnay are lighter and fresher and, hopefully, more generous in fruit flavours.

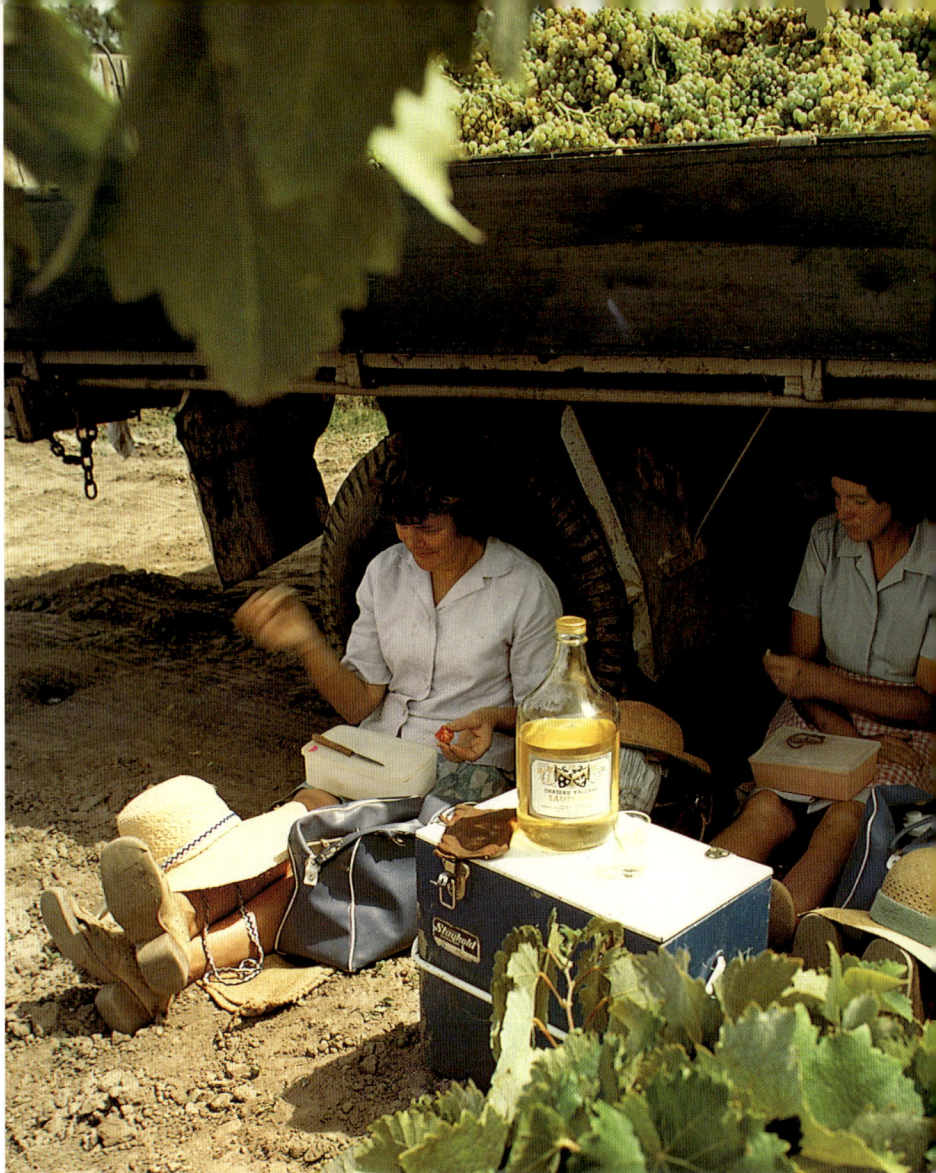

Some very good chardonnays are now being made in Australia, but you need to shop around and try various types until you settle on one or two you really enjoy.

Some should be keeping prospects, too. Avoid the temptation to drink the better (again, usually more expensive) ones now and you will see them change and improve. But there are not too many that should be kept more than three to five years. There are also some very expensive quality wines, including makers such as Petaluma, Mountadam, Mt Mary, Coldstream Hills, Woodstock, Piper's Brook and Mosswood, to pick a few, that are all good wines to cellar and worth trying if you can afford the ticket — usually between $15 and $25 a bottle.

There's no doubt that chardonnay is the quality white wine of today and the future, in Australia and elsewhere, because of the very pleasing blend of fruit and wood flavours. A lot of chardonnay vineyards have been planted in recent years by grape growers and wineries who saw prices soar for the variety as export markets soaked up fruit. That is continuing, but there is a lot of chardonnay in the ground, some of it still to bear worthwhile crops, and prices seem to have stabilised to a large extent.

Chardonnay is also one of the three major varieties the French use in Champagne (the others being the red varieties pinot noir and pinot meunier).

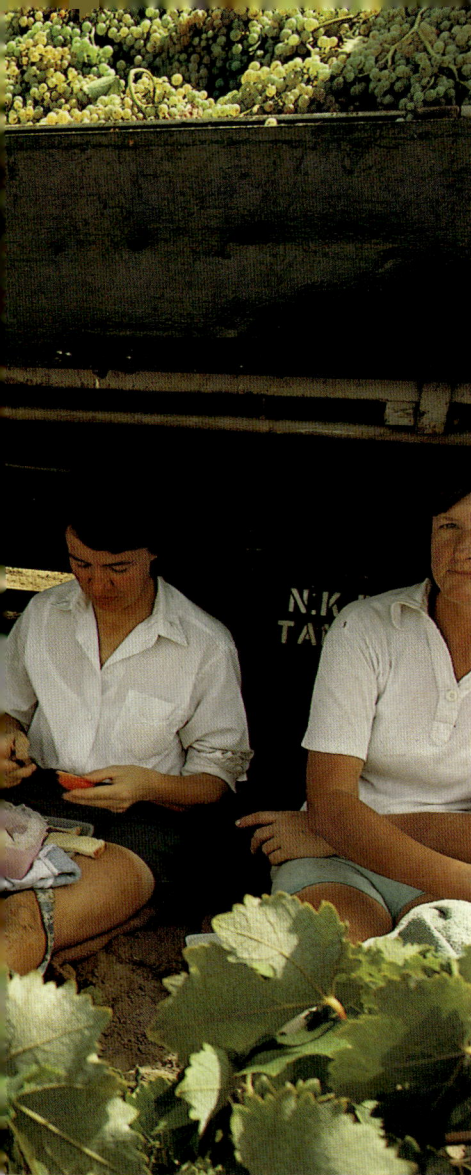

A lunch break during the vintage, and last year's finished product washes down the sustenance for the grapepickers to continue harvesting the crop for next year's wines – in this case chardonnay white grapes.

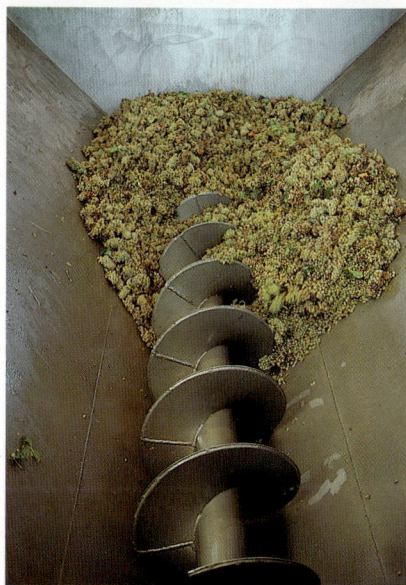

The last of a batch of white grapes go through the crusher on their way into the winery.

This practice is now increasingly being adopted by Australian sparkling wine makers to make really good bubblies, often with the chardonnay component identified on the labels (try the more upmarket wines from Seppelt/Great Western, Orlando Carrington and their Trilogy brand, Yellowglen or Tyrrells.

A personal view: chardonnay as a dry white wine is a very nice drink, when you find a good bottle. Yet it's not a 'quaffing' drink (as perhaps riesling is) and is more of a food wine, one to go with poultry dishes, lighter meats and heavier seafoods. A little tends to go a long way, especially if the wood flavours are very obvious.

SEMILLON

Semillon is another dry white variety, though it can be used to make good sweet "stickies", as it is in parts of France. It's grown in a number of areas in Australia, including South Australia and the Riverland areas, in quite large volumes. Much of that disappears into casks and other blends.

It's left to the Hunter Valley of NSW for semillon, originally described as "Hunter River Riesling", to find its best form as a dry white wine of distinction. Hunter semillons are often somewhat neutral when young, even dry and high in acid. With some bottle age they should acquire a deeper, pleasing golden hue and rich, honey-like flavours and a "toasty" smell. Most of the Hunter makers produce and sell semillons, notably Tyrrell, Tulloch, Hungerford Hill, The Rothbury Estate and especially Lindemans.

The main Hunter market is on its own doorstep, the Sydney/Newcastle areas, and even there it is not easy to sell semillon under any name. That's probably because when young the wines are not as appealing as they are when mature (say three to eight years, and even then many people don't appreciate them), and few people in these frenetic times can be bothered, or can afford, to perform the ageing ritual.

Sometimes semillon is used in a blend

with chardonnay, occasionally producing reasonable wines, but the excuse for doing it (shortage of chardonnay) tells you what the end result will usually be: drinkable but seldom remarkable.

Wood-aged semillons can be pleasing, serious drinks, but also usually need some time to knock off the rough edges.

By the way, I pronounce it as it sounds, that is SEM-ILL-ON, but others prefer the more French "SEM-EE-YON".

SAUVIGNON BLANC

If there is a "rage" grape variety to super-sede chardonnay among the trendies, sauvignon blanc has to be it (though I doubt that will happen). In the Loire Valley of France it can produce some nice wines, with flavours and smells which are often described as "herbaceous". But it is also a difficult variety to grow and, per-haps a bit like oysters or brains, you'll love it or you'll hate it.

New Zealand produces some powerful sauvignon blancs, wines with almost over-whelming smells reminiscent of "grass" or "asparagus". (Don't laugh; good sauvi-gnon blancs really smell like asparagus; if you don't believe me, buy a bottle of Kiwi-made Cloudy Bay Sauvignon Blanc; another widely available Kiwi example is Yalumba's "Nautilus" brand.)

A lot of makers have tried to make good Australian sauvignon blancs, but few have yet scaled the heights. Enjoyable, even very good, ones have been made by Seaview, Tim Knappstein, Wirra Wirra, Shootesbrooke, Lindemans/Buring, Hardy's, Geoff Merrill, Brown Brothers and a few smaller WA and Victorian wineries. For the most part, though, the results have been pleas-ant but not memorable wines.

The main problem is that only certain vintages harness the sought-after herbaceous quality; if they don't have that, the wine tends to the simple and unremarkable.

The term "Fumé Blanc" is sometimes used by makers to suggest that the wine is made from sauvignon blanc grapes. Some of it is, for example by Orlando, who have described theirs conversely as "Blanc Fumé". This is all a marketing attempt to suggest that this is a flavoursome but dry white wine, maybe with "smokey" (i.e. woody) overtones.

Sauvignon blanc can be an enjoyable and different drink, especially at the table.

TRAMINER (or GEWURTZTRAMINER)

Another aromatic variety. Traminer (sometimes called Gewurtztraminer, or literally "spicy" traminer) is also a tough one for wine makers to bring out the flavours and fruit they'd like to get. Really good traminers are delightful, as Alsace's best wines can show us. But again, Aussies seem to have had trouble either growing the right grapes or converting them into wine. An oily, often too-sweet wine tends to be the end product.
The good ones should be fruity yet dry, delicate and spicy to the nose. Orlando is probably the best handler of traminer in this country, though a few other companies occasionally do good ones from certain vintages.
When dry, the wine can be an enjoyable drink with fruit, before or after meals. It goes with dishes which may be slightly spicy or with fruit, for example prosciutto and melon.

CHENIN BLANC

A lesser white grape variety, in the sense that it is not frequently used alone. Brown Brothers, Coriole and Houghton make good examples, among others. Chenin blanc can benefit from wood treatment. In general it is better used in blends with other varieties (it often forms an important part of the blend in "white burgundies") as by itself it tends to blandness.

MARSANNE

A somewhat unusual white variety, grown in the Rhone Valley in France. In Victoria Chateau Tahbilk and Mitchelton make good, dry yet full-bodied whites from marsanne, almost alone among Australian wine makers. It is a wine that will accept bottle ageing and get quite complex and honey coloured (and flavoured!). Otherwise it is a little one-dimensional in flavour, even with the addition of wood ageing.

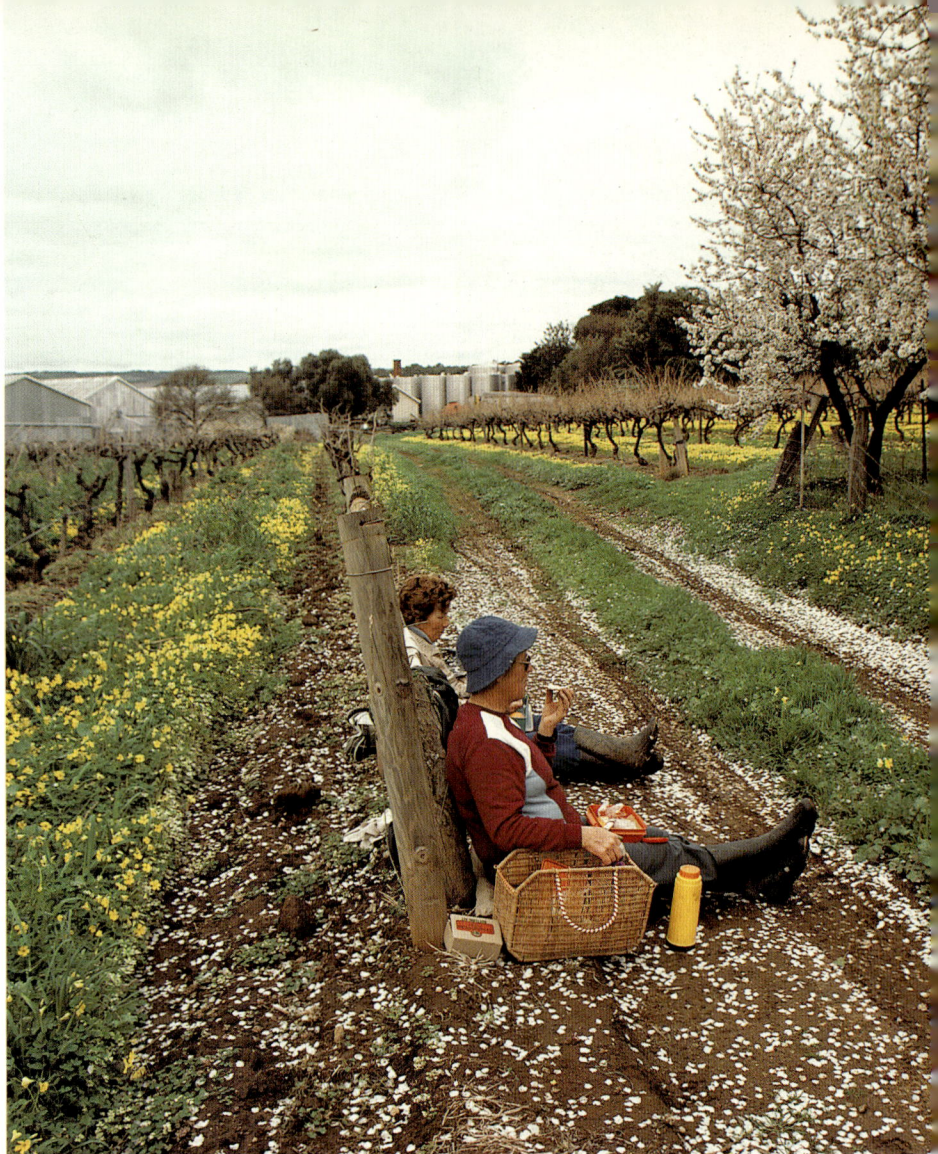

MULLER THURGAU

Another unusual white variety, widely grown in New Zealand and Germany, though not in Australia. It is quite fruity, as it was derived from a cross between the white varieties riesling and sylvaner, so it has riesling-like character.

MUSCAT

Or Muscat of Alexandria, or Muscat Gordo Blanco. A widely grown variety throughout Australia, and a generous-bearing grape vine, especially in irrigated areas. The table wines which generally come from muscat usually show a coarseness of flavour — you can detect it in most cask and many flagon wines. Not unpleasant by any means; think of the difference between eye fillet and chuck steak, if you can, to use a food comparison. You'll eat and enjoy both, perhaps in different situations. Muscat is fruity, and often makes cheaper wines that reflect sweetness, too.
There are white, red and brown muscat variants, making white wines, fortified wines and even sparkling wines, depending on what the wine-maker needs. **Frontignac** is another name for this family, and you will occasionally see Frontignac or Frontignan used on a white wine label (e.g., some very good Orlando and Brown Brothers whites). It is usually at the fruitier end of the spectrum.

SULTANA

Many of the same things said of muscat can also be applied to sultanas, the flavour of which is familiar to most of us who've eaten table grapes. It is widely grown, fairly cheap and again a key component in many casks and flagons. You won't see the word sultana, also known as Thompson's Seedless, on many bottles, as wine makers widely regard it as an anony-

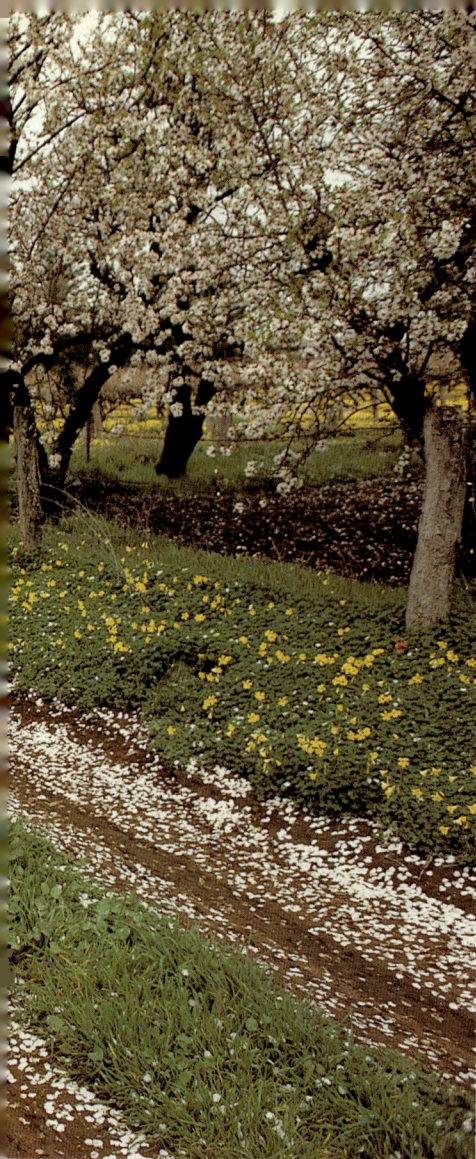

A break in pruning the vines in late winter near McLaren Vale, South Australia. The blossoms come from local almond trees.

mous, multi-purpose, cheap and readily available source of juice for making a wide range of commercial wines. Ripens early, fairly neutral in flavour and so good for bulk use and for distillation into spirit.

VERDELHO

Another unusual one, though quite a bit is planted in Western Australia, making some quite good dry white and not-so-dry white wines.

The Hunter Valley in NSW has taken to it (including Lindeman's and The Wyndham Estate) in more recent years. It's a variable grape variety, appearing in some WA wines with almost "steely" overtones. There's a lot of variation, though, from vintage to vintage and maker to maker.

It has also made some super fortified wines, such as Sandalford's Sandalera liqueur. Verdelho (or Verdelhao) calls the Portuguese Atlantic island of Madeira its home, where it is turned into fortified wines of amazing longevity. (I recently drank an 1854 Madeira, which was dry-sherry-like, though recognisable — think of it, a wine made half a dozen years before the outbreak of the American Civil War, and in the year of the Eureka Stockade rebellion at Ballarat, Victoria!)

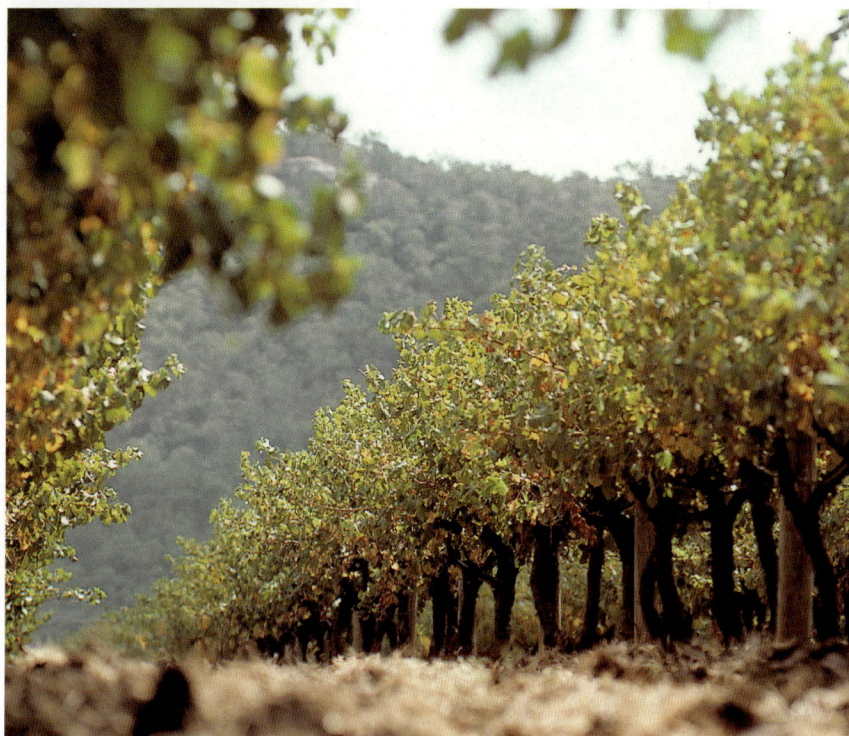

Below: *There are many varieties of white grapevines, yielding so many different wines.*

OTHERS

There are many other white grape varieties: *ondenc,* which was one of the mainstays of Seppelt's Great Western Champagne; *palomino* and *Pedro ximinez,* which made many classic Australian sherries; *muscadelle* (also known as *tokay*) which is, with *muscat* the basis for many superb Australian dessert wines; *colombard* and *crouchen* (or, incorrectly, Clare riesling), which can make some pleasant dry/medium whites.

One maker in particular, Brown Brothers of Milawa in northern Victoria, have some quite unusual varieties, such as Orange Muscat, which make pleasing white wines. Try some of them.

You don't often see a reference to many of the other white grape varieties on table wine bottles, and knowledge of them is not important to the enjoyment of quality whites.

As you can see from the above, knowledge of a handful of premium whites (riesling, chardonnay, sauvignon blanc, semillon and traminer) opens the key to the door of white wine enjoyment. Try, talk, taste, compare and be critical. That's all it takes.

There is certainly no shortage of white wines to try ... as someone once said in another context: So many whites, so little time.

RECOMMENDED READING : If you're interested in grape varieties, Brown Brothers of Milawa put out some excellent advertisements describing the properties of the wide range of white (and red) wines they make. They produce some very good literature too and you can write to them at their Milawa Winery, Victoria 3678.

RECOMMENDED DRINKING : If you haven't tried chardonnay yet, buy a bottle of Lindeman's Bin 65 Chardonnay ($5 - $7) to find out why so many drinkers are going for this dry white variety today.

SPARKLING WINES

*The use of the word 'champagne' sends the French makers
of sparkling wines, from the Champagne area north of Paris,
rushing for their lawyers. Some years ago they took court action
in Australia to try to stop the Spanish calling their sparkling
wines 'Spanish Champagne'. Fearful of a precedent being set,
makers of Australian sparkling wines (such as Seppelt Great
Western) sided with the Spanish, and the French Comité
International des Vins de Champagne lost the case. (Freixenet,
the big Spanish maker of sparkling wine, has advertised
its product with the amusing line: 'Freixenet, the
imported Champagne for every Juan'.)*

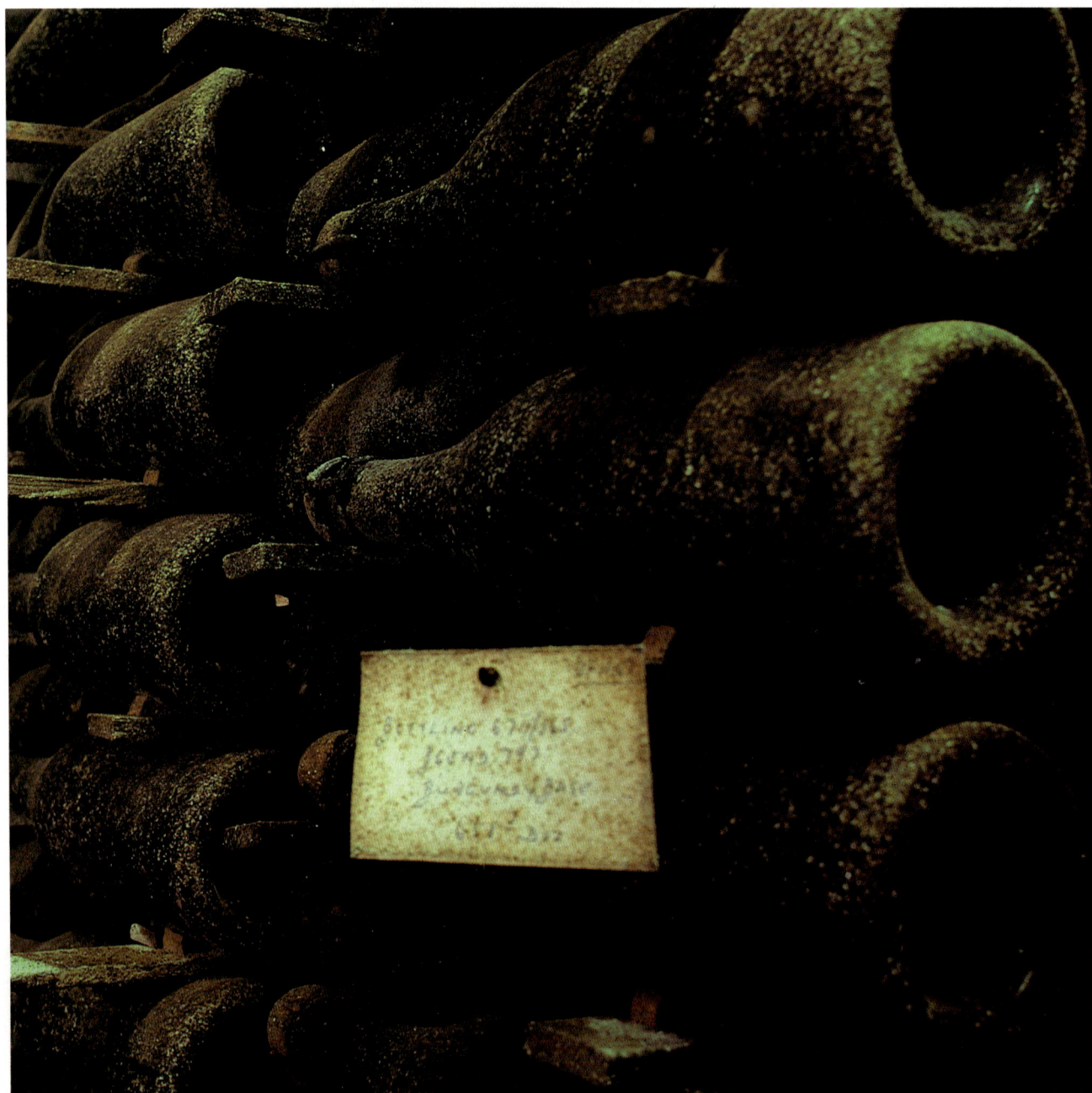

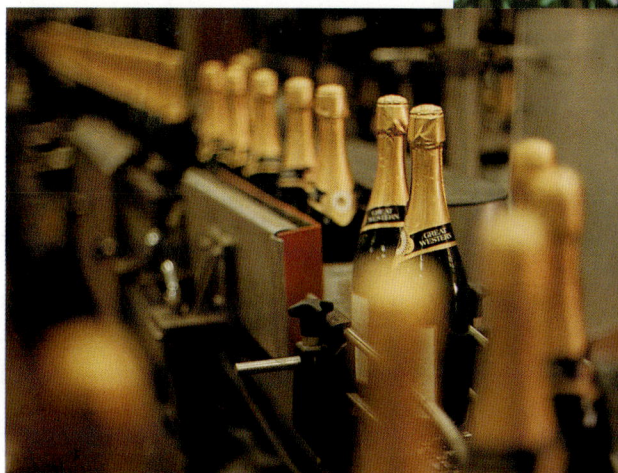

*Champagne is the great party starter, and most of it is uncorked when young, not long after the maker releases it, **right**. But some good champagnes age in the cellar and improve gracefully with age, **left**. From the cellar the wine goes down the bottling line to be dressed and packaged, **below**.*

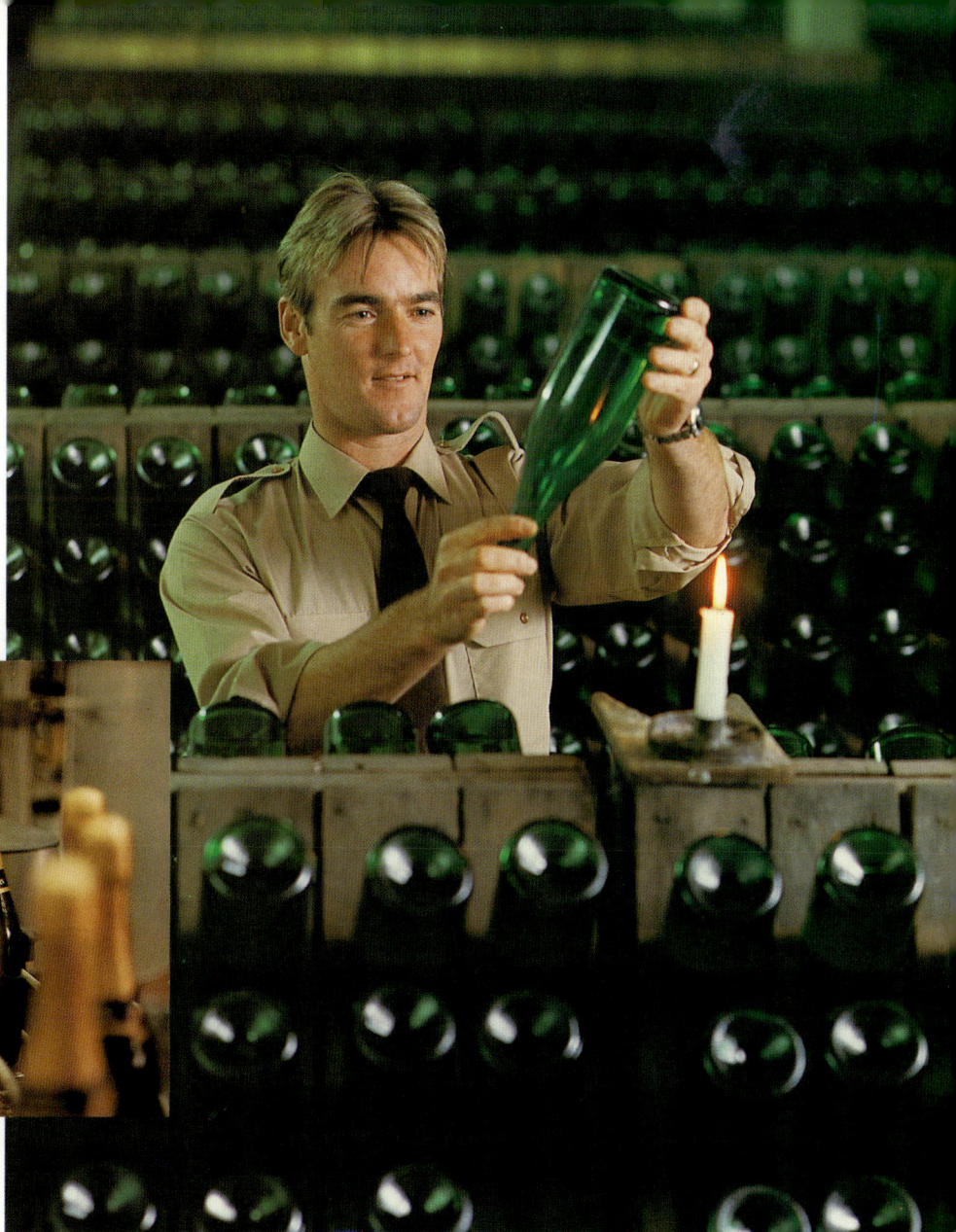

The French are rightly jealous of their name and indeed, there is really nothing quite like the real thing. Although Australian makers are getting closer to the taste, I don't think there ever will be an exact flavour clone of French champagne. That's because of the climate and soil make-up of this cool grape-growing region, 50° north of the Equator.

Good French champagne has a creamy, yeasty, full-flavoured taste to it. Then, of course, there are the bubbles, that extra dimension of taste which also heightens the visual appeal of the drink. That nice popping noise when you draw the cork is so remindful of a special occasion. I don't want to spoil any special regard you may have for champagne, but of course the bubbles and the fizzy nature of the drink and the popping of the cork are simply caused by the presence of CO_2 gas, the same stuff that makes Coca-Cola and lemonade fizzy — it just gets into the drink in a different way.

It's how the CO_2 gets there that makes the difference. You can take a white wine and simply inject carbon dioxide into it. I have never tried it, but you could probably make your own fizzy alcoholic drink by using one of those gadgets that make soda water at home; I suspect the result might be a little disappointing in flavour, but I cannot see any reason why it would not work.

French folklore has it that the Monk Dom Perignon "discovered" champagne. As I mentioned, Champagne is a northerly, cold district of France. Our monkish wine-maker must have either made or stored some white wine that had some grape sugar left in it. What obviously happened was that the oncoming winter stopped the fermentation and left some of the sugar in the wine bottle with the wine. Come the warmer months and the yeasts woke up and started gobbling away again at that grape sugar; the gas generated as a by-product of that second fermentation could not escape from the securely corked bottle, and so the gas was dissolved in the wine. Voilà! Champagne!

The curious monk must have enjoyed the sparkling wine that miraculously appeared when he opened the bottle. What went on inside that bottle demonstrates why champagne is such a special drink in the world of wine.

Rather than look at Dom P's bottle, consider what happens when modern champagne is made. The process is not

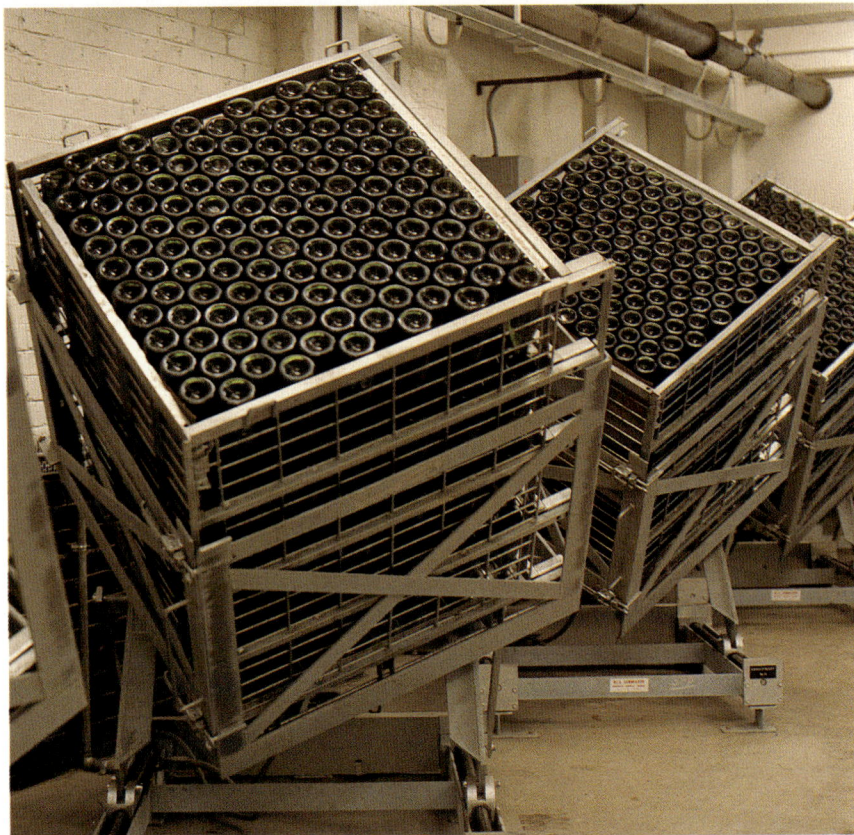

so different from that evolved by the monk three centuries or so ago. First a base white wine is made; as it happens, the white grape variety chardonnay and the red variety pinot noir (sometimes with some pinot meunier, too) provide much of the base for French champagne, which helps account for part of the special and delicious flavour. As with many conventions, these two main varieties were adopted by Champagne for a special reason: they both ripened early and therefore had a better chance of attaining adequate ripeness before the frosts of autumn and winter. Today wine-makers in Australia are turning more and more to pinot noir and chardonnay for their base wine for up-market bubblies.

The base white wine is put into bottles, and a little extra natural grape sugar and laboratory-bred yeasts are also added, and the bottle is sealed, usually by a crown seal (the type used on beer bottles).

So the "secondary" fermentation begins. (The primary fermentation, of course, was the initial conversion of grape juice to white wine.) Exactly the same thing happens: yeasts consume sugar, producing a little more alcohol, plus that vital CO_2 gas, which cannot escape through the crown seal. The yeast cells, having done their job, die. You can actually see them making a fine, cloudy mist, if you shake the bottle. (If you'd like to see for yourself, buy a bottle of Cooper's excellent Sparkling Ale; this South Australian brewer makes the ale by a very similar process, leaving the dead yeast cells in the bottle.)

The yeast cells are important to the process not just because they produce the carbon dioxide, but because they add flavour. You'll sometimes hear people talking about certain champagnes having a "Vegemite" character; after all, the great Australian spread is made from a yeast extract.

Makers of quality champagnes will leave the dead yeast cells (the "lees") in contact with the wine for quite a long time to help pick up as much of its character as possible; two or three years is not unusual.

Then comes the problem of getting the yeast cells out. They're not harmful; just unsightly. They could filter the wine, but that runs the risk of losing some flavour as the delicate drink is rammed through the filter pads under pressure. Some makers do this with the bigger-selling bubblies.

There's another way — the traditional "Méthode Champenoise" — and it's clever. It's also intriguing to watch, should you ever get the chance to see "real" champagne being made or disgorged.

The disgorgement involves taking the bottle after the secondary fermentation, when the wine has spent a suitable amount of time picking up the yeasty flavours, and placing the bottles in special "tables", actually wooden inverted "V" racks, necks stuck in holes, facing downwards. Over a period of some weeks, the champagne cellar hands turn the bottles, usually a quarter of a turn a day, using a chalk mark on the base of the bottles to ensure even turning. As they do so they increase the vertical angle of the bottles. The dead yeast cells slowly fall towards the neck, and finally gather on the base of the crown seal.

This is a natural method of filtering, and when the process is complete, the bottles are carefully removed from the racks and placed with necks still down, in wire crates. The crates are lowered into a very cold brine solution, which quickly freezes the neck and the top centimetre or two of wine, including the unwanted dead yeast cells.

The makers then use an ordinary bottle opener to remove the crown seal; the pressure of the gas inside the bottle blows the little wad of yeast cells out, together with a very small amount of the wine. A bottle from the same batch is used to top the bottle up, a cork is added (the cork's mushroom shape is acquired after being placed into the champagne bottle neck), and the cork is wired into place to ensure it stays there under pressure and movement.

The champagne can either be packaged and sold, or kept to acquire a little more bottle age before being released by the makers.

It's labour-intensive, and expensive if you do it properly, but the purists declare that the "Méthode Champenoise" is the only way to make a top-quality champagne.

There are short cuts and the French have been among those to implement

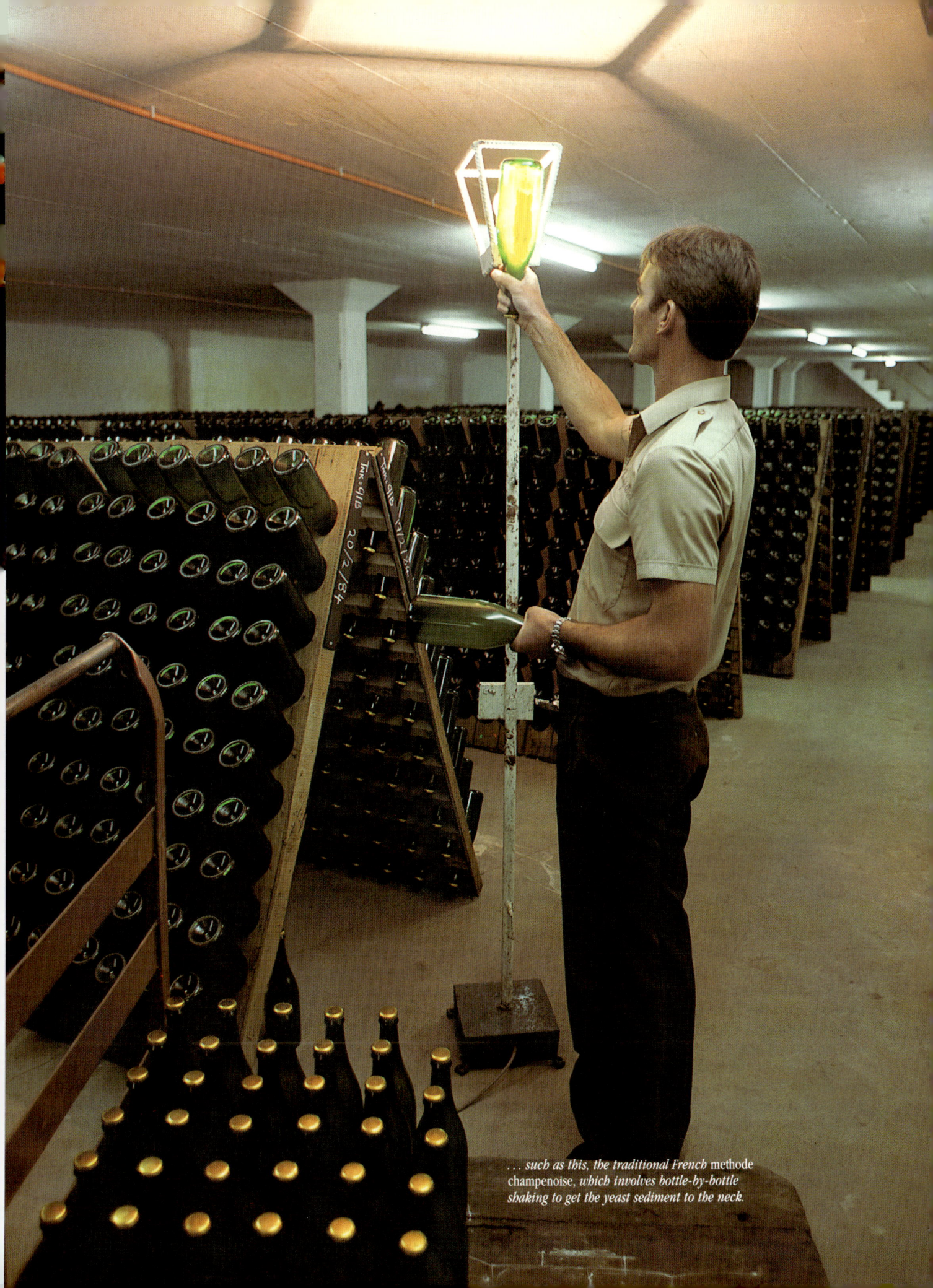

... such as this, the traditional French methode champenoise, *which involves bottle-by-bottle shaking to get the yeast sediment to the neck.*

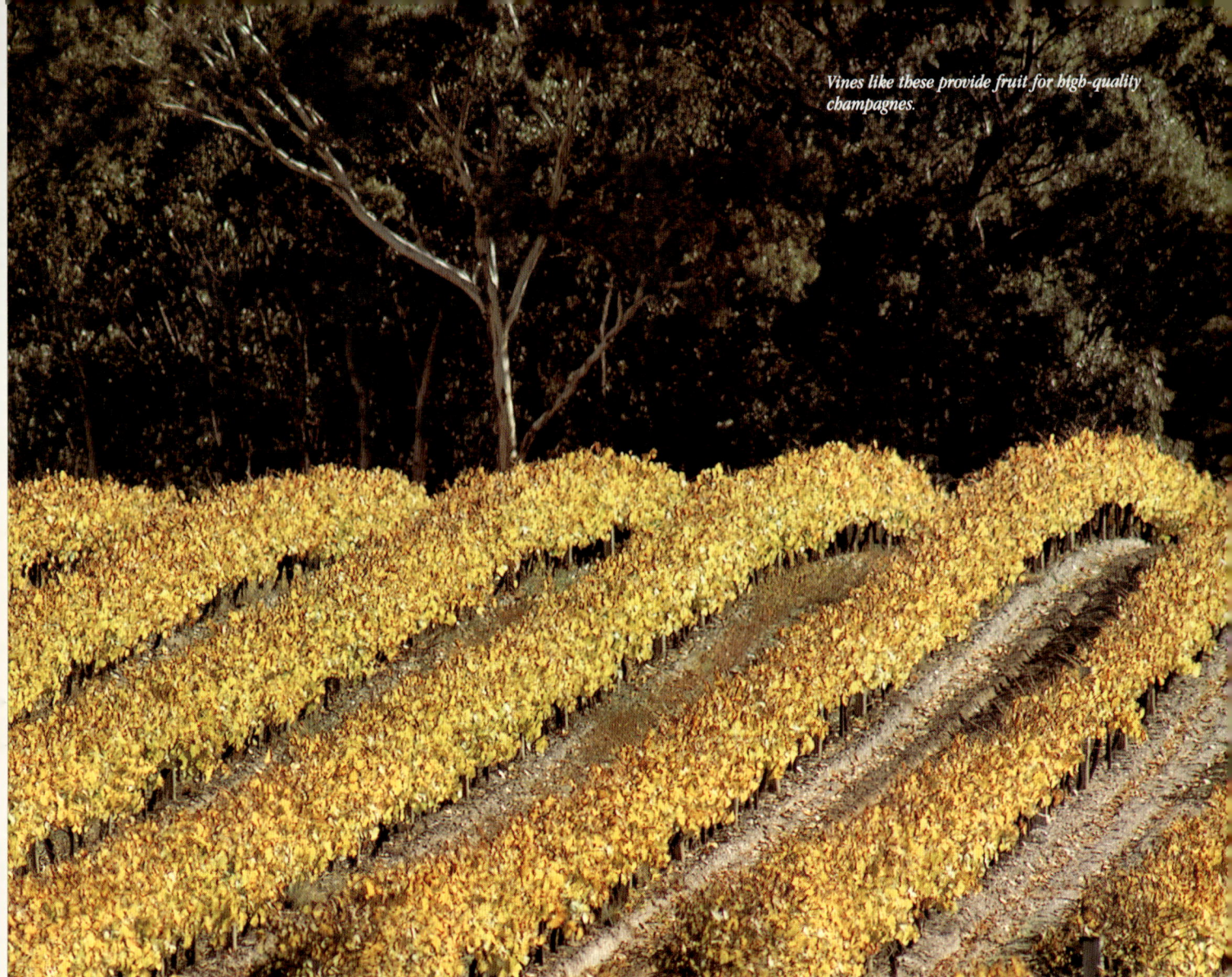

Vines like these provide fruit for high-quality champagnes.

Pink champagnes have become more popular over the past couple of years. This probably has more to do with visual appeal than taste; drinkers are always looking for something new. Thinking pink didn't seem to be cute enough, so we've been treated to names such as Blush. Some of the more expensive pink bubblies are made from the more exotic (and flavoursome) grape varieties, such as pinot noir and cabernet sauvignon. But the medium and cheaper pink sparkling wines often have some red wine added at one stage of the wine-making process.

We all call it champagne, even though some wine-makers are now doing it by implication (bottle shape, neck wrappers and so on) rather than explicitly by name. And no matter what the French do or say, ordinary drinkers will always call it champagne. It is a delightful drink and a great party starter, and at long last, Australian wine-makers are making really good mid- to up-market bubblies, even as the battle for the popular market continues in the discount liquor stores.

Several final suggestions. Alone among the wine drinks, champagne should be served fairly cold. Cheaper ones especially so. Several hours in the fridge or 20 minutes in the freezer or ice bucket will do the trick.

And a final word or two about that cork blasting out. Be careful, as it travels very fast (the pressure inside can be as high as 80 psi.), and a champagne cork is ideally designed to fit in your eye socket. The sound should not be loud and vulgar. The great, late founder of the International Wine and Food Society, André Simon, summed it up perfectly when he said: "The sound of a champagne cork emerging should be like the sigh of a well-contented woman."

The French, as always, know what they're talking about — when it comes to champagne.

RECOMMENDED READING : Seppelt produce some of the best sparkling wines from Australia. Ask for some of their literature by writing to them at Great Western, Victoria 3377.

RECOMMENDED DRINKING: Seppelt Fleur de Lys sparkling wines, or at a more budget-conscious level, Yalumba Angas Brut wines are excellent value. Top end bubblies include Croser, Killawarra Premier Vintage Brut and from NSW, the better sparkling wines of McWilliam's and Tyrrell's.

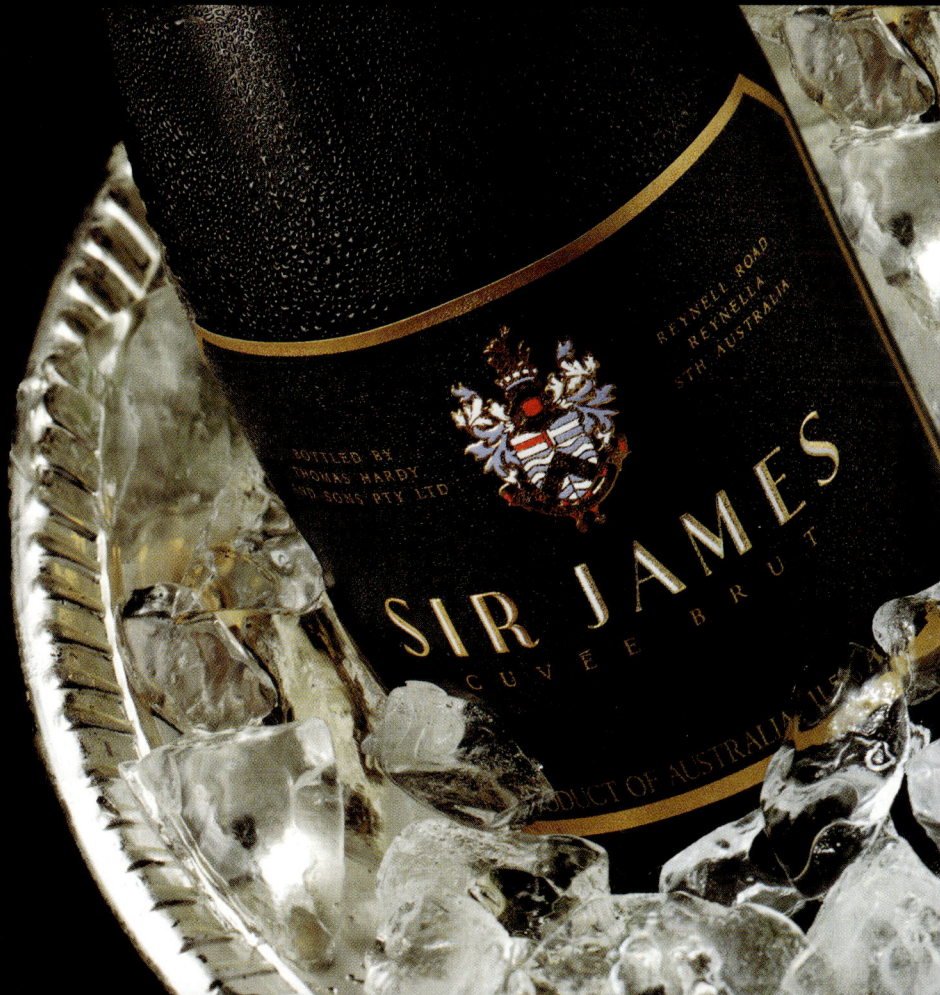

A fine champagne
in anyone's language.

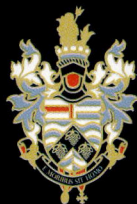

HARDYS

APB 18722-A

RED WINES

"All wines
would be red if they
could."

— SIR JAMES HARDY.

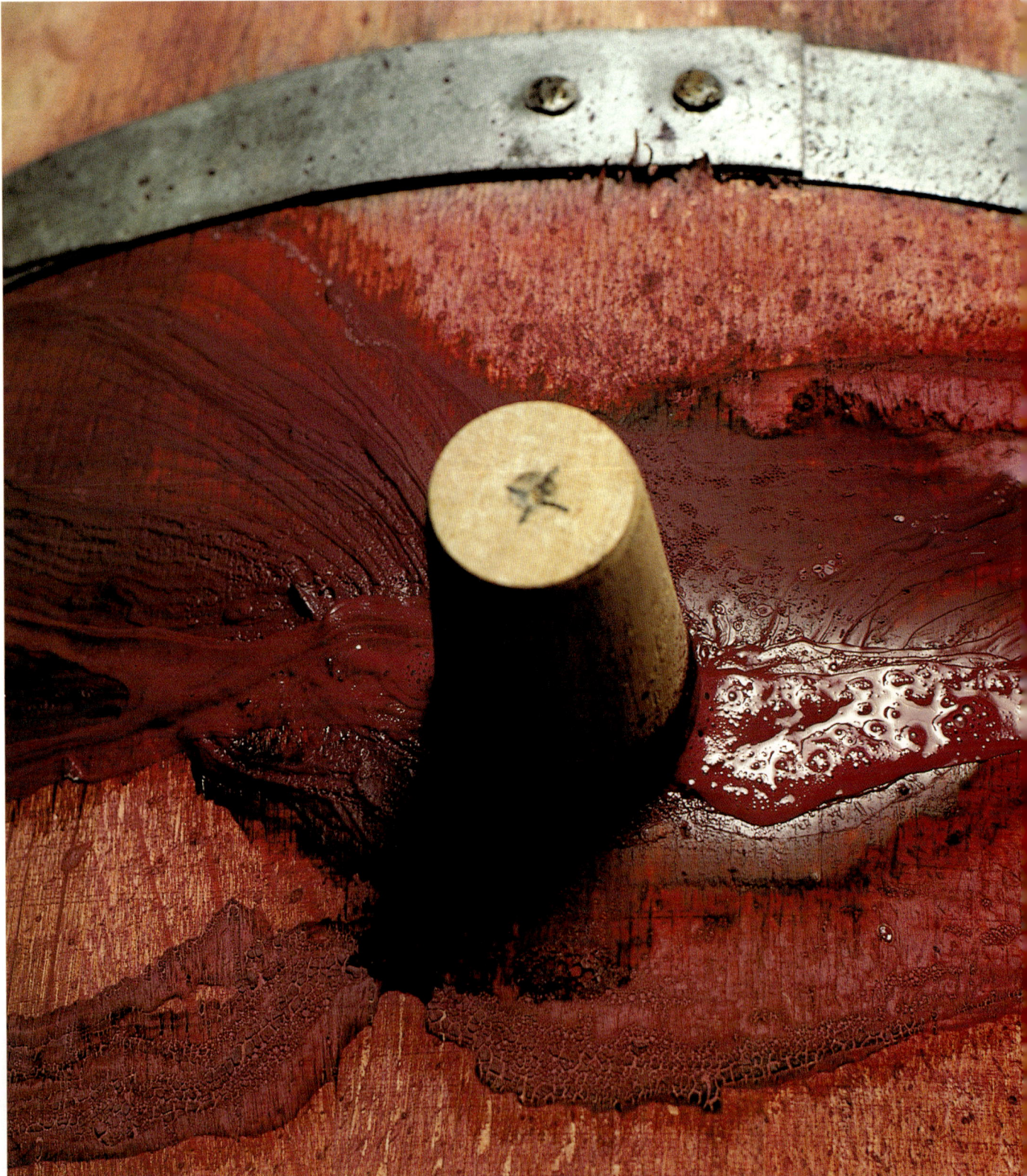

So, there are real differences between red wines and white wines, and if you want to get into a quick argument with a wine lover or wine-maker, tell them that you get worse headaches from drinking red wine than white wines!

Is this really true? I doubted it for a long time, believing instead that it was consumption of absolute alcohol that caused the problems. After all, red wines tend to come towards the end of a chain of drinks, if you have a heavy night out: perhaps a beer, maybe a glass of champagne, some white wines and over the main course and perhaps the cheese, some red wine.

For a while histamines were blamed, but that didn't seem to make sense, as many, many substances have far higher levels of histamines than red wines, and many white wines have them, too. (It's often been noted that a banana contains more histamines than a bottle of red wine.)

However, just before this was written, some overseas researchers announced the results of a "blind" trial using volunteers who drank several different but significant amounts of alcoholic beverages without knowing what they were drinking. Flavoured vodka was one of the forms of alcohol fed to them. The results indicated quite strongly that red wine did give some people headaches and migraine, while the other forms of alcohol did not.

This is not to say, of course that drinking red wine (or even small quantities of red wine) will necessarily bring on a headache. Only some people seem to be affected in this way, though some others (a small proportion) say it happens with only a very small quantity of red wines. Obviously allergies exist in wines, too, as they do with just about everything from housepaint to dust mites.

I suppose all this can be summed up by saying : there is increasing evidence to show that some people are predisposed to headaches of various types by drinking quantities of red wine, or certain types of red wine, in quantities

ranging from a mouthful to several bottles.

Big, gutsy reds (by definition, wines which have higher levels of extractive grape solids and oak extracts) seem to do more damage than lighter reds, which are more fashionable now anyway, such as pinot noir and many cabernets.

So much for the health warning! I am more attracted to the remark made to me by Sir James Hardy: "All wines would be red if they could!" By that he is saying that there is much more satisfaction in red wines ... more complex flavours, more to savour and enjoy. Once again, a little understanding of the wine-making techniques and some knowledge of grape varieties (though fewer than with whites) helps you enormously in approaching the task of selecting wines you will enjoy, now or later.

Essentially reds are made the same way as whites. That is, you pick ripe grapes, crush and extract the juice and then start a fermentation so the grape juice turns into wine. Technology has again played a part and many red wine fermentations these days are done in stainless steel containers with the air excluded as far as possible.

But several other factors come into play with reds. You need to get that red colour, so the skins may be more heavily pressed and returned to the juice or fermenting wine, which "picks up" the colour and the extra tannins from skins, seeds and perhaps some stalks. Some wine-makers (Tyrrell's in the Hunter Valley, for example) still believe in the old method of using open, concrete fermenters and "plunging" the cap of skins and seeds (which float to the surface of the fermenting juice) by hand to increase colour and tannin acquisition. Watching this done as the purple juice bubbles away (remember the CO_2?) is quite impressive! There is an argument that doing this in open fermenters allows too much air to get to the wine — a typically traditionalist vs. modernist approach, but certainly some very good

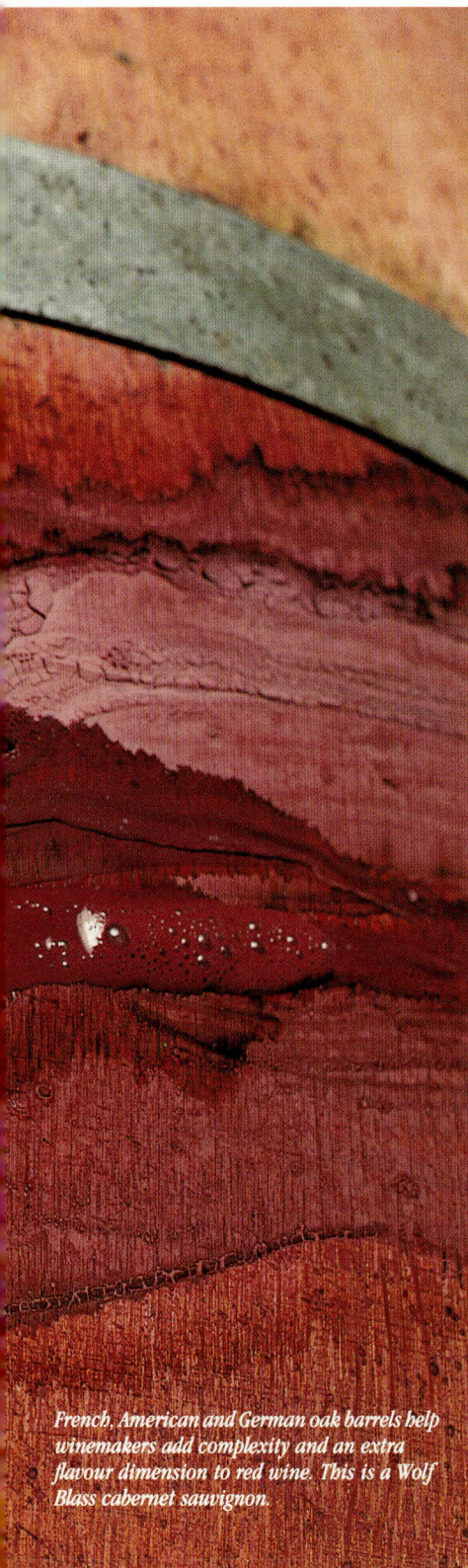

French, American and German oak barrels help winemakers add complexity and an extra flavour dimension to red wine. This is a Wolf Blass cabernet sauvignon.

wines have been made this way over a very long period, both in Australia and elsewhere.

Murray Tyrrell's publicly stated wine-making philosophy is interesting in this context: "Great fruit, commonsense and observant wine-making are the most important ingredients in the production of great wines — there are no substitutes."

Then there is the wood treatment. Many centuries of European wine-making have shown that the right type of red grapes, properly vinified (turned into wine), will appeal more to the palate if lain in barrels made from the wood of certain trees, usually oak from Europe and America. Sometimes these oak flavours add quite startling extra dimensions of flavour — flavour that resembles sweetness. When poorly handled, old or "diseased" wood barrels are used, the wood can impart a bitterness to the wine which can be unpleasant. Wood maturation that avoids this is part of the skill of wine-making.

These days we are enjoying lighter, fresher and more 'elegant' reds. By this I mean they are wines which, compared to their counterparts of the 50s, 60s and even the 70s, have more dominant fruit flavours, less tannins and less wood, as a rule, and are also more in 'balance'. Changing marketplace demands have forced wine-makers to make such wines, and the new technologies have given them the tools to do it. They are, in a few

---

TOP SELLING BOTTLED RED WINES

1. **Orlando Jacob's Creek Claret**
2. Seaview Cabernet Sauvignon
3. **Penfolds Koonunga Hill**
4. **Tyrrell's Long Flat Red**
5. **Matthew Lang Australian Beaujolais**
6. Seaview Cabernet Sauvignon/Shiraz
7. Matthew Lang Cabernet Sauvignon/Shiraz
8. Wolf Blass Yellow Label
9. **Woodley Queen Adelaide Claret**
10. Mildara Jamieson's Run

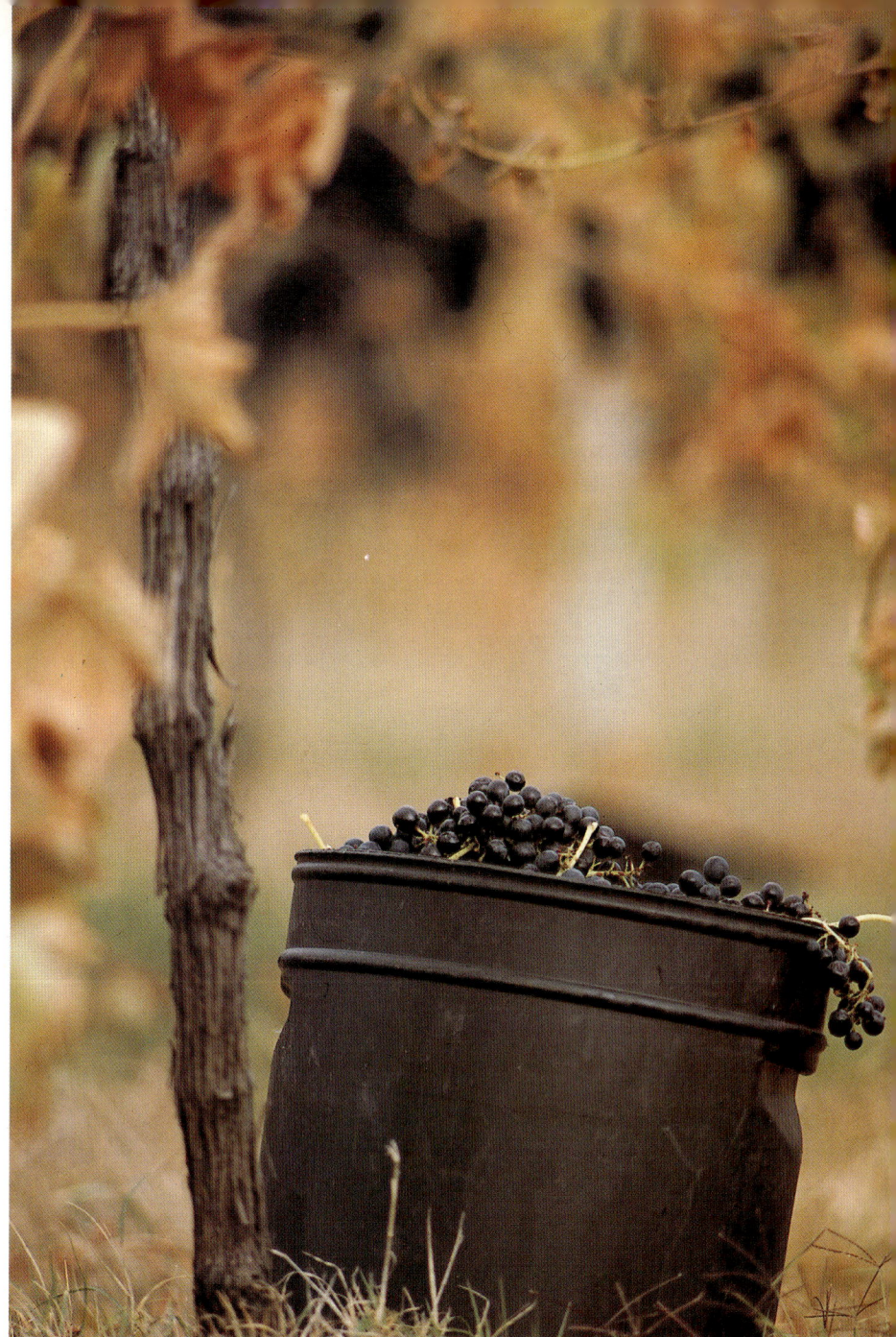

---

words, easier to drink, and sales certainly show that these premium (bottled) reds are increasingly popular in the marketplace.

Stainless steel tanks and temperature control equipment are how wine-makers can offer us these wines, and at reasonable prices. Lindemans, with their Rouge Homme division, were among the leaders in developing these wines in the 1970s, and others either went down the same track or followed soon afterwards. If you want to taste what I mean, try many of the red wines of Penfolds, Seaview, Orlando, Mildara, Krondorf and Wolf Blass, among others.

Price, as always, plays an important part in drinker preferences, and the $5-$10 area is now replete with well-made Australian reds, all from big makers with a dominance of the SA Brewing Holdings' companies (Penfolds, Lindeman's, Seaview, Matthew Lang, Tollana, Kaiser Stuhl, Woodley, Leo Buring and Rouge Homme). Here is my "best-bet" guesstimate of the top-selling reds in late 1992, again with the generic and semi-generic wines in bold.

Another change was the recognition by wine-makers that blending varieties, as the Bordelais have for centuries in France, adds interest by adding complexity. Blass did it with the conventional varieties (shiraz and cabernet sauvignon, for the most part) but

Good wines begin their journey to your lips in the vineyard. Hand picking gets more fruit, in better condition – but at greater cost than mechanical harvesting.

more particularly by blending these varieties from different areas. He (and his wine-makers) have been very clever at this skilful blending and, notably, at their use of wood.

Others, such as Tyrrells, pioneered "new" varieties, such as pinot noir; while at Krondorf, Burge and Wilson blended the varieties cabernet sauvignon and cabernet franc to get wines of very pleasing taste. At Chateau Reynella, Geoff Merrill used yet another technique: he selected three varieties (cabernet sauvignon, malbec and merlot) for one of his best red wines, but blended them at the crusher, as fruit, instead of as juice or finished wine. And so on.

The sweet flavours of well-handled red grapes, good technology, good winemaking and then good wood maturation are today giving us some wonderful red wines.

Again, from all this you can see that it comes back to varieties, and the list you need to remember is again not a long one.

CABERNET SAUVIGNON

Cabernet sauvignon, or just 'cabernet', or to some just plain old 'cab', is unquestionably the most liked and admired of Australian, and probably world, grape varieties used in red winemaking. Many South Australians, by the way, pronounce the variety as "CARBERN-AY" which I think is a historical hangover (so to speak) of a 19th century misspelling of the variety.

From its home in France it has viticulturally marched forth to conquer red wine drinkers in the United Kingdom, where they named it (or at least the cabernets and cabernet blends of Bordeaux) as "claret". Cabernet does have universal appeal, and an almost universal similarity of flavour. This doesn't mean that you can taste one from California and say it tastes exactly like an Australian cabernet. But you almost certainly — if the wine is well made, the usual qualification! — will be able to identify it as being from the cabernet family.

It should have that intense, berry-like flavour, often reminiscent of blackberry or similar fruit, sometimes minty, rich and sometimes tannic. The cabernet grape berries themselves are what you would possibly expect them to look like: small, round and very dark black to purple in colour.

These Australian cabernets tend to be, like their Bordeaux cousins, long-lived wines, especially those from cooler-growing districts. The best come from the Coonawarra area in the southeast of South Australia, but splendid cabernets have come from the Barossa Valley, Clare, parts of Victoria, McLaren Vale and occasionally (though not often) from the Hunter Valley (the Hunter seems so much better suited to shiraz).

Among the better makers of cabernet in Australia are Lindeman's and especially their brand of Rouge Homme; Wynn's (and occasionally their sister company Penfolds, notably their Bin 707); Brown Brothers; Cape Mentelle; Chateau Reynella; Chateau Tahbilk, Leconfield; Geoff Merrill; Petaluma; Ian Hollick; Woodstock; Stanley; Seppelt; Orlando and Wolf Blass. There are certainly many others making good, and occasionally great, cabernets, but most of them tend to do it erratically rather than consistently — and consistency is the mark of a great wine-maker.

Mechanically harvested shiraz fruit goes into bins for carriage to the winery and its crusher.

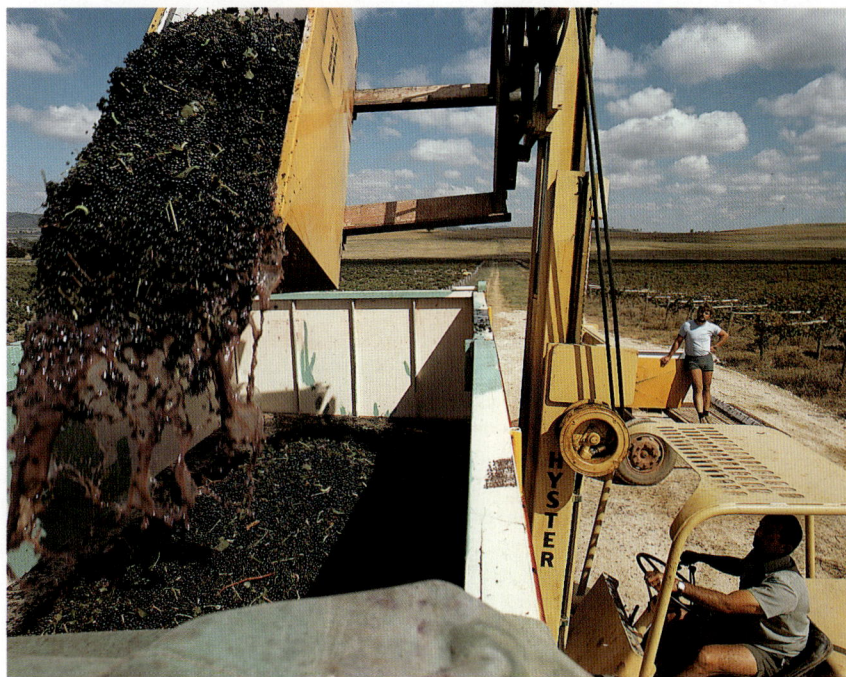

If cabernet has a fault as a variety, it is the very thing which makes it great; the very intensity and often the purity of flavour can get monotonous. To put it in this way sounds somewhat gross, though it is not meant to be: it is almost as if too much of a good thing tires. It is a sipping drink rather than a quaffing drink.

That's perhaps why many makers blend it with something else from the red stable — not to mention cost, as good cabernet sauvignon fruit is becoming expensive, with Australian and overseas drinkers latching onto its quality and relative value.

SHIRAZ

The red variety shiraz has long been the workhorse of the quality end of the red wine market. It grows vigorously, usually bears generously, and at its best produces outstanding red wines of world class, such as Penfold's famous Grange Hermitage.

The good, full-bodied shiraz reds often have a peppery, intense taste to them, generous flavour and plenty of body and colour.

Hermitage, the other name for shiraz, comes from the Rhone area of France, where it also produces wines of great distinction.

Shiraz can make wines right across the quality/price spectrum. Usually sourced from the irrigated areas, it supplies quite a lot of the cask and flagon

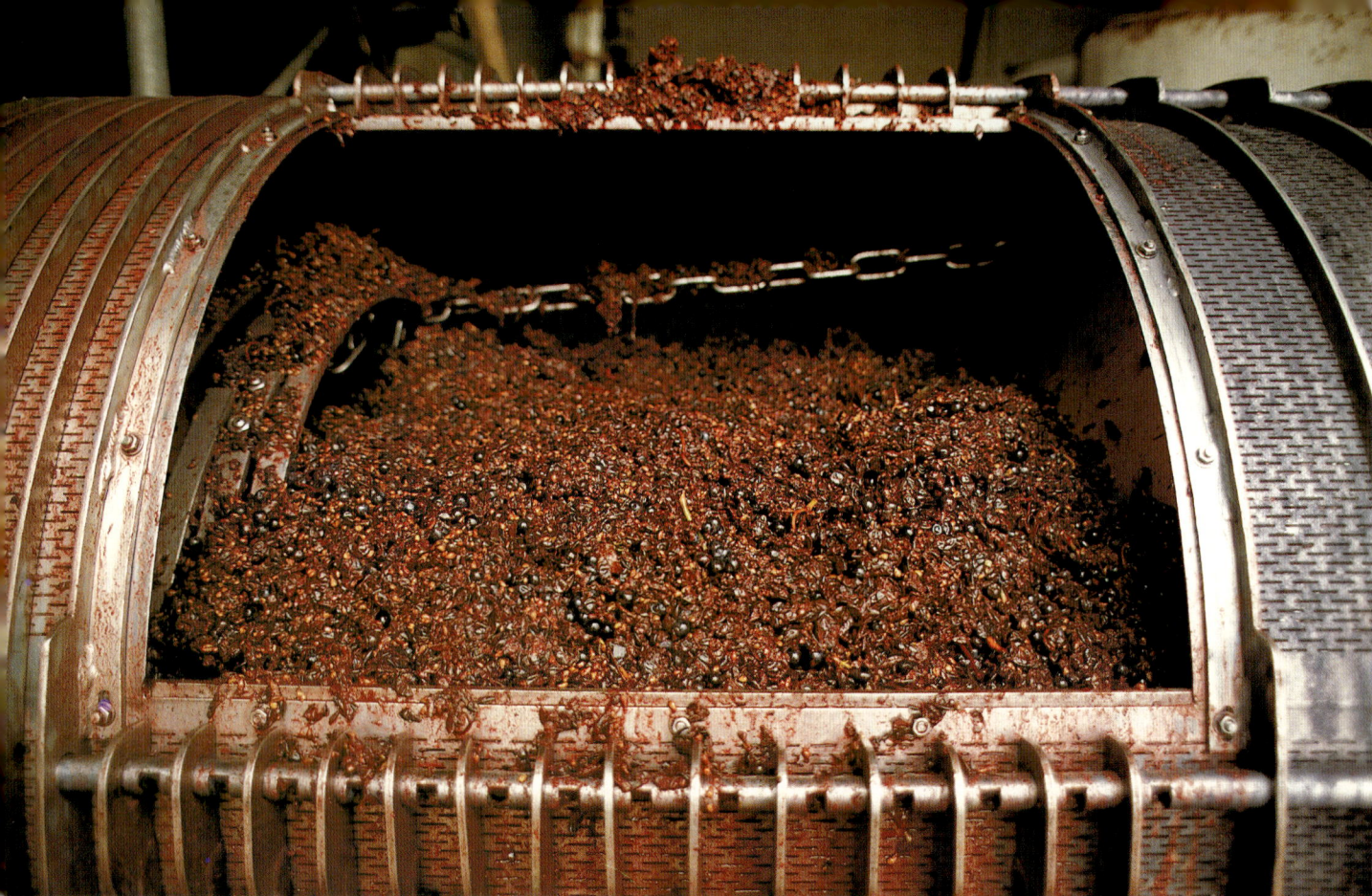

Red fruit is pressed to extract maximum juice in this mechanical press.

reds we drink. Depending on how it is treated, it can make light and fresh reds all the way through to wines of heroic proportions which can last for decades.

Its styles and flavours vary quite a lot more than do those of Australian cabernets and indeed it can sometimes be quite difficult to differentiate from a cabernet. Victorian shiraz wines seem to have a 'mintyness' about many of them which adds to this confusion. As I write, a resurgence of shiraz popularity seems to be happening. This is undoubtedly a good thing, as some supremely good (and often grossly underpriced) reds have been made from shiraz over the years.

In the Hunter Valley of New South Wales, shiraz (often called hermitage) is the red on which most of the locals hang their claim to red prowess. Here as with a few other districts, a certain "earthiness" often creeps into bottles of shiraz. "Sweaty saddle" is a term used from time to time, which amuses visitors, but seems to summon up the right imagery for those wines so blessed. Frankly, I don't like earthy flavours in wines, though some people do.

It is difficult to summarise about shiraz. It can be all things to all people, from light, fresh, unwooded reds (sometimes sold as Soft Red and designed to be slightly chilled) through the F.A.Q. (Fair Average Quaffing) range to better wines (say as a part of the blend of our biggest selling bottled red, Orlando's Jacob's Creek Claret), and so on. It also provides the likes of Wolf Blass and Penfold's with sturdy and reliable components for the big-selling wines they market as Yellow Label and Bin l28 respectively. Shiraz also provides Penfold with Grange Hermitage and Hardy with their best red, the Eileen Hardy Dry Red.

Shiraz makes reds of powerful flavours, combines neatly with most oak types, has plenty of colour to contribute, and can gracefully age in the bottle for many years if it gets the right treatment.

A generalisation, certainly, but shiraz is usually at its best when blended with another variety — unless very high quality fruit is used. Most makers of shiraz seem to have grasped this thought.

Shiraz is a red wine grape for all seasons, whose best vintages in Australia may well be yet to come.

PINOT NOIR

If a varietal wine can be seen to be streaking towards the top-of-the-trendy-pops in Australia, it has to be pinot noir. However, because it is a red grape variety and because it is a difficult and intransigent grape to grow and to vinify, its rush to trendiness has been slower than, say, chardonnay or sauvignon blanc.

Pinot noir is the classic variety of the French district of Burgundy which, if you'll allow me another sweeping generalisation, makes some of the best and the worst red wines in all of France!

Here in Australia there has been a search for the pinot noir Holy Grail, with very mixed results: more poor than great wines have been produced. Some of the big companies (Lindeman's, Hardy's, Orlando) have produced nice to very good wines; others have not been so good. A few small companies (Mountadam, Yarra Yering, Coldstream

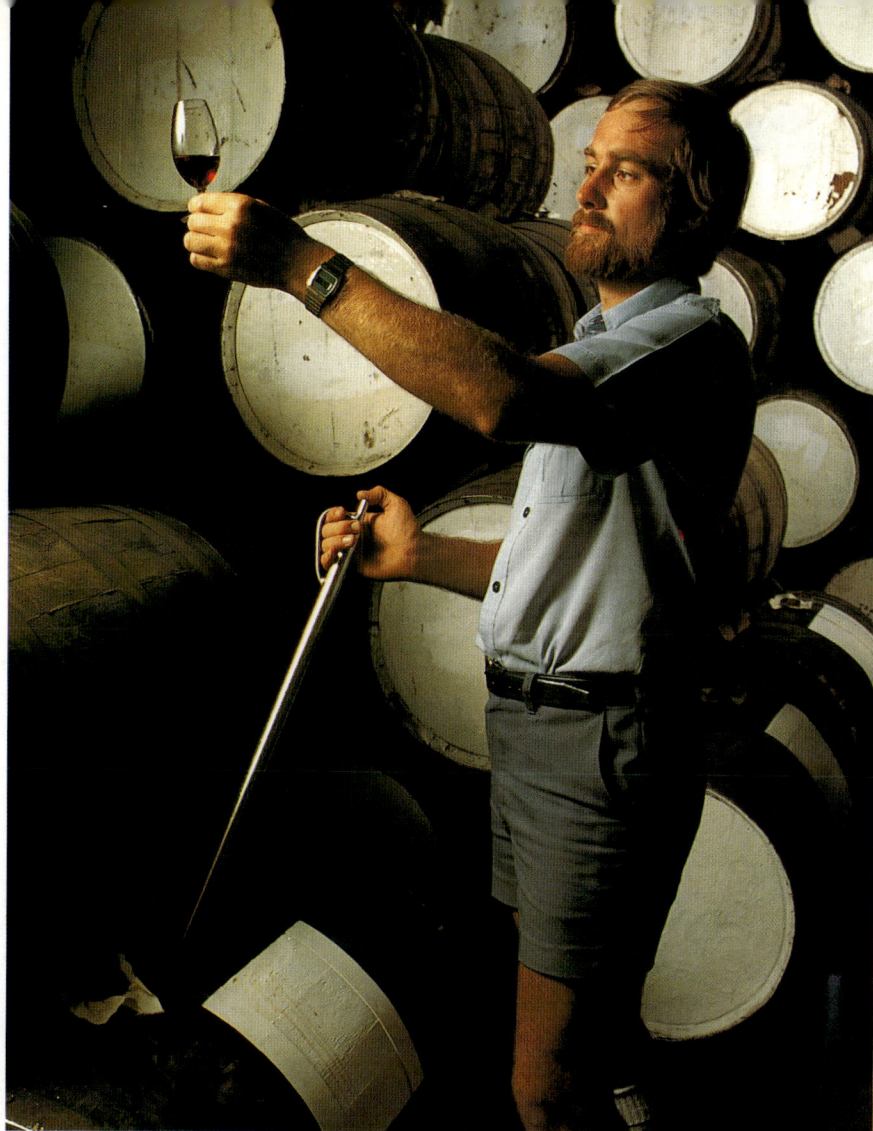

Wood and time are the factors that act on wine to change its quality. Winemakers, such as Don Buchanan, must monitor their wards to observe, protect and decide when to bottle them.

OTHERS

There are a number of other red grape varieties, all of which are grown to some extent or another overseas. For example, barbera and nebbiolo are quite common in Italy but are little seen here. (Montrose grows them in Mudgee, as it was once owned by an Italian consortium.) Zinfandel is to California what shiraz is to Australia, but not much is grown here at all and varieties which were once widely grown for reds, such as mataro, grenache and durif, have fallen from grace as the "aristocratic" varieties, such as cabernet and pinot noir, have become better understood.

There are others to add to the list, but those mentioned above provide enough to give you a working knowledge of the language of red wine.

Obviously there will continue to be plenty of experimentation with red grape varieties, and especially with blends, as wine-makers seek out that extra benefit of 'complexity' in reds. But a simple and economic example stands out : Orlando's supremely successful Jacob's Creek Claret, which is a blend of shiraz, cabernet sauvignon and malbec. If you want a wine to launch yourself into the delights of red wine drinking, try this first.

Red wine is an endlessly interesting subject, with so many variables. That's why wine buffs talk about it so much, compare notes, save and cellar various wines to see what happens to them over a period of years — and generally get a great deal of satisfaction from consuming good reds with food.

RECOMMENDED READING: *Vines, Grapes and Wine* by Jancis Robinson, RD Press. All you ever wanted to know about the hundreds of red and white grape varieties by a world authority on grapes and wine.

RECOMMENDED DRINKING: If you've tried Jacob's Creek Claret, the next step up the ladder is a value-for-money varietal red wine from the same maker — Orlando's RF (for Rowland Flat, their Barossa Valley winery) Cabernet Sauvignon.

Hills, among others) have produced good and once-in-a-while brilliant wines. But much remains to be done and the pursuit of a really good and reliable pinot continues.

Such a wine should be comparatively light in style, though with that pronounced "berry" flavour that hits the tongue straight away, and remains on the palate. The wood treatment should be gentle and not too obtrusive.

At its best (and they are getting better, though I believe there's a long way to go), a lovely drink with poultry, lighter meats, stronger fish and some milder types of cheese. Don't confuse pinot noir, which is a true red wine, with rosé wines; rosé will not have wood treatment, will be lighter and fresher.

MALBEC AND MERLOT

These two red grapes are seldom seen by themselves, because they tend to be uninteresting. ("One dimensional" is a term which may not mean much, but expresses the general feeling about their flavour structure.) They are increasingly seen in blends, sometimes containing as many as four red varieties. Lindeman's Jimmy Watson Trophy-winning Pyrus (a vineyard at Coonawarra) wine of a few years ago was such a blend, containing proportions of cabernet sauvignon, cabernet franc (a cabernet relative, emanating from Bordeaux in France), malbec and merlot. The result, properly grown, made and blended, can be fascinating and produce complex flavours.

These varieties, including cabernet franc (which I happen to like very much in blends with cabernet sauvignon), add extra dimensions of flavour and complexity, and we'll see a lot more such quality red wines as the varieties become increasingly available from Australia's spreading vineyards.

FORTIFIED WINES

Be careful — they give you more bang for your buck!

FORTIFIED wines are just how they sound — stronger! Therein, of course, lies a warning for the unwary. And probably because they do contain considerably more alcohol than 'ordinary' table wines, people are tending to shy away from them today.

First let's define a fortified wine, and it's a simple definition. A fortified wine has extra alcohol added during, or after, the partial or complete fermentation of the natural grape sugars in the wine.

Fortified wines are usually rich and generous in their flavours, sometimes luscious and, at their best, very complex. You drink them to work up an appetite, for tasting pleasure, for good conversation or company after dinner, to go with chocolates or because there's a fire going — or maybe because you're in the Officers' Mess. (You pass the bottle of port anti-clockwise, by the way!) They are wines to be taken seriously.

These are not wines to be consumed because you're thirsty!

The key fortified wines include these styles:

Ports of various types — the two main ones being Vintage Port and Tawny Port.

Sherries, including dry, medium, sweet and cream sherries, plus some specialised sherries such as Flor Fino, Amontillado and Olorosos. Usually made from a white wine base.

Vermouths, sweet through to dry. Mixer or on-the-rocks aperitif drink.

Muscats. Old and rich, usually.

Tokays. A bit lighter than muscat, but ditto.

Speciality fortifieds — such as madeira, sauvignon blanc and some others.

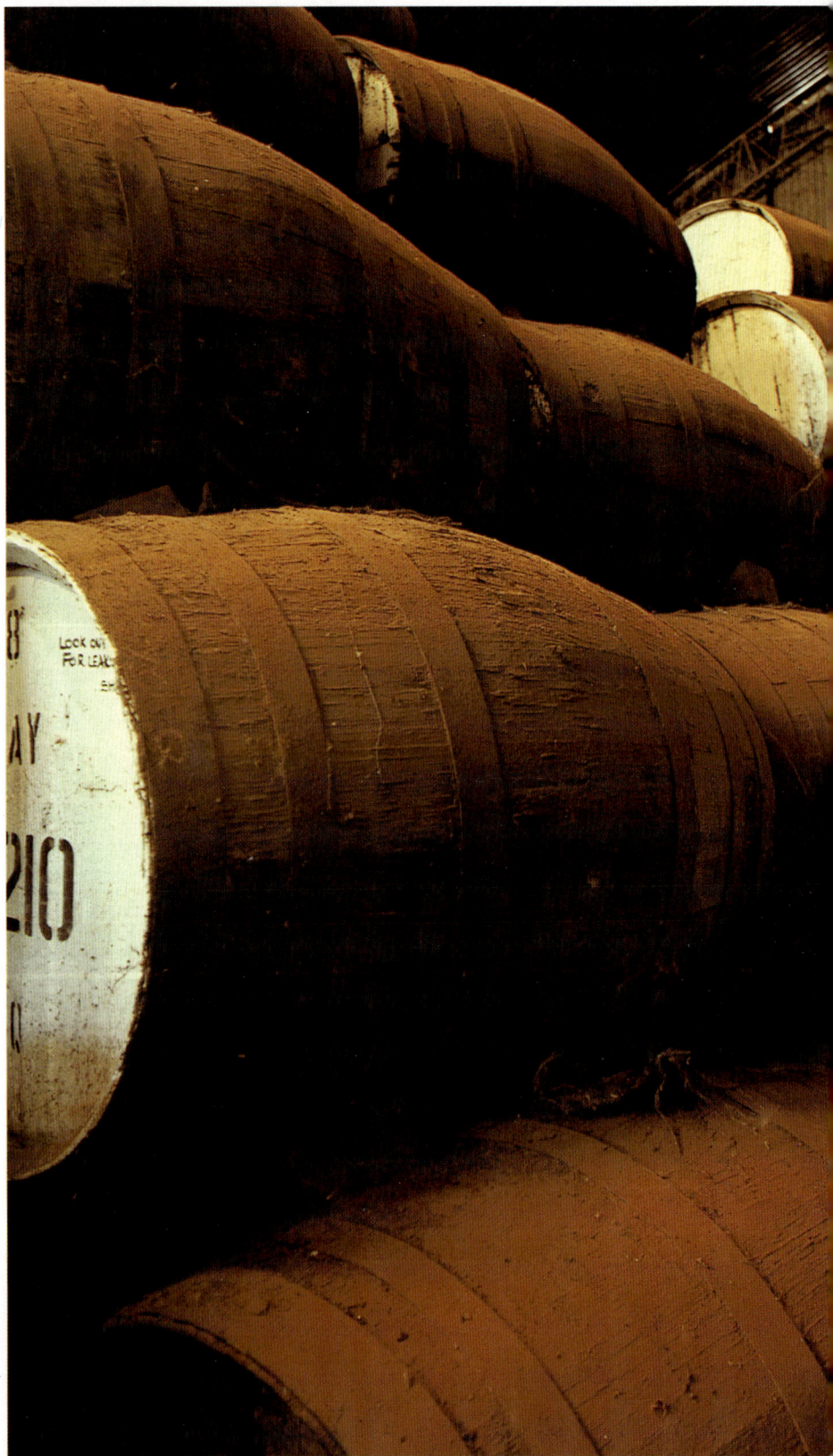

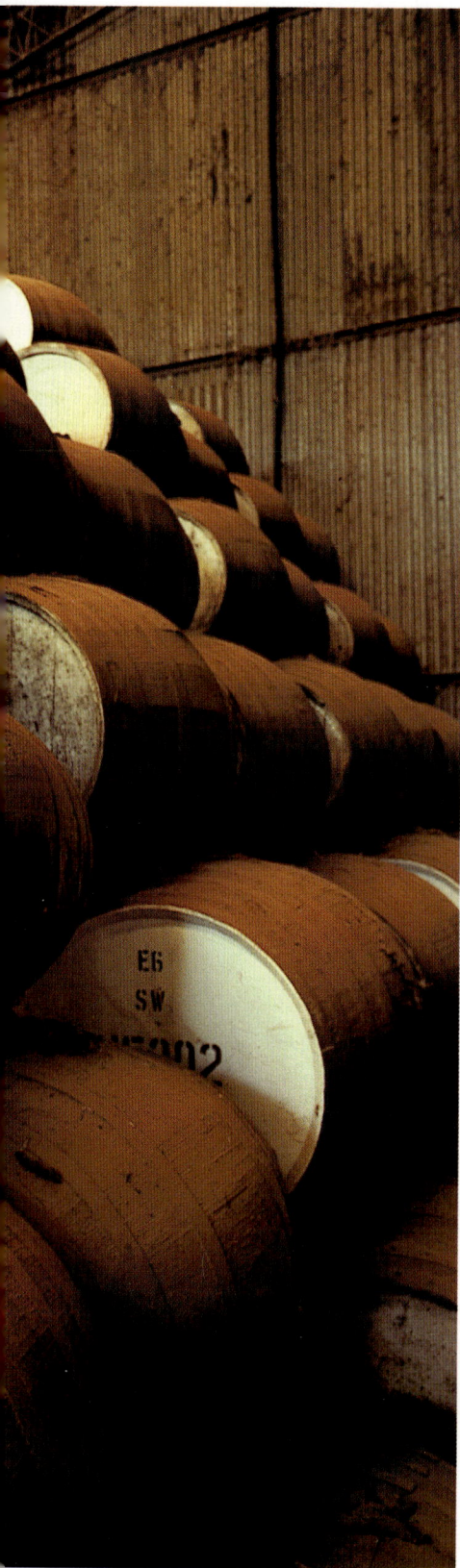

The way it used to be, **right:** *McWilliam's have long been and continue to be the biggest sellers of fortified wines, such as their famous Cream (sweet) Sherry.* **Below:** *Fortified tokay gathers age and lusciousness in wood barrels in the winery.*

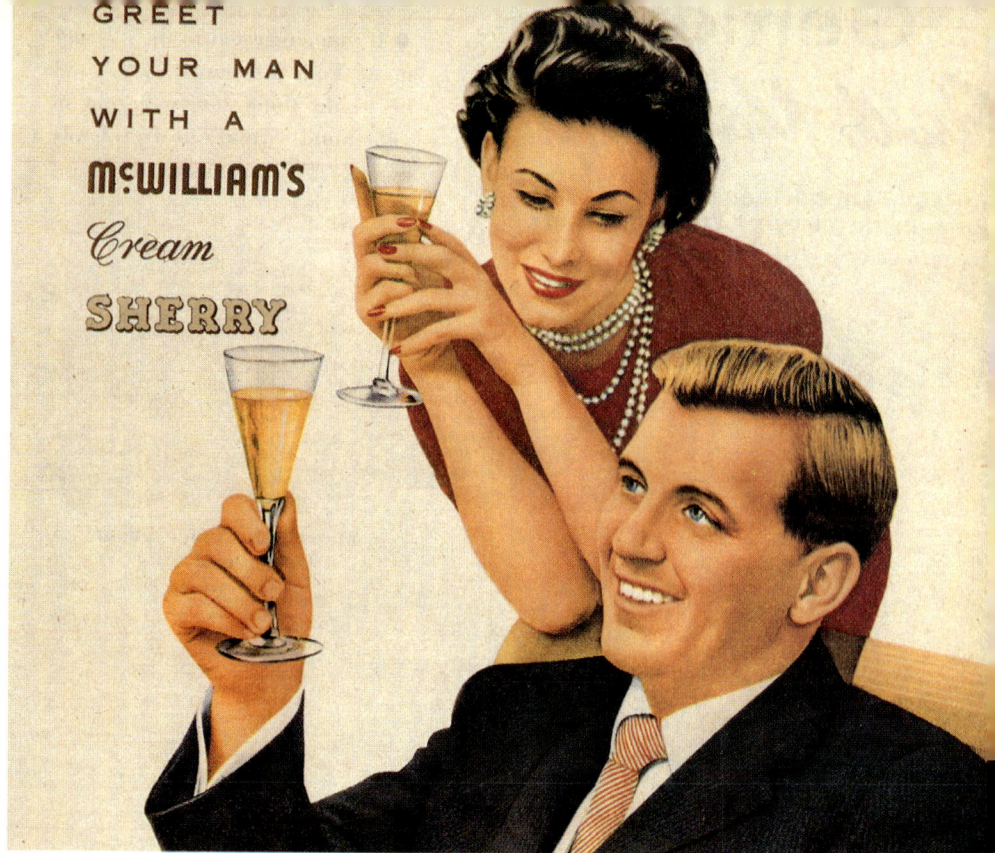

GREET YOUR MAN WITH A McWILLIAM'S Cream SHERRY

Our wine industry grew up on, even began with, the production and consumption of fortified wines. There were several reasons for this, among them that a fortified wine will usually remain in better condition than table wines (because of the preservative presence of extra alcohol) and, in times when bacterial spoilage was not fully understood, and technology not available to help, the production, transport and sale of fortified wines was a safer proposition.

And if you were looking to a market with a sweeter tooth, not to mention one whose palates may have been educated in England on the pleasures of the wines of Oporto (Ports), then fortification was one simple way of retaining sugar in the drink. Remember that without temperature control of the fermentation it's difficult to stop it to leave some natural grape sugar in the finished wine. But if you dump a large dollop of brandy spirit into a partly fermented vat of red (or white) wine, the remaining sugar is stabilised and the fermentation is stopped. That's why many ports are quite sweet — and why dry sherries are really dry, because the additional alcohol is added after the fermentation has continued through to dryness.

Large volumes of fortified wines were made from the beginnings of commercial wine production in Australia, say about the 1820s to the 1850s, and until the 1960s. In fact at the turn of the decade Australians started the big switch from fortifieds to table wines, initially red table wines, and fortifieds have been in decline ever since.

The boom years were the 1920s to 1930s, when huge volumes of cheap, sweet red wines, often of a rough-as-guts port style, were made in South Australia and parts of Victoria and irrigated New South Wales. Empire preferences and soldier settlers with blocks of grapes ("blockies") produced oceans of cheap wines which, with the high prevailing sunlight levels, had a high sugar content and were therefore ideal for conversion into high-alcohol reds for the English market.

The resulting bad image has remained with Australian wines in some overseas countries to this day, and Australians flinch when they hear we are still exporting fortified wines under the "Emu" brand to Canada. (In fact the Emu Australian Wine Company was bought from its British owners in 1976 by Thomas Hardy and Sons and now exports good commercial fortified wines under this label, particularly to Canada.)

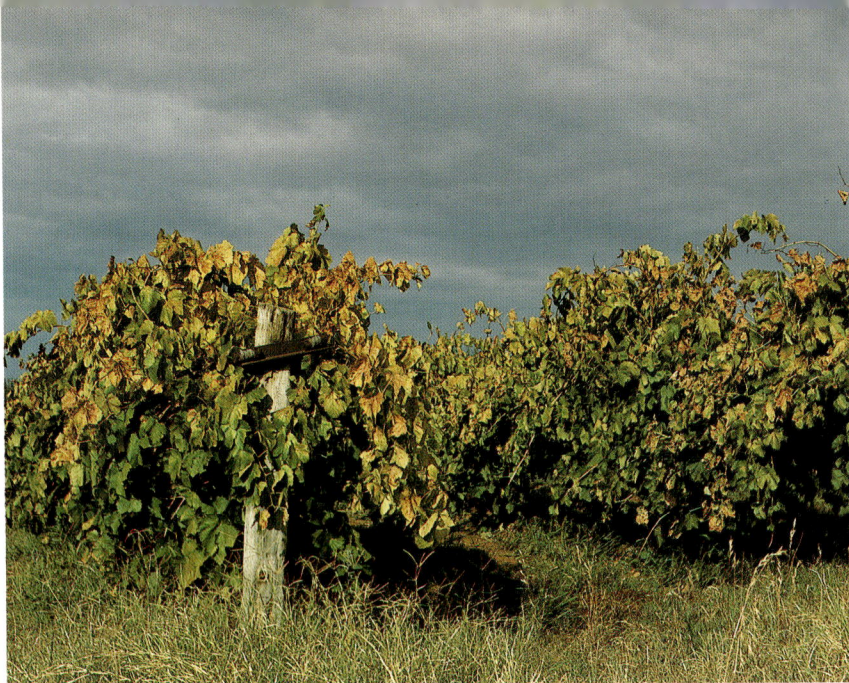

The vines head towards autumn after yielding their grapes for fortified wine in the Hunter Valley, N.S.W.

PORTS

There is obviously a lot of confusion about port wines, which I hear when listening to people talking about them, and from time to time when I've been on the receiving end of talk-back radio shows.

The key to understanding and enjoying ports is to appreciate the essential differences between **vintage port** and **tawny port.**

Vintage port is, as the name suggests, a fortified wine made from one particular year's grape harvest. It is made from a red wine base and then spirit (often brandy spirit) is added during the fermentation process. The fermentation stops and the wine can either be put into wood, or straight into the bottle. The essential difference between vintage and tawny port is that with vintage port the wine-maker expects you to do the ageing necessary to make the wine mature and enjoyable; with tawny port the wine-maker does the maturation for you and it is ready when you purchase it.

Australian vintage ports can be quite extraordinarily long lived: I tasted a 1901 (Hardy's) vintage port at age 83 years (the wines' age, not mine!), and I can report that it was drinking very nicely! Such wines may 'throw a crust', that is some of the grape sediment may settle on the bottom of the bottle, and to get rid of it you may need to decant it or pour it very carefully, leaving the (harmless) deposits at the bottom of the bottle. If you really need to impress, put a lighted candle or another light source behind the bottle so you can see when the sediment bit comes close to the neck of the bottle!

On the whole, most Australian VPs need at least five to eight years' bottle ageing, and 10 to 15 years or more is usually desirable. Keep these wines on their side in a cool, dry place free of vibration, if possible. Half bottles will mature faster, though not dramatically so. Magnums (two bottles, or 1.5L) more slowly.

Australian vintage ports are among the few of our wines that can, with some reasonable level of assurance, be bought in a child's birth year and kept for him or her to enjoy on their 21st birthday. Good makers include Seppelt, Penfolds,

In many ways it's disappointing, though understandable in the age of random breath testing, that the sales of fortified wines are still dropping in Australia, because without doubt we have made and can still make some fortified wines to equal the world's best.

They include the wines of Morris of Rutherglen, among others (Muscats and Tokays), Seppelt (sherries and ports), Hardy's and Chateau Reynella (ports), Penfolds (ports) and McWilliam's commercial sherries — indeed the 'Happy Monk' sherries of McWilliam's are the major sherry brand in this country today and have been for many decades.

Fortified wines are not, of course, intended for guzzling. Nor are they intended for all-day (or all-night) drinking. They are garnishes to the main affair — appetisers, dessert accompaniments and (rarely) an adjunct to a part of the main meal.

I once had a meal at a function at the Melbourne Regent Hotel at which all of the dishes were accompanied by fortified wines and, while it was a fascinating experiment where the chef nobly did his best to match the foods to the wines (rather than the other way around), I must say it left me and a few others (a) feeling like we'd just been feasting, nay gorging, indulging, quaffing and wenching like some modern-day Falstaffs, and (b) begging for a glass of ordinary table wine, preferably red!

The richness of the foods required to match all types of sherries, ports, muscats and tokays, contributed to our post-pran-

dial feelings, as they included things like roast kangaroo. (If you haven't eaten kangaroo you have missed one of the great table delicacies, and it is entirely free of cholesterol.)

I am a passionate advocate of Australian sherries, and I believe that they make exceptional aperitifs or appetiser drinks. One or two small glasses before dinner have a very rousing effect on the appetite. Most of the traditional makers, such as McWilliam's, Seppelt (with their appealing Solero sherry range), Mildara's 'Supreme Dry' and 'George' sherries, and a number of others, are worth exploring until you find something you enjoy.

Below I run through the types and styles of the principal fortified wines, but a word of caution may be useful. The alcoholic content of most of these wines speaks for itself. All bottles these days carry the level of alcohol-by-volume, and most of these wines have between 17 and 20 per cent alcohol — up to a fifth of the content is pure alcohol. At the end of a meal at which other forms of liquor have been consumed, a few glasses of tawny port can catch up with you pretty quickly! And, I have to admit, some of these fortifieds have spent time in wood, sometimes many years, picking up the wood flavours and providing a complex and — if you drink too much — potent recipe for a hangover.

Many of our best fortified wines are superb drinks, in the right context, and really worth exploring in a pre- or after-dinner context, but they need to be consumed with respect.

McWilliam's, Hardy, older Chateau Reynella wines, Lindeman, Yalumba and Mildara, and some of the Rutherglen makers such as Morris and Chambers.

There was a boom in special vintage ports a few years ago, commemorating racehorses and other equally unlikely namesakes. Their long-term worth is very debatable, even though many of the ports (especially from makers such as Yalumba) were excellent. Whether they will be worth heaps when they're very old is highly questionable, as many thousands of dozens were packaged up for the America's Cup, the Grong Grong Picnic Races and even Government awards and other unlikely events. My advice is to drink 'em on a special occasion, and enjoy the wine for its own sake.

Remember one last thing that has to do with the wine's durability after removal of the cork — they don't keep in the opened bottle as do tawny ports. Hence the adage: pull the cork on a bottle of vintage port, and throw the cork away!

Tawny port -Tawnies (so called because of their colour) are 'drink now' propositions. The wine is made in a similar way to vintage port, but then transferred to oak barrels (usually older barrels, hence the wood influence is less sharp) for some time, perhaps some years. The ageing process continues here before bottling, at which point the wine is ready for sale and consumption.

Tawny ports are often blended wines — blended from different varieties, barrels and vintages. The skill of the tawny portmaker is to blend in small quantities to get the right compromise between age, mellowness, fruit, spirit, wood age and, of course, economy.

The older a port the more expensive it is. Australia's top commercial tawnies, wines like Seppelt's Mt Rufus, Penfold's Magill, Yalumba Galway Pipe, Hardy's Show and and Saltram's Mr Pickwick, have ages varying from 10 to 30 years. Clearly, keeping a wine so long has its cost, and this is reflected in the price of these and similar wines, though I must say that they are still remarkably good value for money.

At another level, say around five years' average age (meaning that some of the

blend could be seven years and some could be three years old) you can still get good tawny Australian ports, at very reasonable prices. Making port is a skilful business, requiring dedication (Seppelts, for example, have been making and keeping the stuff for well over 100 years), so a large maker's name will help you get value.

Tawnies *will* keep for some time after being opened, if recorked, though the presence of air inside the bottle does cause slow deterioration, as it does with any wine.

OTHER PORT STYLES

Ruby port -A halfway house between TAWNY and VINTAGE PORTS. Young and ready to drink early. Few now made in Australia but very easy drinking, if you like the style. The name is a reference to the wine's colour.

Late Bottled Vintage (L.B.V.)-A VINTAGE PORT that has spent some extra time in wood — part of the way to being a TAWNY

PORT. Again, not much in evidence these days in Australia, as the general port market diminishes.

SHERRIES

As I indicated above, the key difference between sherries and ports tends to be when the spirit is added to the fermenting wine. If the wine-maker wants the wine sweet, the spirit is added as it is fermenting, to retain sugar. For medium dry (or sweet), leave a bit longer. A dry sherry? Then add the alcohol when all the sugar has gone and it'll stay dry!

In fact, of course, it's always a bit more complicated than that. The mechanics of sherry-making don't matter, though perhaps it's useful to know a little and appreciate how things get that way.

Sherries do vary a lot, and dismissing them out of hand as yesterday's wines is a pity. They can be fascinating pre-, post- and during-dinner drinks and they're something fascinating to add to the food

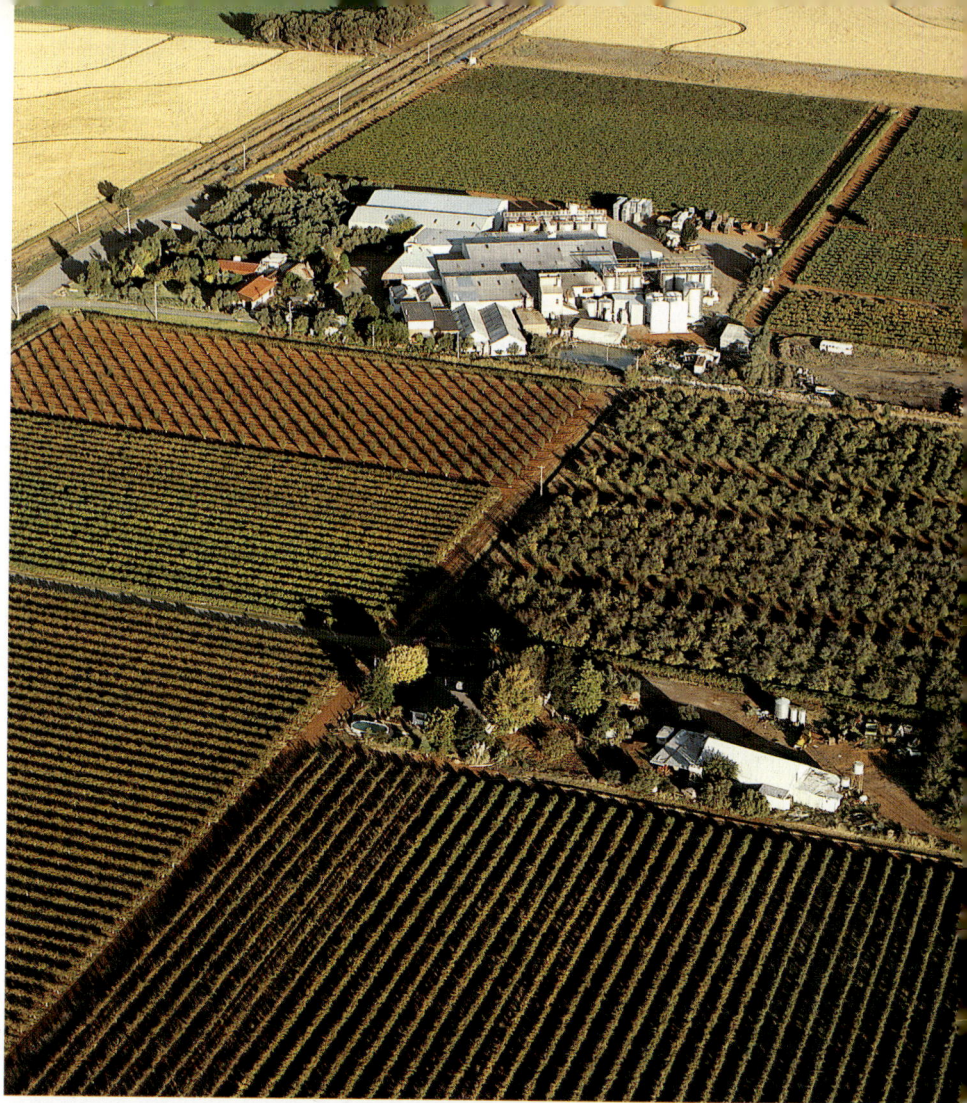

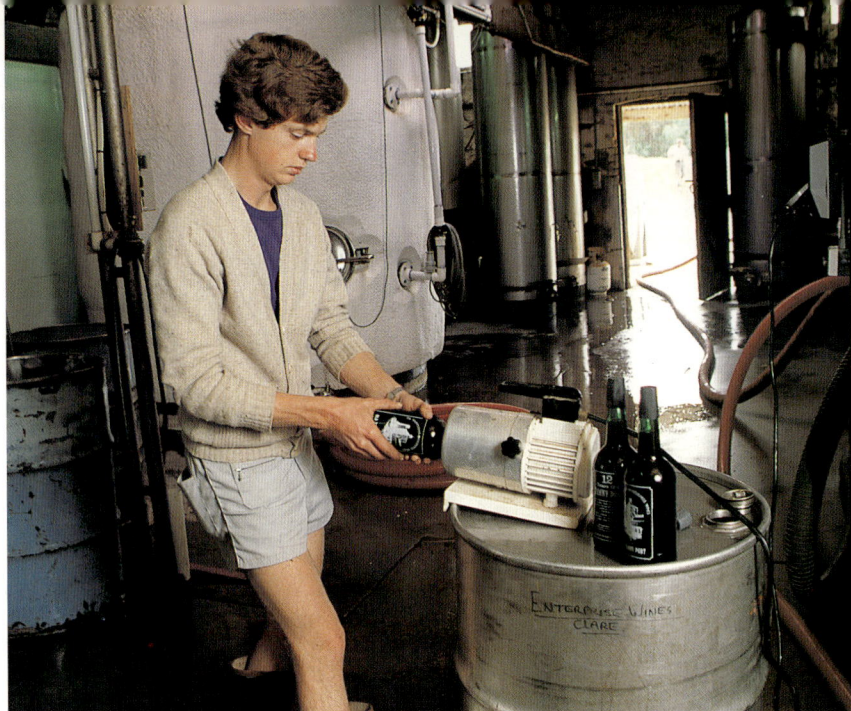
The small winemaker has to do it all by hand. Here lead neck capsules are being added to bottles of port.

— for example to soups, in particular. I always do so in my weekend soup brews; I add a splash to gravy and often put another splash or so in some marinades for meat, chicken and some seafoods.

Sweet sherries are, well I guess, just sweet. They are enjoyed by many, but they do dull the appetite.

It's the medium and dry sherries that provide the really attractive differences in flavours. The flor fino sherries, made in barrels by allowing a yeast bacteria to grow across the top of the sherry, adopt a nutty, crisp and altogether delicious flavour. These are the Australian sherries that most keenly rival the wines of this type from Spain, and they really do challenge the Spanish supremacy with sherries. (The word 'sherry', by the way, is a bastardisation of the Spanish town name Jerez, *Pron. Hare-Eth*).

They tend to be very dry, even mouth-puckering to the uninitiated. You'll like them or you'll hate them, but if you don't try them, you'll never know. A number of good ones are recommended above, and in the Glossary at the end of this book. The others include some exceptional wines, ranging in price from cheap to expensive, but their consumer appreciation is so limited these days I won't describe the other styles further here.

By the way, don't hesitate to chill them in summer. Even an iceblock is not out of place in a quaffing sherry — it cools *and* it dilutes. Alternatively, keep the bottle in the refrigerator, though good fino sherries should be served at (low) room temperatures to enjoy them.

VERMOUTH
Essentially the basis of a mixer drink, though in this case wine-based rather than spirit-based. Made by starting with a red or a white wine and adding alcohol plus various herbs, flowers and roots so that the end result is quite a complex drink. They come in sweet, medium and dry styles and the big makers are Cinzano and Angoves (with their Marko brand). Rather out of fashion, but can make a very nice, refreshing, long, summer drink with the addition of ice, soda or lemonade.

MUSCATS AND TOKAYS
Very rich and usually quite old fortified dessert wines. At their best, absolutely superb after-dinner drinks in place of port. The finest examples come from some of the older wineries around the Rutherglen/Milawa/Glenrowan areas of north-east Victoria. Some of the best come from Morris, Chambers, Campbells, All Saints, Brown Brothers and Lindeman's. People like Mick Morris work with base material which has been stored in casks for up to 80 years and which has a consistency like treacle. They blend them up with younger, fresher fortified wines and market the results as 'Liqueur Muscat' and 'Liqueur Tokay' (to differentiate them from the cheap, under-the-bridge brown-paper-bag fortified muscats).

North-east Victoria is a hot grape-growing region, as is Western Australia's Swan Valley, from whence come some super fortifieds also, notably Houghton's Liqueur Tokay and Sandalford's Liqueur Sandalera.

Wonderful wines with deep colours and luscious aromas and flavours for after-dinner enjoyment.

MADEIRA (and other special fortifieds)
Madeira is an Atlantic island 650 km west of Morocco, which is famed for its luscious fortified wines, some of them very old. The (white) grape varieties, verdelho and sercial, are widely used and the wine then fortified and aged in wood.

Australian versions are not now popular though they went through a long period of popularity. Sweet, rich and woody wines.

OTHERS
A number of other fortifieds are made in Australia in addition to those mentioned above, though in fairly small quantities and as specialised wines. One unusual example is Hardy's Fortified Sauvignon Blanc. This is again made from a white grape variety, and could be called a 'white port', though the wine is old and the colour has deepened to a rich caramel colour after wood ageing. A very unusual and enjoyable dessert wine — excellent over rock melon and ice cream.

Our fortified wines look like going the way of the Dodo, so enjoy the better ones while you can.

RECOMMENDED READING : Mark Shield's *Australian Good Wines Companion* (Penguin).

RECOMMENDED DRINKING: A bottle of Mildara Supreme Dry Sherry, or if you are really into mouth-puckering dryness, try their "George" sherry before dinner one evening. For a port, Hardy's Show is a very nice Tawny Port, and Morris Liqueur Muscat is irresistible if you want something rich, luscious and lingering.

Choosing Good Wines

All about wine labels. Some useful tips on choosing wine. A vintage chart.

Because there are so many wine labels around, choosing isn't always easy — and the wine companies don't try as hard as they could do to help you wade through the confusion.

Nevertheless, after some decades of confusion, I believe that the Australian wine market is settling into a period of relative stability, at least in consumer tastes. The wines we will be drinking in the years to come are likely to be those in vogue today — chardonnay, semillon, riesling and dry white blends, cabernet, shiraz, blends and perhaps pinot noir if and when we start making better and more consistent pinot noir reds.

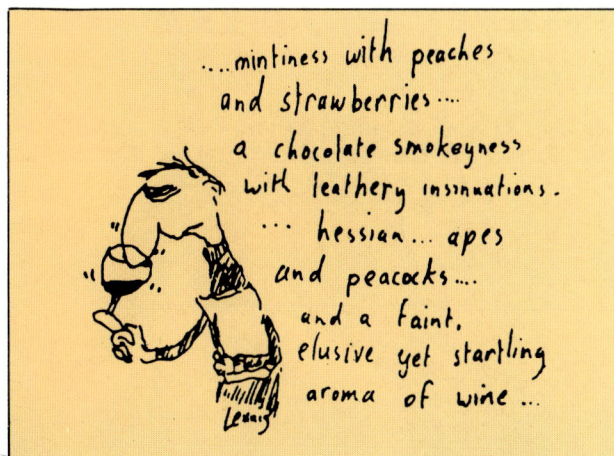

...mintiness with peaches and strawberries.... a chocolate smokeyness with leathery insinuations. ... hessian... apes and peacocks.... and a faint, elusive yet startling aroma of wine ...

Michael Leunig

We've been through varietal and generic wines, and your knowledge of these is your most important key to enjoyment. Another important key is a knowledge of makers (because good makers seldom make duds, and they're usually consistent). Area knowledge is also helpful. All of these things are touched on elsewhere between these covers.

Actually reading and understanding the labels is also important to enjoyment. You can easily make mistakes — such as picking a sweet wine when you want a dry wine; I've done this by glimpsing a label and spotting the word "riesling", only to find on tasting it that on top of the grape variety was a smaller word that said "Spatlese" or late-picked, hence a sweet white wine.

Over the past few decades, Australian wine label designs have changed enormously. From the plain-type labels (which you can still see on some of the Leo Buring DW and DR wines/Penfolds Grange/Hardy's Siegersdorf labels, and so on), which were once almost universally used, we have progressed to vividly coloured and more visually appealing designs. There have been paintings (Andrew Garrett, Hardy Collection, Leeuwin Estate, Mitchelton), birds (Hardy's and Geoff

Merrill, among others), illustrations of the winery of one kind or another (Rothbury Estate, Mildara, Chateau Reynella, Yalumba, Wynn), grapevines (The Rothbury Estate again), war-like eagles (Wolf Blass, whose label designs were amusingly referred to in the wine industry as the 'Ben Hur' style), wildflowers (Houghton) and abstract paintings (Belbourie) ...

In fact, just about every shape, form and design you can think of, so many that I often wonder if there are any fresh ideas left. (There must be, because they're still thinking up new designs for postage stamps!) Change is endemic as competition continues to be so intense, and many companies change at least one set of labels every vintage. It is hard to keep up.

If one was sufficiently cynical, one would think that there was more in the packaging than in the wine quality, and to

a point I think this is true. A number of Australian wine companies have succeeded by putting wines of very ordinary, sometimes sub-standard, quality in eye-catching packaging, and hyping up the marketing and advertising, and selling it successfully. I'd like to think they'll come unstuck, and some have.

Fortunately the shonks are the minority, and the majority make wines of good to excellent quality. As I've said elsewhere, the competition is too intense, especially among the big makers, to allow mediocrity to succeed.

I have talked elsewhere about varietal and generic terms on labels and it's important to look at these descriptions carefully to ensure you're getting what you want. If you are seeking a chardonnay, be careful of a wine that is advertised or labelled as a "SEMILLON/CHARDONNAY" or "CHENIN BLANC/CHARDONNAY"

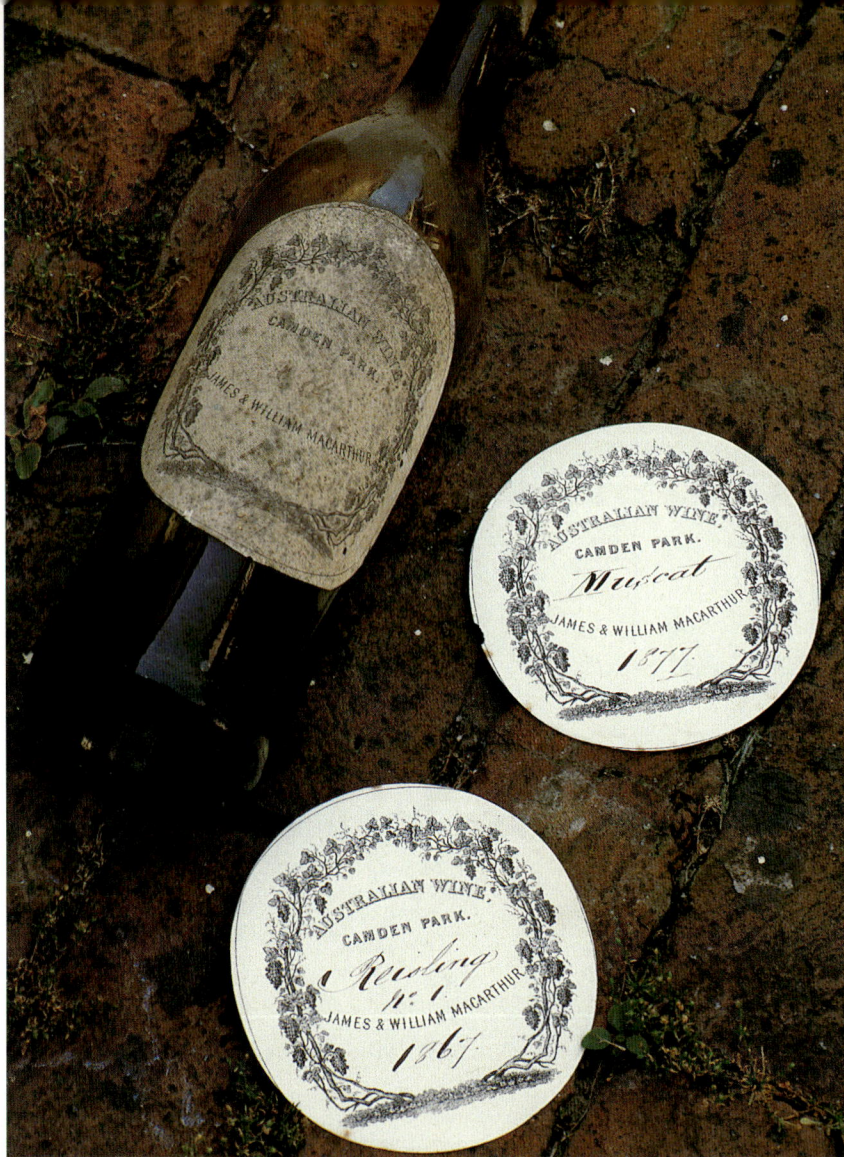

Were they good wines? Nobody left alive knows, for these wines from the Macarthurs' winery established at Camden Park, south of Sydney, came from vintages of the 1860s and 1870s.

or whatever — the maker is trying to s-t-r-e-t-c-h those chardonnay grapes available with something else, and suggest to you that you're getting chardonnay alone.

HOW TO STAY INFORMED

The best way is to taste as many wines as you can as often as you can, but that takes time, effort and money, and for most of us that is not practical advice. Nevertheless, do try to taste a variety of wines and make a mental note if not a written note as to whether you enjoyed the wine.

If you can't taste many wines, one way is to read what's written about wine quality·and buy on that basis. Again, if you do

this, try to experiment as much as possible, by all means using recommendations as a buying guide.

There are many thousands of words written weekly about wine. Just about every newspaper, and many magazines, have wine columns. Unfortunately, there is and has been for some time a prevailing attitude that writing a wine column is a bit of a lurk and there's plenty of free wine to go with it, so anyone can do it. The quality of some wine columns and the adequacy of the advice to readers suffers greatly as a result. The main problem is that most wine writers tend to write for wine people, not ordinary drinkers.

"Ordinary drinkers" — people like you

and me — drink wines they can afford and that they know they'll enjoy. That often means cask wines and economic bottled wines. Sometimes of course we'll drink a better bottle of wine on a special occasion. But we won't be quaffing the wines the wine writers are talking about daily, more often than not.

Among the wine writers are certainly some who know what they're talking about and aim at an everyday palate. You'll have to make up your mind which do by comparing what they recommend with what you like.

Several of the better newspapers go around the discount shops and let you know what's good. The Sydney Morning Herald, The Age and the Melbourne Herald-Sun all have good wine columns and sometimes do this.

One of the best ways to get wine advice is to read a wine magazine. Winestate (bi-monthly) tastes most wines commercially released in Australia at regular "blind" tastings, using a blend of wine-makers, professional palates, retailers and others, in order to make recommendations to readers. I believe the magazine conducts its tastings scrupulously and honestly, and its endorsement usually constitutes good advice.

These magazines and newspapers often use a star system, which is sometimes equated with cost, so you know where you stand, and you can identify the wine simply because many of the wines recommended have the labels reproduced in colour.

Another way to explore is to buy mixed dozens. There are now quite a few of these, including one operated by American Express and another by Cellarmasters, and their buying power can give you value for money.

One hitch in buying some of these dozens is this. Wine retailers hate seeing wine sold by mail order, for fairly understandable reasons — it hits them in the cash register. To keep their retail trade happy, many big wine makers offer their wines in special labels to the mail order sellers such as Cellarmasters. The wine may be exactly the same wine as a big branded product, but you often won't be

YEAR	1980	1981	1982	1983	1984	1985	1986	1987	1988	1989	1990	1991	1992
Barossa Vlly	6/4	4/3	6/5	2/3	5/6	6/5	4/5	5/6	5/6	5/6	6/7	6/6	5/6
Clare	4/5	5/6	5/6	3/4	6/7	5/6	4/6	6/6	5/6	4/5	5/6	5/5	4/6
Coonawarra	5/7	5/6	5/6	2/2	5/6	6/6	5/6	6/5	5/5	5/6	6/7	5/6	5/7
Padthaway	5/6	5/4	4/5	2/3	5/4	6/5	5/5	6/4	5/6	4/5	6/5	5/6	6/6
McLaren Vale	6/6	4/5	5/6	3/4	5/6	6/5	5/6	6/6	6/6	5/6	4+/6	5/6	5/5
Hunter Vlly	4/5	5/6	5/5	4/5	6/5	5/5	6/5	5/4	6/5	5/4	6/7	5/5	6/6
Mudgee	5/5	5/5	5/6	5/5	5/6	6/5	4/5	4/5	5/6	6/6	5/6	5+/6	5/6
Swan Valley	6/5	5/6	5/5	7/6	5/6	6/5	6/5	5/4	5/6	7/5	6/5	7/5	6/5
S. WA	4/5	6/7	6/6	6/7	7/7	7/6	5/6	6/5	5/6	5/5	6/6	7/5	6/6
Central Vic.	5/6	5/5	5/6	5/6	5/5	6/2	5/5	6/6	6/7	6/6	6/6	6+/6+	6/6

This, then, is a wine-maker's guide to what should be good around Australia from the last decade or so. Vintages are assessed out of a possible maximum of seven points, with consideration given to both the year itself, plus some weight to how the wine might be now. Bear in mind that a wine made in 1970 will be, by the attrition of time, very different to a wine made in 1980.

Two points is a shocking vintage, three points is a poor vintage, four drinkable, five enjoyable, six very good, and seven outstanding. The first figure is for white wines, the second for red wines.

able to find the same label at your retailers, even though the same wine may be there behind the branded label.

One very interesting and high-quality dozen is the annual offering from the Adelaide paper, the Advertiser, which offers a mixed dozen late each year, picked from prizewinning wines at the Adelaide Wine Show in late October.

The Australian also offers two separate dozens each year to its readers, as does the Australian Wine Society, and all of these are reliable buys.

But in the end the choice is yours. I'd simply urge you to be a little adventurous.

AUSTRALIAN WINE VINTAGES

In spite of the general conception that Australia's sunny climate provides unfailingly good vintages, they do vary. The variations are caused by seasonal changes (for example, 1983 was a rotten vintage in South Australia, and in several other areas), by human failings, by lack of experience and, indeed, by acts of God. I would like to think that God was (is?) a wine drinker. (His son certainly was.)

In general I do not put great trust into vintage charts. They are at best a broad generalisation. Nevertheless, there are certain guidelines about Australian wine vintages that can be of help to wine drinkers and collectors. Vintage charts such as the one above are not intended as infallible guides, but rather as an indication of wine quality in one area in a particular year. It is a fallible guide, because in some poor years some makers will make good to very good wines (for example, there were some quite reasonable reds that were salvaged from '83 in South Australia). Of course in some great years, some makers will slip.

And not all areas are covered, as that would consume too much space and really not help anyone a lot as the ones missed are small, and variances are considerable. There also seemed little point in including the main irrigated areas (the Murrumbidgee Irrigation Area, the South Australian and Victorian Riverlands) as they generally don't make wines to keep, rather wines to enjoy early which, as I've mentioned elsewhere, is a realistic approach to modern wine consumption habits.

RECOMMENDED DRINKING : Tollana TR 222, a blended South Australian cabernet sauvignon, again from the Penfold stable — wonderful, below-$10 red of exquisite flavour and balance.

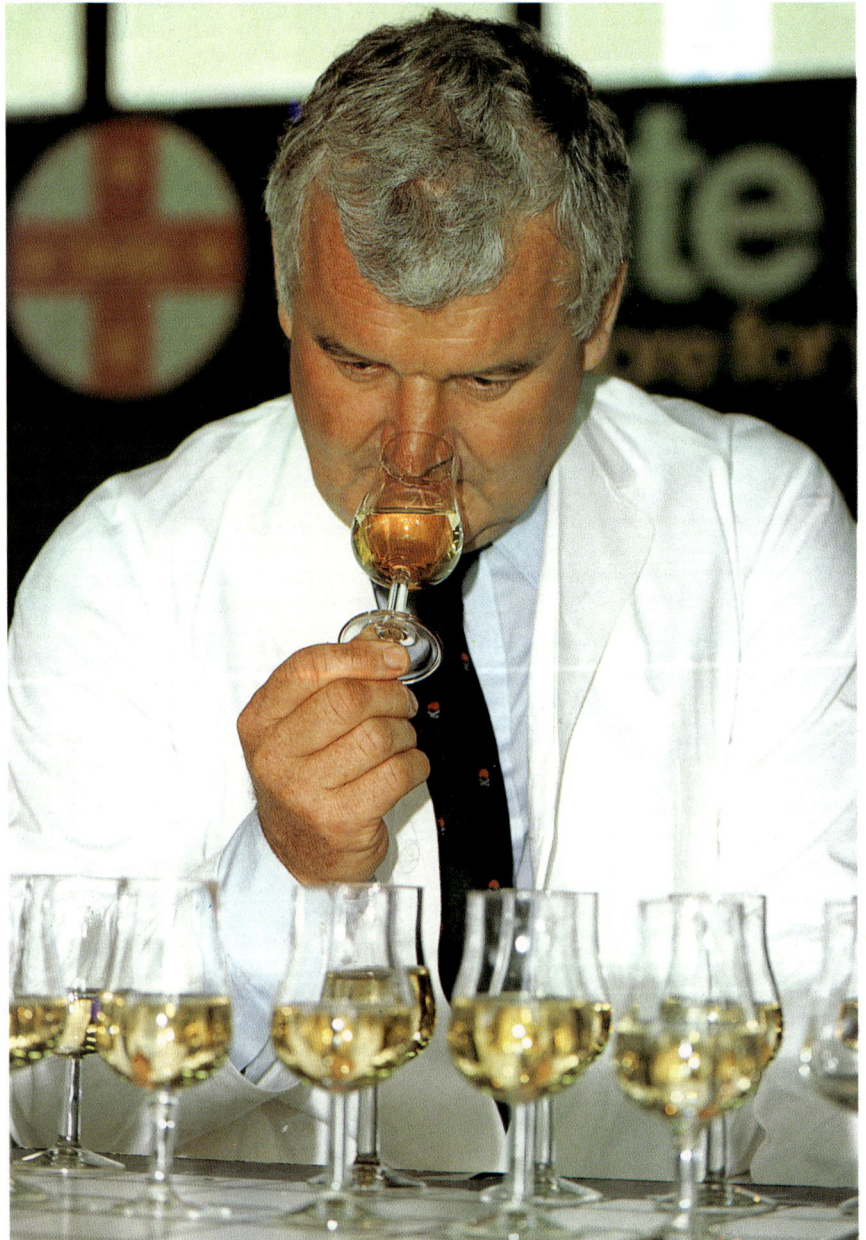

WINE SHOWS

... and how they can point you in the right direction

Wine shows are probably the most misunderstood — or perhaps least understood — competitions in Australia. This is despite the fact that hundreds of people give up thousands of voluntary hours of their time annually to judge most of the many thousands of wines produced.

"Wine Show" is a bit of a misnomer, as they could be more accurately described as "wine competitions". I'm talking here mainly about the capital city wine shows, but there are also many regional shows. For example, the Hunter and Barossa Valleys have their own wine shows each year, and regional shows operate in a similar way to the major shows.

Chairman of Judges at the Sydney Wine Show, Len Evans, at work.

Wine shows are conducted in all Australian capital cities, including Canberra, by the respective State agricultural societies. The Sydney Wine Show, which is the first each year (in February), is organised and run, and the judges are selected, by the Royal Agricultural Society of New South Wales. Anyone can enter wines, provided they are Australian wines (except for the so-called National Wine Show in Canberra, where New Zealand wines can be entered), and they conform to the rules of entry.

And, make no mistake, while a minute proportion of the population, let alone the wine-drinking population, understands how they work and what they mean, wine shows are important if you want to know where to look for the good wines.

What judges attempt to do at wine shows, and usually successfully, is to reject wines with wine-making faults, or lack of wine flavour, and then cull from those remaining. The object is to find the "best" wines, although in theory every wine entered could win a gold medal. In practice, however, very few do, as the judges at most shows are hard critics.

For example, at the 1992 Royal Adelaide Wine Show, there were 1,984 wines entered and the judges, chaired by Brian Croser (whose full-time occupation involves making the brilliant wines of Petaluma) awarded a total of 27 Trophies,

83 Gold Medals, 211 Silvers and 539 Bronze Medals.

The capital city shows are hard work for the judges. That's no exaggeration when you consider how many wines they have to taste and assess. Most modern wine shows attract at least 1,500 entries each year, and 2,000 is not unusual. The judging conditions are often less than ideal. Walking into a large, non-air-conditioned hall at breakfast time to be faced with 150 very young red wines is enough to daunt most. And while at least they don't have to actually swallow the stuff — they usually sniff, savour and spit the wines — some alcohol is absorbed by the mouth and tongue anyway.

If you believe that smelling a wine is pretentious, note that most wine judges, and indeed just about anybody else, can detect a poor or badly made wine just by a careful sniff. Many judges run through the range of wines presented to them and simply push back the glasses which don't attract or which have obvious faults. Then they'll taste and more carefully assess the rest to locate the good to outstanding ones.

The usual method of judging is a simple one. The judges operate by a system which gives a wine a maximum of 20 points. In theory, any wine which got 20 points would be the perfect wine and, while it has happened once or twice, it is exceedingly rare.

The maximum of 20 points comes from three areas of assessment: a maximum of three points for colour and condition; a maximum of seven for bouquet (smell) and a possible 10 for taste. Any sound commercial wine should get the three points for colour and condition; getting six for smell is common and seven out of ten for taste. That's a possible 16 out of 20, and such a wine would be awarded a bronze medal.

There isn't much room for error if you want to make an award-winning wine. The medals are awarded on the following basis: 15 to 16.9 points gets a bronze; 17 points to 18.4 for silver; and 18.5 and above for gold. As you can see from the Adelaide Wine Show example cited above, less than 5 per cent of the entries were considered deserving of a Gold medal.

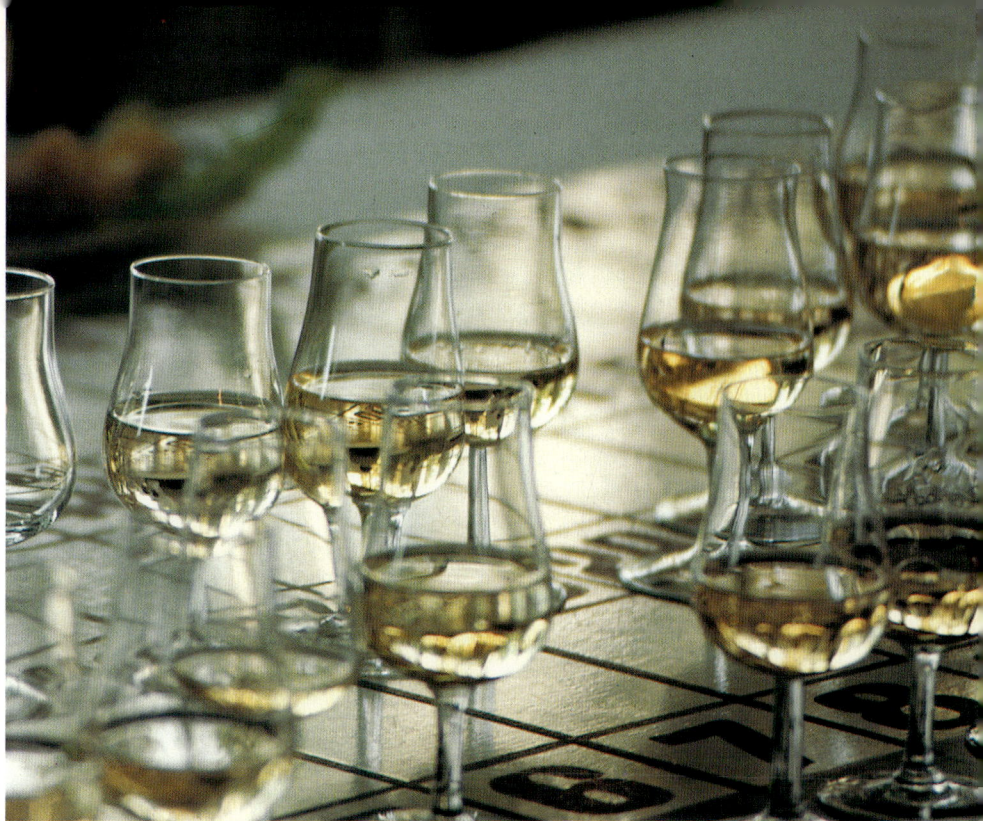

Young white wines sit in ordered, numbered yet anonymous rows as they are assessed at the Sydney Wine Show.

Wines are entered in different classes so that the judges can compare apples with apples — or more accurately, rieslings with rieslings, and cabernets with cabernets and so on. There has been much debate over the years about the actual "show specifications". The problem was well identified some years ago when at one major wine show, the exact same wine won a gold medal in the Claret class and a gold medal in the Burgundy class! This example mainly serves to identify the problem existing in this country with the generic use of European names, such as claret and burgundy. Today, in general, the wine show organisers have got a large measure of agreement as to what should be compared with what, and what constitutes wines of gold, silver and bronze quality.

The people who judge the wines at most of the capital city shows are very experienced wine men and women. At the top shows, including Sydney, Melbourne, Adelaide and Canberra, they represent wine judging experience and standards comparable with, and probably better than, anywhere else in the world. Visiting overseas judges have almost invariably been amazed at the time, trouble and skills brought to wine judging in this country. It's more amazing when you consider that Australian judges do it for nothing in their

own time (or sometimes their employer's time).

It may take four complete days of hard slog for the 8 or 10 fully qualified judges, backed by about half a dozen or so "associates" and a group of "stewards" (in effect, apprentices), to wade through the 1,500 to 2,000 wines and weed out the good ones from the mediocre and the duds. They'll judge from breakfast time to early evening, and be back at it, probably judging an entirely different class of wines, the next day.

Different shows and different chairmen of judges work in different ways. But often the chairman, the most senior and experienced of them, will put judges and associates together in groups of two or three and ask them to "look at" (taste) various groups of wine. The wines will be lined up in numbered positions and poured by stewards. This is called "blind tasting" and simply means that the judges don't know whose wines they are assessing. All they know is that they are judging wines belonging to, say, the "Cabernet Sauvignon — Two Years and Older" class. Against the backdrop of their own experience and expectations for this style of wine, they look, smell and taste. They usually, if they're wise, roll the wine around in their mouths and then spit it out into buckets of sawdust. They will try to reach

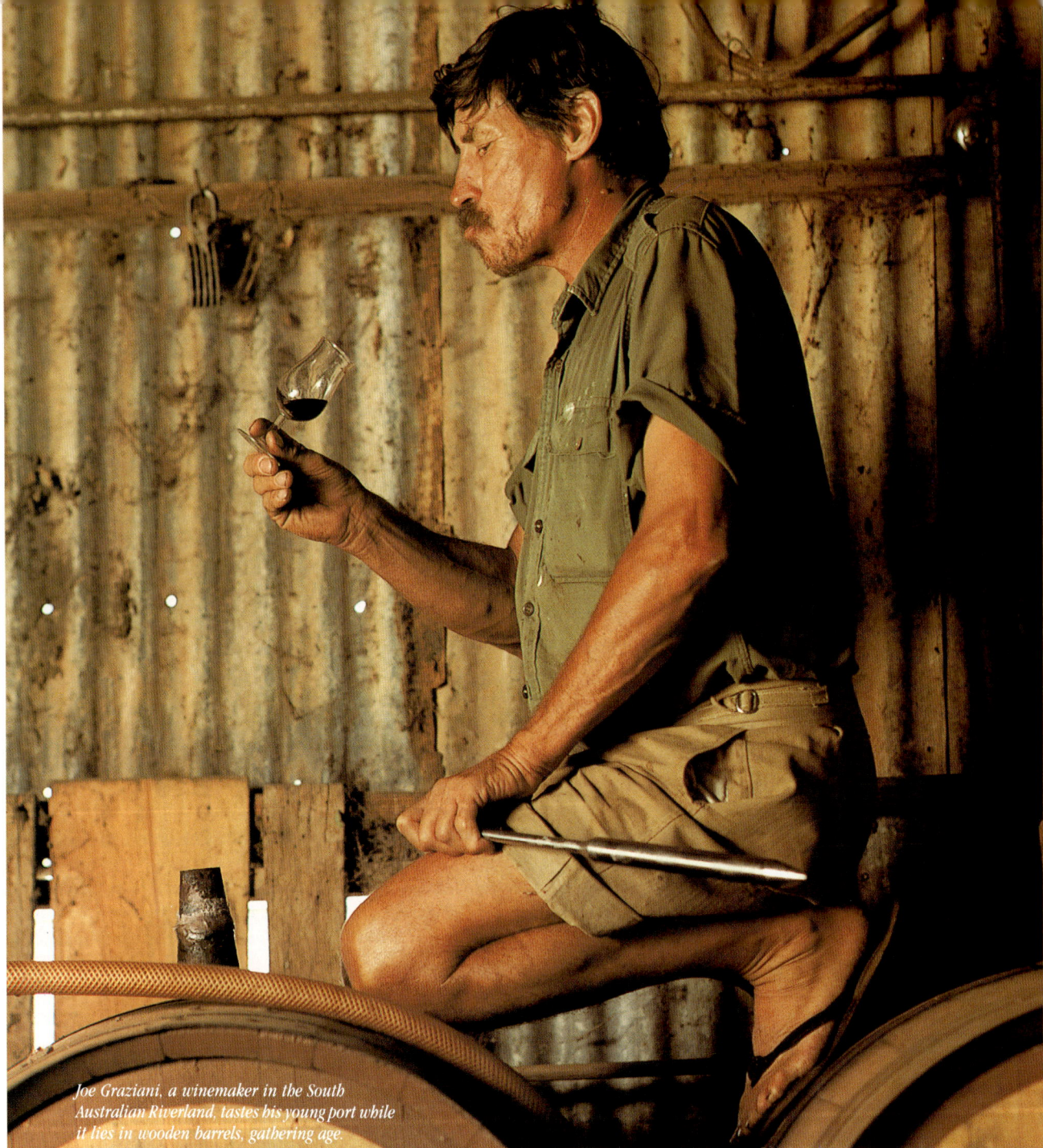

Joe Graziani, a winemaker in the South Australian Riverland, tastes his young port while it lies in wooden barrels, gathering age.

agreement by consensus about each wine: which ones are rejects, which are bronze standard, which deserve silvers and which gold medals.

It's fairly unusual but it can happen that a whole class of wines can be considered below bronze standard and so none gets an award. It is quite common for none in a class to get a gold.

If there is an irreconcilable difference of opinion among the panel of two or three, the chairman will be called in and will resolve the stalemate by assessing and coming down on whichever side he believes is right.

It's by no means a perfect system, and undoubtedly injustices are done from time to time. But I believe, and I think the wine industry at large believes, that it works well and generally fairly.

Here is what's important about Australian wine competitions for the consumer.

Gold medals awarded at recent capital city wine shows, particularly the major ones, do mean you'll get a good wine. Bear in mind that it may not necessarily be a wine you like; but it will be a very good wine indeed, judged

against its fellows and by the standards of some of the world's most experienced and dedicated wine palates. "Even" a bronze medal indicates a pretty good wine, certainly one worth buying at a fair price.

The regulations of most of the wine show societies are quite strict, not just about entry standards (to ensure that a wine competes fairly against its opposition) but also about how a successful wine-maker can promote a prize-winning product. You cannot, for example, put a sticker on a bottle of wine and blurb: GOLD MEDAL AT SYDNEY WINE SHOW. You have to be specific and say

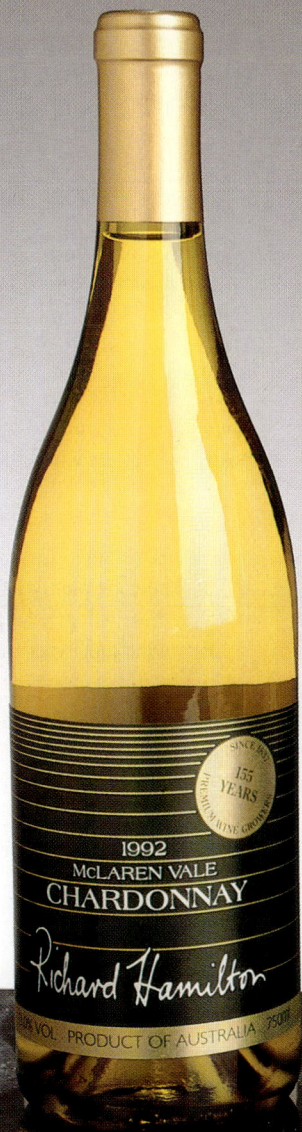

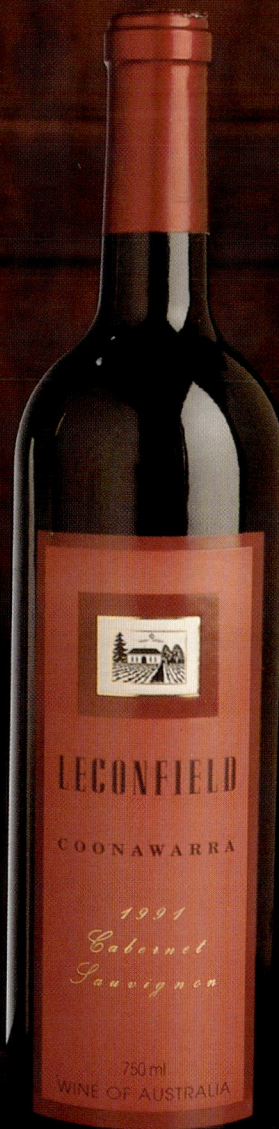

RICHARD HAMILTON WINES
Main Road, Willunga, S.A. Telephone: (085) 56 2288

GOLD MEDAL / 1988 SYDNEY WINE SHOW / CLASS 16. Therefore beware of generalised advertising claims which say things like: OUR CHATEAU OUTBACK CHAIRMAN'S SELECTION RANGE HAS WON 103 MEDALS! That means that a range of products so designated by the maker has, or may have, won gold, silver and bronze medals on some, perhaps all, of the Australian wine show circuit, possibly including local wine shows in their district. But it could be over a 20-year period. They may not have won anything significant for quite a few years, and it certainly doesn't necessarily mean that the company's present vintage of these wines is anything out of the ordinary.

There have been attempts to delineate the boundaries for each style of wine, and the following few examples are drawn from the Australian Wine and Brandy Corporation guidelines for their export inspectors. The Corporation, which is the Australian Government's Statutory wine authority, licences all wine exports and then tastes and authorises, or rejects, each individual wine destined for shipment overseas. They are not looking for gold medal winners, but simply for what are described as "sound and merchantable" wines.

DRY WHITE TABLE WINE
Should be in brilliant condition, pale to light straw in colour, preferably with a slight greenish tinge, light to medium bodied, medium to high acidity and yet soft, with a fresh and flowery bouquet and a clean aftertaste, free of bitterness or lingering sweetness.

DRY WHITE TABLE WINE — FULL BODIED
Should be in brilliant condition, light to medium straw in colour. Medium to full bodied and yet delicate with medium acidity and a fresh bouquet. Its aftertaste may be a little more pronounced than in dry white table wine even with a very slight bitterness but no lingering sweetness.

MEDIUM DRY WHITE TABLE WINE
Specification similar to dry white table wine but with some sweetness.

LIGHT BODIED DRY RED
Colour light to medium red. A blue or purple tint may be present. Aroma and

bouquet-varietal aroma may occur in varying degrees. It should be fresh and fruity and in harmony with the body and flavour of the wine. Palate soft and light without being thin, and rounded in the mid palate. Body should be light and the acidity in balance with the body of the wine. Finish clean and crisp with soft astringency.

FULL BODIED, FIRM FINISH, DRY RED
Colour medium to deep red. According to age, a blue or purple tint may be present in a young wine or a light brown edge may be present in an aged wine. Aroma and bouquet — varietal aroma may occur in varying degrees. It should be fruity and in harmony with the body and flavour of the wine. The bouquet may show evidence in older wines of maturation in oak vessels and/or the bouquet to mature with bottle age. Palate soft, rounded and generous in the mid palate. Body should be full and acidity in balance. Finish, clean and with a firm astringent grape tannin. With or without the flavour of oak, tannin from the maturing wood should not predominate.

AUSTRALIAN CHAMPAGNE
Colour should be pale to light straw. Should have good acidity and not be too light in body. Bouquet should be fresh, fruity but without particular varietal flavour, and should indicate some years in

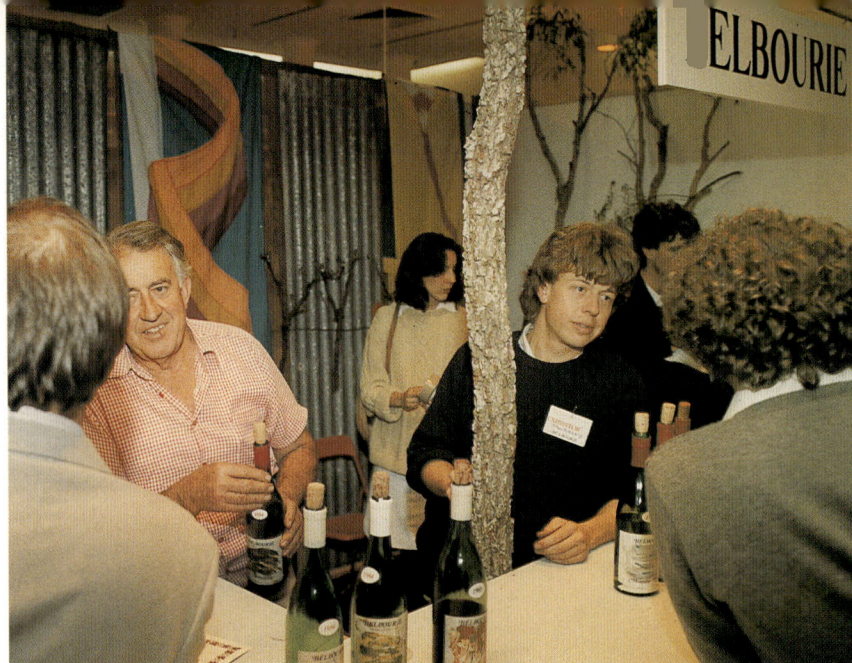

Above: *Hunter Valley winemaker, Jim Roberts, shows interested drinkers his wines at a Sydney exhibition.*

Right: *Wine exhibitions are held regularly in most capitals and are a good opportunity to taste for yourself.*

bottle. The wine should be fairly dry but show no astringent finish. Bone dry or excessively sweet wines should be penalised. Bubbles should be fine and persistent.

There are plenty more examples but these will give an idea of how the wine judges set their parameters. (The use of certain words needs explanation: "brilliant" refers to colour and clarity, not to wine quality; "fine" as in the reference to bubbles above means "small".)

Here is the very thing that frightens many people about the subject of wine: the mumbo-jumbo that often goes with it.

There is also the problem that those of us who write about wine strike all the time: wine is for drinking and enjoying, of course, and it is difficult indeed to talk about how something actually tastes. Wine is the quintessential example, and many, many people have wrestled long and hard with the problems of communicating wine tastes in print. That's why catchwords like some of those above have evolved, words like "body" and "soft". Wine has no "body", of course. It is not a living thing. But it can be thicker or thinner according to how many constituents are in it.

It is a pity that some of the wine show organisers, the Royal Agricultural Societies, do not make greater efforts to publicise successful wines, particularly widely available commercial wines, to the

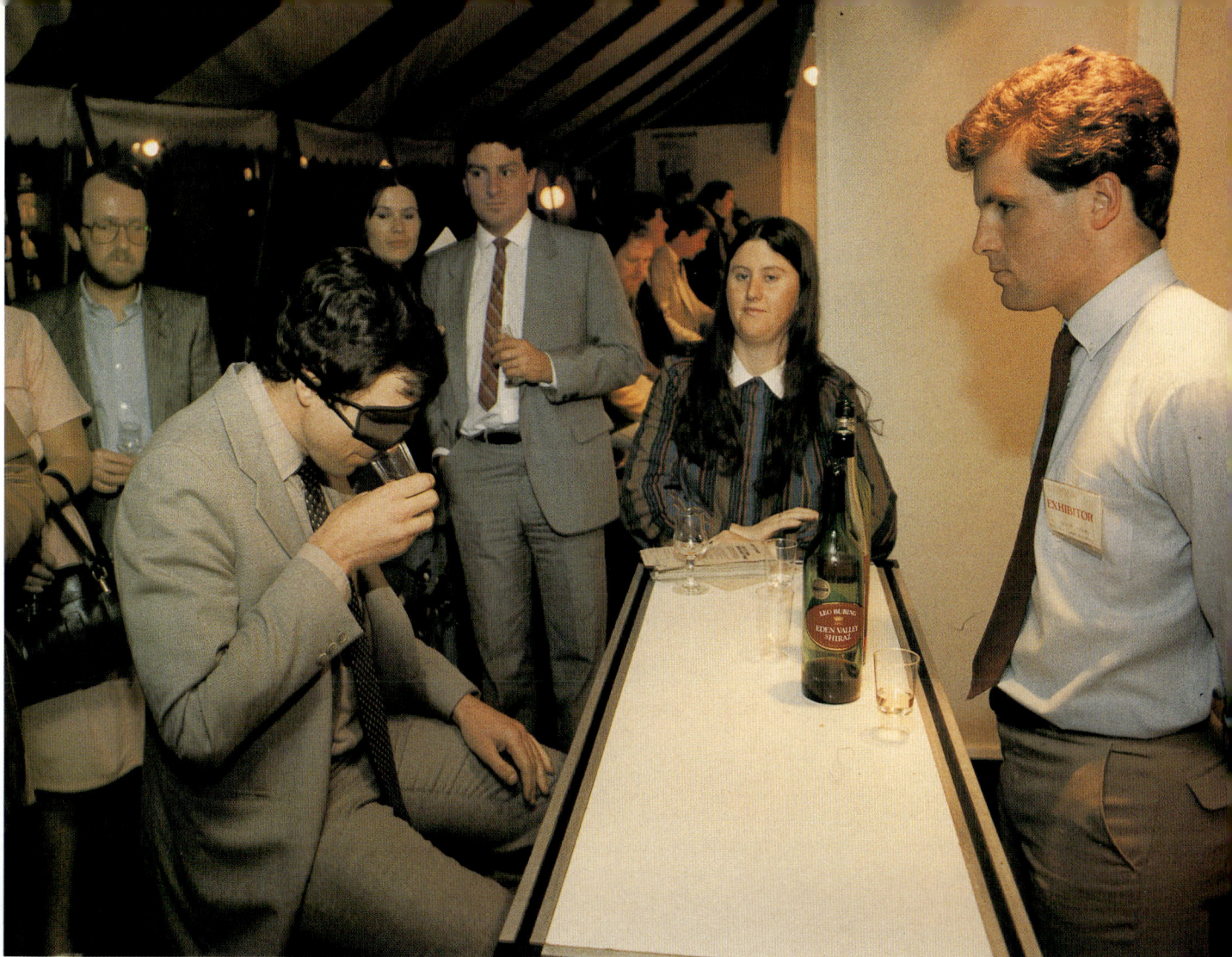

public. They print the results in a booklet form and you can get these results from the various societies. But the results are meaningless unless you know how to decode them, and our newspapers seldom pay much attention to wine show results and what they mean to us wine consumers.

Some companies will amass high-quality wines in their "museum" in order to be more successful at wine shows. Show organisers usually specify that a company must have a certain volume of a wine in order to be eligible for entry in a particular class — it may be 1,500 litres in older classes or for smaller producers; it may be 22,500 litres for more "commercial" lines. But no one says you have to put these wines on sale. It happens sometimes that the company will keep the wine and never release it for sale, winning medal after medal in order to reflect credit on the producer or their other non-medal-winning products.

The wine show "circuit" is a highly competitive one, and a handful of the big companies have dominated it over recent years: first Orlando, then Lindemans and Seppelt slogged it out for the "Most Successful" trophies. Who's top depends on which way you look at it — but it does help consumers a great deal to know that wines from Seppelt, Lindeman, Orlando, Hardy's, Wolf Blass and so on are consistently good.

One recent development I welcome came at the 1992 Adelaide Wine Show. For the first time in Australia, wines in the commercial classes were assessed in classes of "Above $10 a bottle" and "Below $10 a bottle". These are the main retail price point distinctions in our present wine market, so if you know what won medals at this show in these classes, it gives you a reasonable idea of what is value for money. I suspect other wine shows will follow suit.

Another welcome development is classes for aspiring wine judges conducted regularly at the Australian Wine Research Institute at Urrbrae, Adelaide. To be eligi-ble you must already have a working knowledge of what it's all about. This system, instigated by the Wine Committee of the South Australian Agricultural Society (organisers of the annual Adelaide Wine Show) is designed to train associate (or junior) wine judges for the show.

Our wine judges do a good job for consumers like us. Take heed of their advice and you'll drink good wines.

RECOMMENDED FURTHER READING : Dr Bryce Rankine, a distinguished wine scientist, has written several books about wine and wine-making, though they enjoy limited circulation. If you're interested in knowing more, you can contact him through the Society of Wine Educators, telephone (08) 364 1122.

RECOMMENDED DRINKING: A regular medal winner is Jim Barry's Clare Valley Rhine Riesling — a quintessential, top-quality Australian dry white.

WINE AND FOOD

The combination of wine and food is one of the few marriages made in heaven, as the menu below might suggest:

Iced Rock Melon	**Lindeman Montillo Sherry**
Kangaroo Tail Soup	**Madeira Lindeman**
Tasmanian Lobster on Shell	**1924 Kirkton Chablis**
Asparagus	
Riverina Black Duck & Salad	**1924 St Cora Burgundy**
Iced Bombe	**Lindeman Extra-Dry Champagne**
Dessert	**Raisin Liqueur Muscat**
Coffee	**Lindeman Macquarie Brandy 1922**

The menu above was used in 1930 by Lindeman's Wines at the commemoration of the Centenary of their Kirkton Vineyards in New South Wales, planted in 1830. Some of the wines used came from the original vines. (Note the extensive use of European and generic names some 60 years ago.)

Clearly, tastes have changed since then, partly through changing attitudes — I don't think you would have walked hungry away from this opulent repast! — and partly because the availability of foods has changed.

It's interesting to note that Lindemans didn't try to match a wine to the asparagus. This has always been one of the great wine/food puzzles, as asparagus (and chocolate, the other Great Challenge) assault with such pungent flavours.

It has been said a million times, of course, in the past decade or two: there are no hard and fast rules in the combination of food and wine — disallowing, perhaps, asparagus!

But so much would not have been written aboutWhich-Wine-With-Which-Food if a lot of people didn't have strong views about the subject. More positively, a great

number of people feel strongly that certain types of wine are best served with certain styles of foods. Some people go to a great deal of trouble, and of course there are clubs and societies (for example, the Beefsteak and Burgundy Clubs, the Escoffier Society, the Chaines des Rotisseurs, the Wine and Food Society of Australia). These people take their food very seriously, in planning, preparation and consumption. They usually take their wines very seriously, too, going to great trouble to "match" the wines to the food — or, occasionally, to match the food to the wine or wines, usually done if a very special wine is available to consume. The most notable occasion I had to do this was with a bottle of 1864 Madeira; out of interest we served a consommé (thin soup) with the old wine, and before and afterwards had table and dessert wines made from the same white grape variety as the Madeira, namely verdelho. The old wine was pretty good, too!

These days you aren't going to get many people raising their eyebrows if you serve a white with a meat, a port with the lobster or a chardonnay with the cheese. True, most people who like food and wine

Lindeman's Centennial celebratory menu reflects times when a meal was nothing if not satisfying! The Kirkton Chablis would have been a dry wine, probably with little fruit, the St Cora a rich, heavy red and the muscat ultra luscious and sweet.

would probably prefer to have a red of some sort with the meat, a chardonnay or lighter red with the lobster and a red or sweet white wine with the cheese. But things are pretty relaxed in the eating and drinking world now, and most of us would shrug and go along with your preference without complaint.

You will find, though, if you haven't already, that your own tastes will probably be best served by roughly sticking to the "rules", that amorphous folklore about wine and food that has grown up over the past few hundred years or so, mainly in Europe because it is the home of modern wine.

The flavours, the colours, the smells and the subtleties of wine are almost as diverse as the differences in flavour, texture, colour, aroma and other variations of foods.

The harmony that comes from linking an oyster to a glass of riesling, a wood-treated semillon to a plate of cold turkey, a complex and fruity cabernet sauvignon to a piece of grilled, lean steak, or the delight of a big, somewhat older shiraz red to a rabbit casserole, are essentially delights of the senses. What improves these combinations particularly is the company of good friends — who will also hopefully enjoy the combination of what is put on your table.

It needs to be said often: wine and food are about enjoyment. Much of that enjoyment has to do with the visual senses (sight) as with the other senses of smell and taste. Something that looks good, usually will be good. And if what appears before you is diverse, then you have the interest of your companions, and you are also probably more than halfway to an enjoyable meal.

That is why, if you wish to build a cellar, try to vary your choices somewhat between wine styles. I am constantly surprising myself these days, when fossicking around in the shed that passes for my cellar, looking for something to have over a weekend lunch, and coming across a bottle that makes me say: "Hell! I'd forgotten I ever put that one down here. Could be just the shot with the barbecued prawn dish" (more of which below).

The rules of dry-with-dry, red-with-red and sweet-with-sweet were certainly made to be broken and fortunately they often are broken, and need to be broken. But only

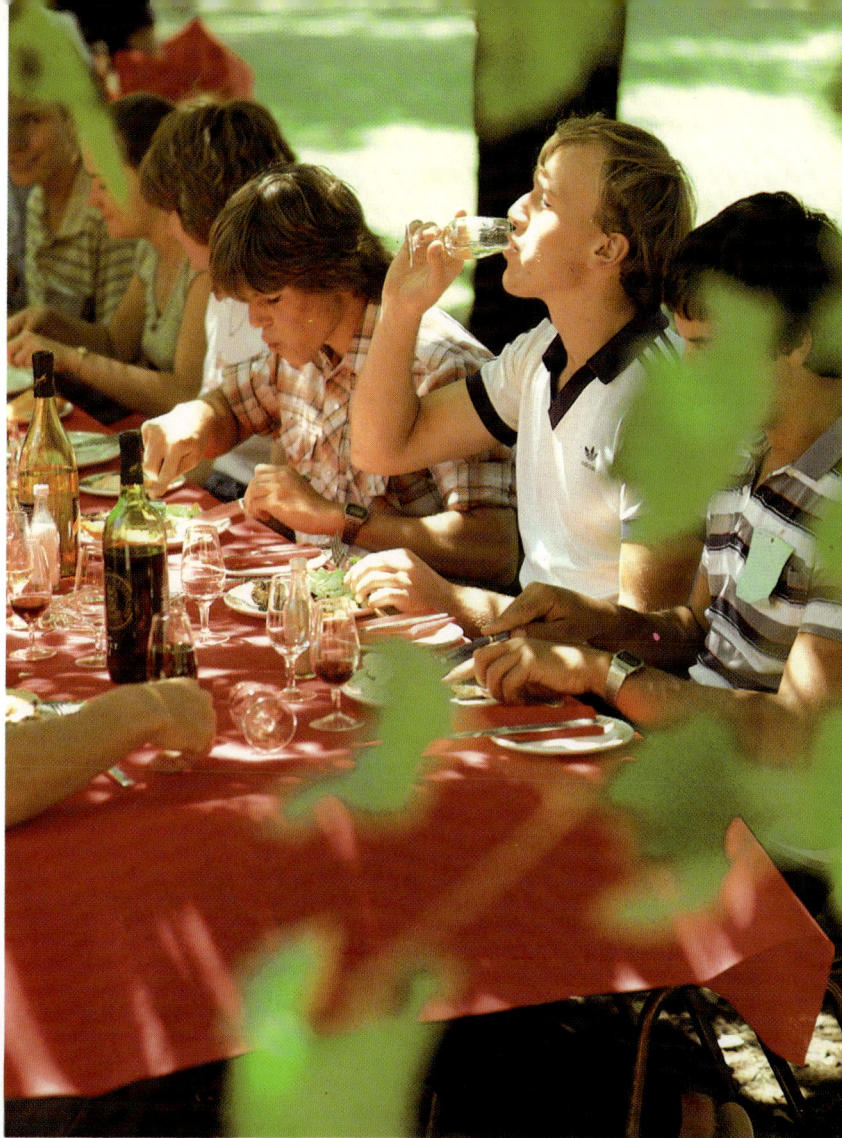

These winemaking students are enjoying an outdoor meal and tasting.

within limits. You must know where those limits are, for you and your guests.

Start with the food selection, almost invariably. Then think what you would like to try to drink with each course. Bear their interests in mind (if you know them) and work out a course of action. Then find, or buy, your wines. Serve them in reasonable but not excessive quantities. At the right temperature. And in the most appropriate glasses available.

Too few wines is better than too many. Unless you are sure of yourself, don't go for very old or unusual wines. Bad wines are easier to spot than mediocre ones!

In regard to food, the emphasis today (other than that on fast food) is on simplicity. In other words, good ingredients which are then interfered with as little as possible by the person in the kitchen. Your wine selection needs to harmonise good wines with these sorts of ingredients, and increasingly of course this means dry table wines (white and red), more than the fortified wines of decades gone by, bigger bodied reds and our constantly improving sparkling wines.

Tables of what-to-drink-with-what are generalised views of the eating and drinking business. But they serve the purpose of making you think about things ... always bearing in mind that it is harmony you should be seeking.

So what is harmony? A little hard to say (like writing a prescription for a harmonious marriage). But, like true love, you'll know it when you've found it.

A FEW SUGGESTIONS

PRE-DINNER WINES *Champagne (brut, semi-brut)*
Dry or medium-dry sherry, such as flor fino
Dry white, perhaps a riesling

HORS D'OEUVRES

Antipasto	*Medium-dry Rhine riesling, sauvignon blanc*
Avocado dip & crudités	*Light red or rosé*
Cheese in puff or filo pastry	*Champagne, sparkling burgundy, any good chilled wine with some residual fruit*
Cheese puffs	*As above*
Pâté	*Shiraz, cabernet, hermitage, beaujolais*
Sesame chicken wings	*Dry white, semillon, chardonnay blend*

SOUPS

SOUPS *Don't serve too much liquid with soup!*

Summer chilled soups *Any of the following will complement soups, but generally sherry can be served with most soups; other suggestions below:*

Consommé	*Medium-dry or amontillado sherry*
Gazpacho	*Pinot noir, dry white*
Cucumber & yoghurt	*As above*
Tomato & basil	*As above*

Hot soups

Consommé	*Medium-dry or amontillado sherry*
Creamed vegetable soups (leek, pumpkin, potato)	*Sherry, chardonnay, chablis, sauvignon blanc*
Minestrone, hearty beef soups	*Shiraz, cabernet*
French onion with melted cheese	*Pinot noir, shiraz, cabernet sauvignon*

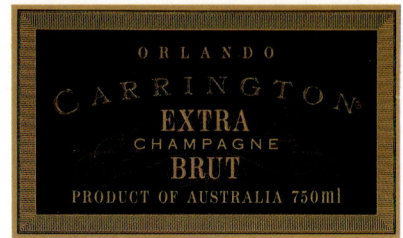

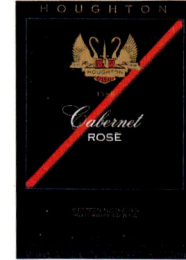

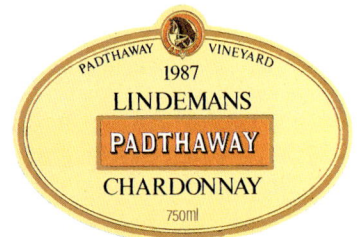

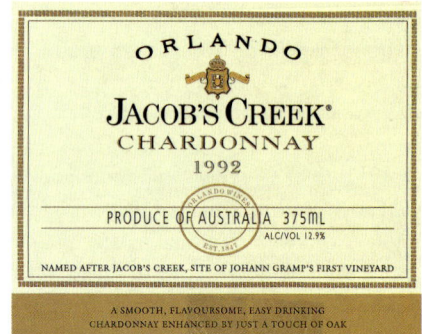

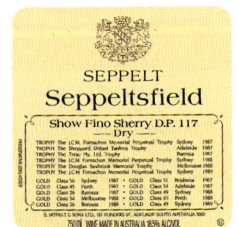

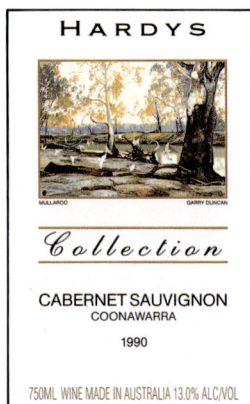

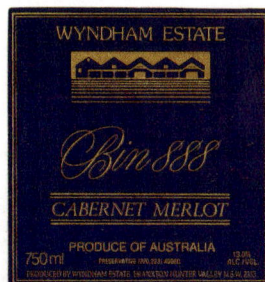

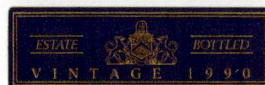

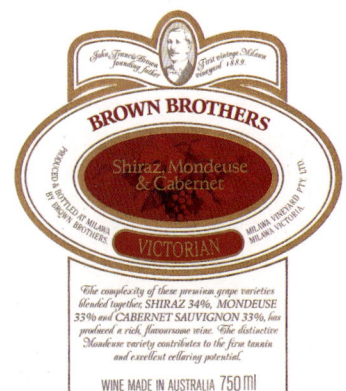

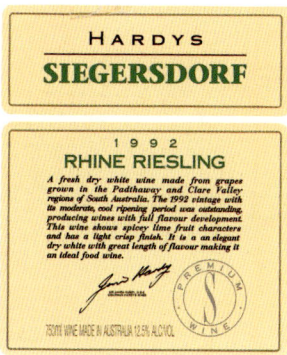

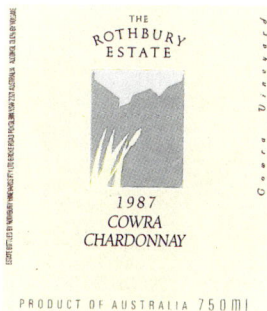

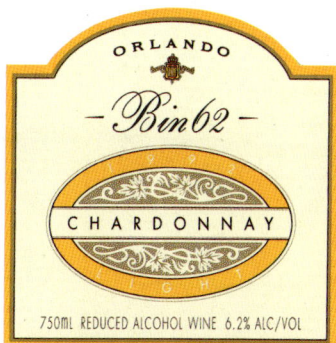

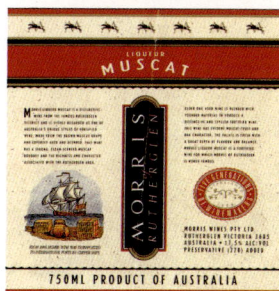

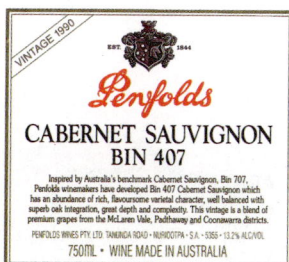

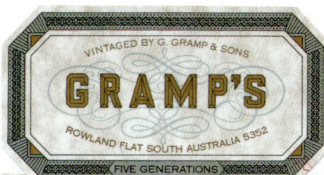

FISH

Baked or grilled whole (snapper, trout, salmon)	*Rhine riesling, white burgundy, chardonnay*
Baked in filo pastry	*Fumé blanc, full-bodied white, semillon, chardonnay*
Fillets in tomatoes & basil	*Rhine riesling, sauvignon blanc*
Crumbed or battered (in beer!)	*Beer – or any of the above*
Ocean trout or salmon	*Dry riesling, or other dry whites*
Poached in white wine with a cream sauce	*Rhine riesling, sauvignon blanc*
Whiting	*Chenin blanc, sauvignon blanc*
Raw fish (*sashimi*)	*Riesling, or a drier white such as Hunter semillon*

SEAFOODS

Calamari, fried	*Sauvignon blanc, Rhine riesling*
Calamari in rich sauce	*Fumé blanc, chardonnay, semillon*
Crayfish salad	*Champagne, riesling, semillon*
Crayfish in rich sauce	*Champagne, white burgundy, chardonnay, or lighter reds if preferred*
Garlic prawns	*Dry whites*
Mussels in tomatoes & basil	*Cabernet/shiraz, pinot noir*
Oysters, natural	*Riesling, chardonnay, chablis, dry champagne*
Oysters, baked	*Chardonnay, semillon*
Smoked salmon	*Chablis, gewurtztraminer*

POULTRY

Chicken breasts in rich sauce	*Dry white, chablis, chardonnay*
Roast chicken	*Chablis, Rhine riesling*
Coq au vin	*Shiraz, cabernet sauvignon, or a blend*
Cold chicken	*Riesling (dry or fruity)*
Crumbed chicken	*Riesling or a light red*
Duck and goose	*Cabernet sauvignon, a red blend such as cabernet/merlot/malbec, or some fuller-bodied whites such as verdelho or a Hunter semillon*

MEAT

Steak, grilled	*Cabernet sauvignon, shiraz*
Steak with béarnaise or other rich sauce	*Young dry red*
Steak hamburgers	*Young shiraz, Coonawarra cabernet*
Grills	*Light to medium reds, shiraz, cabernet, or full-bodied white (chardonnay)*
Beef, roast	*Hermitage, shiraz*
Liver	*Young red, perhaps a pinot noir, lighter shiraz or cabernet*
Kebabs	*Coonawarra reds, rosé*
Veal, roast	*Cabernet sauvignon, cabernet shiraz, pinot noir*
Veal, crumbed	*Dry rosé, light red, medium-bodied chardonnay*
Pork, roast	*Young red or dry white*
Ham, baked	*Burgundy or lighter red*
Ham, cold	*Dry whites (perhaps older riesling)*
Lamb, roast	*Semillon, shiraz, Cabernet sauvignon*
Venison	*Hermitage, cabernet sauvignon, full-bodied red*
Rabbit	*Any good red, cabernet sauvignon, or a cabernet blend*
Cold smoked meats	*Chardonnay, semillon or a light beaujolais-style red, and dry whites*
Pâté, liver-based	*Spätlese (late-picked) Rhine riesling*
Pâté (if served on its own)	*Pinot noir, beaujolais, light red*

BARBECUES

Just about anything !

OTHER DISHES

Pies, meat-based	*Lighter reds, shiraz*
Pies, white-meat-based	*Dry whites, dry riesling*
Chiko rolls	*Frontignac, fruitier whites*
Pasta	*Depends very much on the sauce, but generally dry whites with many seafood-based sauces, reds with meat-based sauces (though it's up to your preference), and light reds are usually good with most pasta dishes*
Soufflé, savoury	*Light dry white or light dry red*
Quiche	*Rosé or dry riesling*
Curry	*Beer is probably best, but if you must drink wine with curry, try a very cold traminer, spätlese or dry rosé*
Chinese food	*Dry Rhine riesling, white burgundy, or possibly champagne*

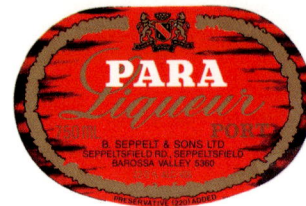

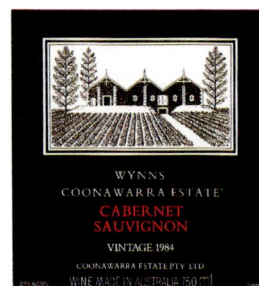

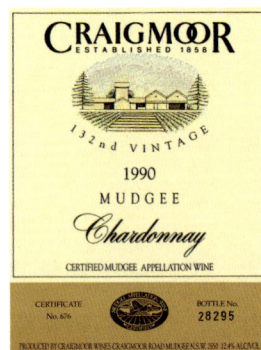

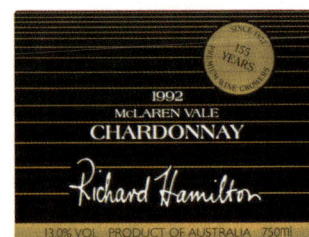

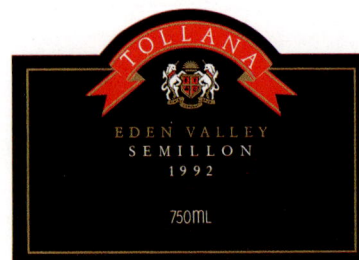

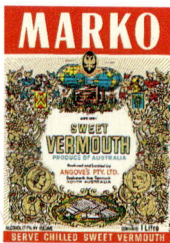

VEGETABLE DISHES

	Mainly whites – not-too-flavoursome good Rhine riesling, lighter dry whites low in (or without) oak ageing
Asparagus	*Try a dry white sauvignon blanc with this 'great challenge'*

(Generally, most luscious sweet wines are excellent with a dessert, and the range is quite extensive. Don't overlook a good old-fashioned muscat or tokay, especially if chocolate is involved in a dish. Lighter ports, or fortified verdelho or sauvignon blanc, are great with rockmelon and ice-cream. The Australian trend towards botrytis-style wines is growing and there is a remarkable range available, particularly from some of the smaller wineries.)

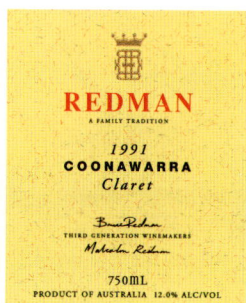

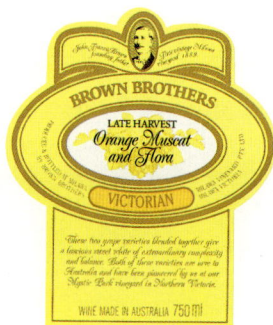

DESSERTS

Soufflés	*Champagne, spätlese Rhine riesling*
Fruits, marinated	*Sauterne, auslese Rhine riesling*
Fruits, fresh	*Dry or medium champagne*
Pastry tarts	*Sweet champagne, botrytis Rhine riesling*
Tortes & trifles	*Spätlese lexia, botrytis Rhine riesling*
Puddings (such as Christmas)	*Vintage or tawny port*
Sorbets or fruit ice-creams	*Spätlese Rhine riesling*
Rich ice-creams	*Difficult to accompany, but try a fruity champagne*

CHEESES

Camembert	*Dry Rhine riesling, semillon*
Fetta	*Dry Rhine riesling, semillon*
Brie	*Soft red, pinot noir, shiraz*
Fruit cheese	*Spätlese Rhine riesling*
Blue-vein	*Cabernet, port, even a good dry sherry*
Gouda	*Shiraz, cabernet, hermitage*
Emmentaler	*Rhine riesling*
Edam	*Chardonnay, semillon*
Gruyère	*White burgundy*
Mozzarella	*Fumé blanc, chablis*
Romano	*Shiraz, cabernet sauvignon*
Pepper cheese	*Cabernet sauvignon, chardonnay*
Leicester	*Burgundy or similar red (a better pinot noir)*
Mild or semi-matured cheddar	*Any good red, such as cabernet; or a dry white*
Vintage cheddar	*Hermitage, cabernet; or a good, strong white like chardonnay or semillon*

It has been more common in Europe than in this country to accompany cheese with a variety of wines; just as it has been to serve cheese and port before a dessert, rather than as the final course. I have a preference – to drink a red through the main course *and* with the cheese.

In Australia there has always been a tendency to accompany cheeses with ports or red wines. However, times are a-changin', and a dinner-party host is more likely to experiment with something completely different, maybe a sweet or more strongly flavoured white wine – a once unheard-of practice! That no doubt has something to do with the decline of the big, rich dessert, often in favour of the cheese-and-fresh-fruit platter – in which case a botrytis-affected 'sticky' white could be a good middle course to steer.

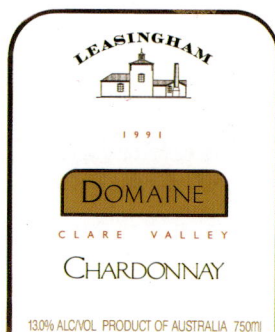

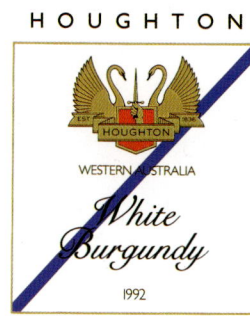

COOKING WITH WINE

Wine is a valuable, even priceless, accessory to cooking. It can be used for tasks as diverse as making dressings (even as the key ingredient in a vinaigrette), adding to stews and casseroles, marinating various foods, on barbecues, in soups, in desserts, on fruit and in fruit salads – in a thousand different ways.

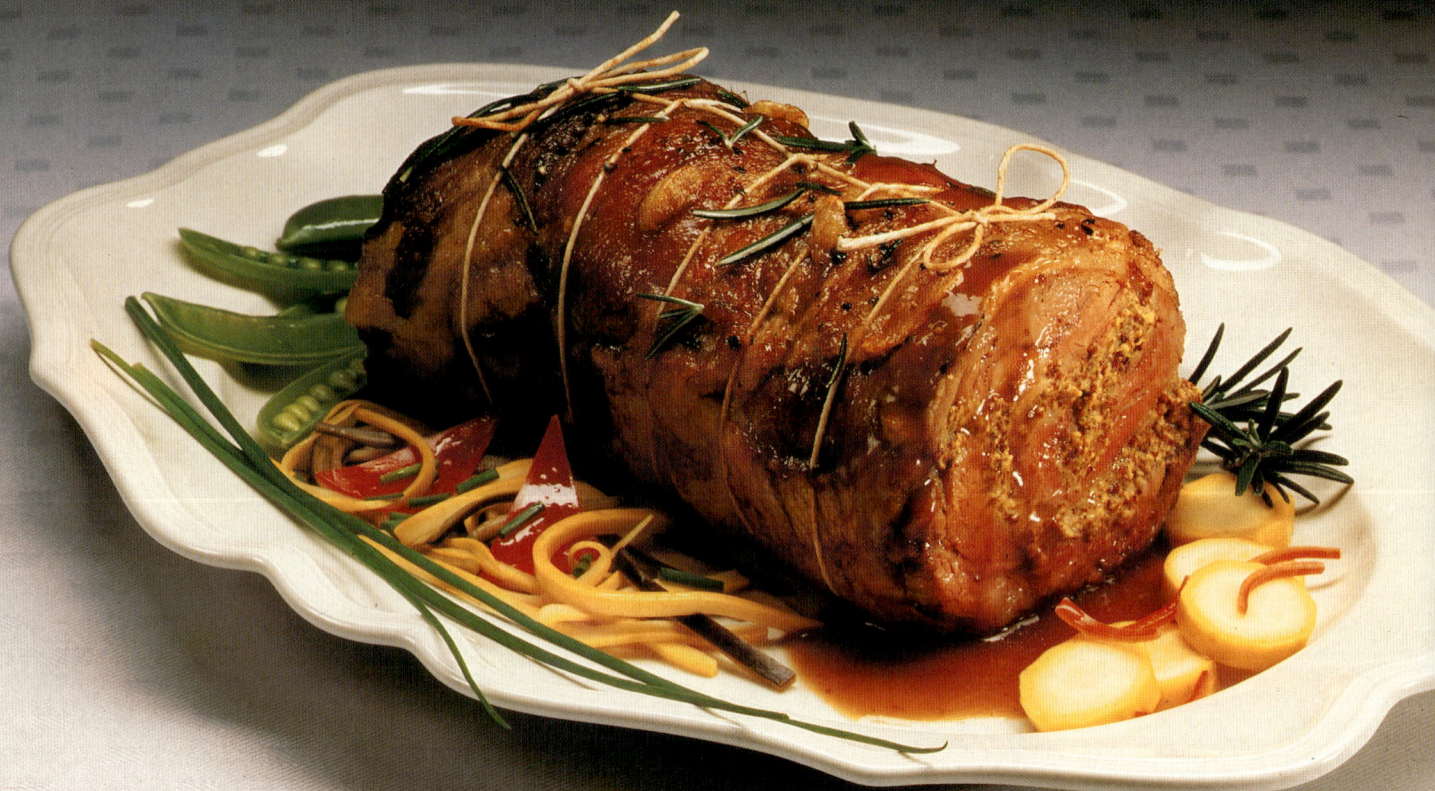

With Beef Wellington, a red wine with a little olive oil and a little onion. (Australian Meat & Live-stock Corp.)

It adds to many dishes, most notably the stew family, an indefinable element of sophistication and 'zing' (as the Italians or French might say with a kiss of the lips!) by the mere application of a small amount of the liquid to the dish at hand.

Using wine to marinate (soak) food is an old, old practice. It has a beneficial effect on the flavour and texture of many dishes, particularly meat dishes.

Marinating in wine tenderises many meats, fish dishes and others — and then goes on to enhance the flavour of the dish as it cooks.

The most common use is to splash some red into casseroles and similar stews, or some white into chicken or veal stews. This is a simple way of noticeably changing both the flavour and the smell of the dish — very much for the better.

It's important to remember several key points, however :

1 The alcohol evaporates quickly in a dish at or near boiling. You are not therefore increasing your alcohol consumption by marinating or adding wine to a dish that is cooking, or about to be cooked. You're only changing (hopefully improving) the flavour outcome. The boiling point of alcohol is considerably lower than that of water, so if your dish is sim-

mering, the alcohol vanishes quite rapidly, leaving the flavour constituents behind.

2 In stews, red wines or sherry or port can be used. Gravies too — they're not a bad graveyard for slightly stale, slightly empty bottles of port!

3 Don't overdo it. Half a cup of wine in most stews is plenty.

4 Splash a little wine (reds on meats, whites on white meats and some fish) on the barbecue plate when cooking. It also enhances flavours.

5 Marinate for as long as you reasonably can; a few hours is better than half an hour. Casseroles can be marinated overnight, in the refrigerator, before being put in the oven (or into the crockpot). And a wee splash of wine, just a tablespoon or so, in the last l0 minutes of cooking, seems to lift the flavour of most dishes.

6 As I've said elsewhere, quality of wine in cooking is important. But most Australian cask and flagon reds are good enough for most cooking purposes. The occasional leftover bottle ends can also be kept (in the fridge, for a few days) and used for cooking. One of the best hints I ever picked up was to add a few drops of cooking oil to a nearly-empty bottle of wine: the thin film of oil which then covers the surface of the wine acts to insulate the wine from further oxidation, so it can be safely used in cooking some days or even a week later, especially if refrigerated.

A little from a bottle you may have chosen to go with your meal is also an easy and practical way of using wine in food; if a bottle holds six good glasses of wine, then half a glass in the cooking (if in fact as much as that is necessary) will not be missed.

Overdoing the amount of wine is a common mistake — too much wine will make many dishes too rich, too wet or will spoil other delicate food flavours. Be careful, too, about the use of woody wines in some delicate foods. Rieslings are often the safe way out with most dishes calling for white wines.

Brandy is one indispensable form of wine that every chef should have in the kitchen cupboard. You don't need a lot, half a bottle (375 ml) is plenty — it will keep for quite a long time, as it is very high in alcohol (almost 40 per cent by volume). And not much is required in most dishes which specify its use.

Brandy is used in many forms of casserole and elsewhere when flaming (flambé) is required, adding a piquancy and richness of flavour which is quite unlike anything else in cooking.

Think about how you can use leftover wines, in the cooking tasks that you have coming up, or can make come up by planning. Just about any wine styles, from dry whites to sweet whites to champagne to fortified wines such as ports, may enhance a dish. For example (just because I happened to look up to my bookshelf and open at random Roger Verge's *Cuisine of the Sun*!), that half bottle of flat champagne left over from last night's party could help make "Cockles with Still Champagne", or the quarter bottle of leftover White Burgundy could help prepare "Rabbit in Jelly from the Moulin de Mougins", or then, of course, the two glasses of Pinot Noir from today's barbecue could make the delicious "Fricassee of Chicken with Wine Vinegar" .... Ah!

Let me pause here to give you an outline of one of the dishes that best encapsulates the advantages wine can bestow on food.

This is a simple yet absolutely delicious dish for a special occasion — perhaps as an entreé or even at a barbecue. I first saw it cooked at The Rothbury Estate by Peter Meier, then Len Evans' right-hand person. It is a little expensive but you don't have to make it as a main course, and it again amply demonstrates the power of wine (or its cousin, brandy) in cooking:

FLAMBÉ PRAWNS IN BRANDY

Buy some green (uncooked) prawns, preferably fairly large ones if you can. Four or five large prawns per person is an ample entreé. Shell them but for the tails, and clean them under running water

Dice some shallots or spring onions, and/or other green vegetables. Get a packet of fresh snow peas and top-and-tail them. You'll also need garlic powder,

chicken cubes and freshly ground pepper.

Use a gas wok or a hot, clean barbecue plate, if you can, otherwise a hot frying pan, smeared with a little margarine or oil, and throw in the diced shallots, then the greens, and cook them quicky. After a minute or two throw in the prawns and season to taste, including the ground pepper and crumbled chicken stock powder.

When the dish is almost done, which takes less than five minutes, toss in a quarter cup of brandy and ignite immediately with a match.

Stir, and when the flame dies down, serve quickly, preferably on white plates to highlight the pink of the prawns and green of the snow peas. (You can also add a little sliced red capsicum to the dish to accentuate the colours, and I like adding either fresh, diced chilli peppers or some chilli paste, but that's up to you.)

The cooking aromas are splendid. Your guests will cheer this bravura — but oh-so-simple — piece of kitchen theatrics!

RECOMMENDED READING : The Australian climate makes outdoor cooking pretty popular with most of us. I use a Weber barbecue kettle, but there are plenty of similar devices around. A very good cookbook and guide for these wonderful gadgets is *The Complete Australian Barbecue Kettle Cookbook* by Ross McDonald and Margaret Kirkwood (sponsored by Weber, printed by Griffin Press, Adelaide).

RECOMMENDED DRINKING: The Penfolds/Wynn/Seaview conglomerate launched two fresh and summery wines in late 1992 — "Alfresco" (a white) and "Pinotfresco" (a red), to be served chilled. These two heavily advertised quaffers take over where Portugal's Mateus Rosé left off (and it's a much over-rated wine). If they're too sweet for you, try a bottle of Peter Lehmann Chardonnay from the Barossa Valley.

WHAT YOU NEED TO ENJOY WINE

Other than a bottle of wine and a modest thirst, you don't need a lot of paraphernalia to enable you to get pleasure from a mouthful of wine. Most of the things you need to enjoy it come as part of your normal bodily equipment, and your tongue and olfactory tastebuds will let you know whether you like the wine or not.
That's why, sometimes, people swill the stuff around in their mouth before swallowing it. It heightens the pleasure, and you'll taste the wine again as it reaches the back of your mouth and the top of your throat (the 'back palate'). That's the simple part, and it comes naturally.

Certain pieces of additional equipment, though, will help you get more pleasure from drinking the stuff, especially in a social environment where most wine is consumed.

Corkscrews and other types of wine bottle openers are the first need, otherwise you won't get a drink at all. The diagram shows the major types of opener now commercially available. The simplest is the T-shaped corkscrew, but you'll often need a lot of force (as high as 80 pounds) to yank the cork from the bottle neck. If this sort of opener happens to be one of those that have the spike at the end to help remove the neck capsule, be careful the sharp bit is facing away from you when you rip the cork out!

Better still is the waiter's friend, so called because it was designed to fit into a waiter's cummerbund or hip pocket. It provides you with the leverage to help you get that cork out.

The best cork extractor is undoubtedly the patented Screwpull, which simply twists with a one-way turn rotation of the handle, and features a plastic-coated and long, computer-designed thread. It almost never fails, even with old and crumbly corks, but is expensive ($25 or so). There is also now a range of Screwpull devices, including a folding Pocket Screwpull model, though it's rather bulky for true pocket use.

Wine glasses are foremost among the necessities for the civilised wine drinker. There's no doubt that good wine glasses will enhance your enjoyment, and you don't need to spend a great deal of money on elaborate glasses.

When you find a good, sensible set of wine glasses you like (preferably, these days, ones which will take some heavy washing up treatment), I think it's wise to buy as many as you can afford. If you think the maximum number of glasses you'll normally use (other than for a big party) is eight, buy a dozen or so; if the number is a dozen, buy 18. Why? Because you will break them or others will help you break them. It's a hassle replacing them six or 12 months down the track, and they may well be superseded by another design so that you can't get them again.

I keep two dozen good wine glasses in my kitchen cupboard, and some special ones in the dining room for extra-special occasions. And some roughies for outdoor use. These days, too, you can buy plastic wine "glasses" which are shaped and feel very much like the real thing, except they won't smash around swimming pools and patios.

Wine glasses come in a wide variety of shapes and sizes. Of them all, though, I prefer the International Standards Organisation's recommended wine-tasting glass. It is classically simple and is fine for serving red or white wine and even champagne. It looks good, is simple and elegant on just about any table and performs the task for which wine glasses were designed: to show the wine off to its best advantage and to let you drink it enjoyably and easily.

Sherry and port glasses should be smaller and can also double up for both purposes. Champagne is best consumed from taller 'flutes'.

Simple is best with wine, so the wine can do the showing off. But your own preference is what you should follow, as everyone has different tastes in glassware, as in just about everything else. I'd only make a couple of points about enhancing wine enjoyment from glasses. One is that most wine glasses show wine off best to the eye, the nose and the mouth if they are slightly or heavily tulip-shaped. This shape allows you to gently swirl the wine around before tasting, concentrating the aromas for you to smell (a pleasurable habit) before tasting and then drinking. That's why wine judges use these for judging wines.

And, most vitally, all wine glasses should be made of clear, transparent glass, not coloured glass. Colour is part of the attraction of all wines, providing a window by which you can assess its age, health and general appearance. Therefore coloured glass should have no part in wine assessment, appreciation or drinking.

Various types of corkscrews

Endless ingenuity has been applied to the mechanical problem of grasping a cork in a bottle and pulling it out without exertion. A straight pull with the bottle between your knees is neither dignified nor necessary: all you need is some sort of leverage against the rim of the bottle. Out of a catalogue of thousands of devices, these are some of the most popular and effective in current use.

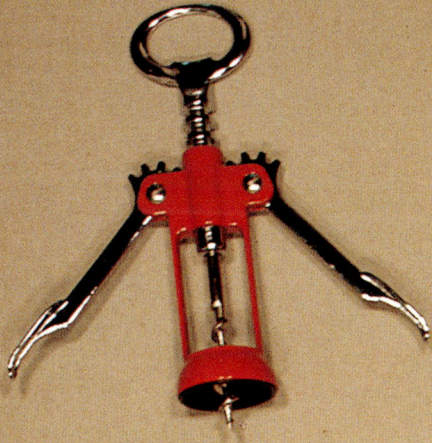

Butterfly

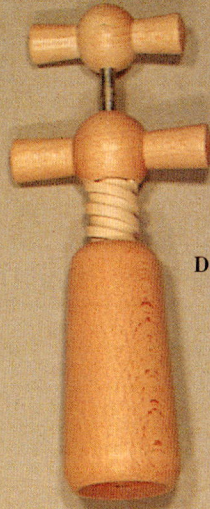

Double-action wood

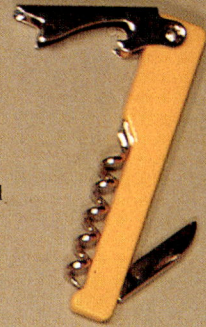

Waiter's friend

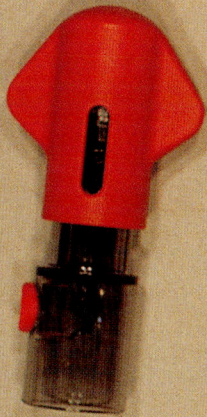

Victorian double spiralled

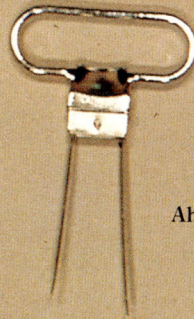

Ah-So

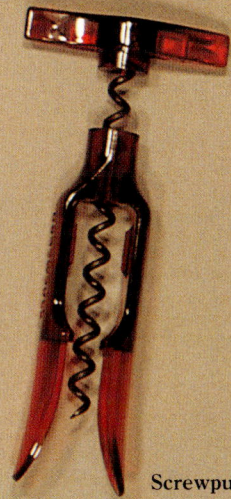

Screwpull

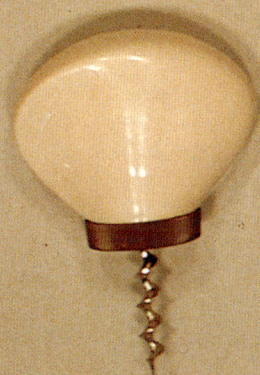

Corkscrew

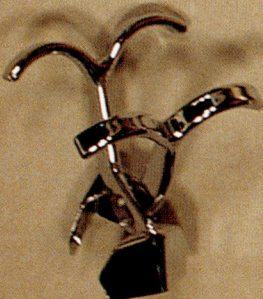

Champagne cork remover

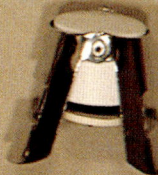

Champagne stopper

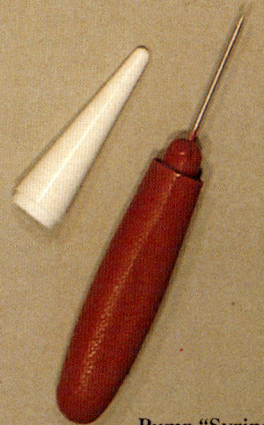

Pump "Syringe" cork popper

Various glass shapes, including the

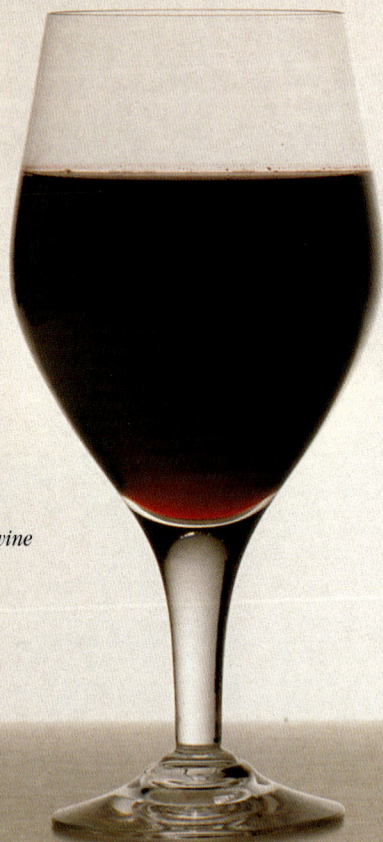

Red wine

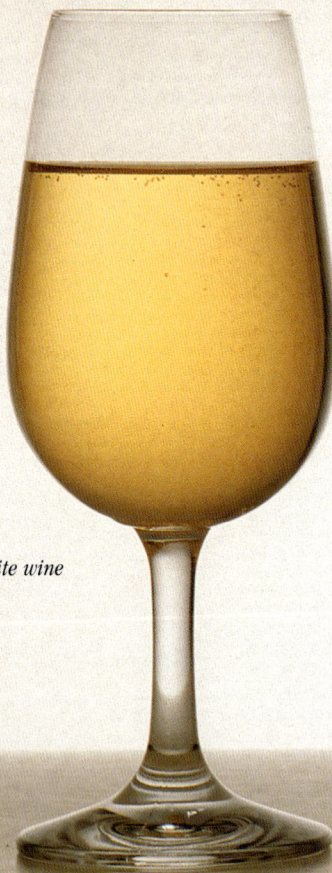

White wine

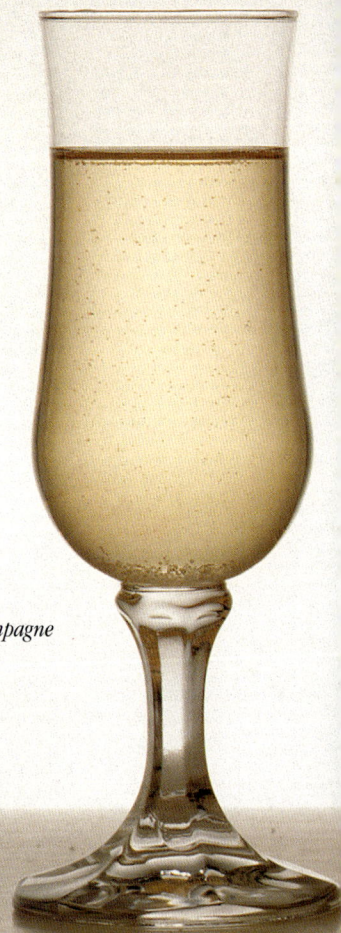

Champagne

SHOULD I DECANT MY WINES?

Decanting is the practice of carefully pouring wine from one bottle to another (perfectly clean) bottle, carafe or decanter. The purpose is to remove any sediment in red or port wines, and to "aerate" the wine. Put simply and straightforwardly, it is seldom necessary to decant, even if a heavy crust of harmless sediment is left in some wines. Leaving the bottle to stand overnight or even for a few hours will enable the sludge to settle to the bottom, and careful pouring will leave it in the bottom of the bottle. I don't subscribe to the idea that wines need to "breathe", though I can't see much harm in letting them do so, either. But some people strenuously disagree with this, especially for older, high-quality wines.

HOW MUCH WINE SHOULD I SERVE — AND HOW?

Never fill glasses of wine more than two-thirds to three-quarters full. Don't refill people's glasses until the glasses are under one quarter full. No one objects to the bottle sitting on the table these days. But perhaps not the cask or the flagon. You can wrap a napkin around the neck if you want, but careful pouring should avoid dripping and spilling. Informality is pretty much the note at today's entertainment. Pass the bottle, please!

WHAT IS THE BEST WAY TO KEEP WINE COOL?

Ice buckets keep them too cold, usually. The modern trend seems to be towards plastic, metal or pottery containers which hold a blanket of cool air around the wine bottle, and these work quite well. It is a fairly unusual bottle of wine that stands on a table for more than half an hour unconsumed, and these will keep it adequately cool if it was brought from a refrigerated cabinet.

champagne 'flute' and the 'tulip'

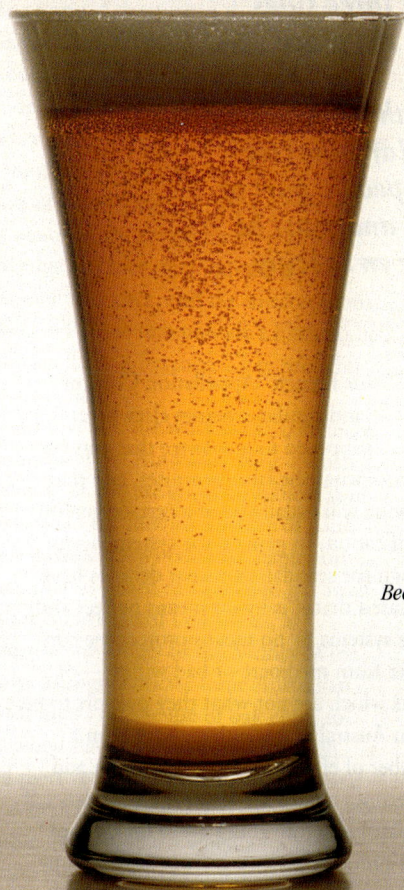

Beer

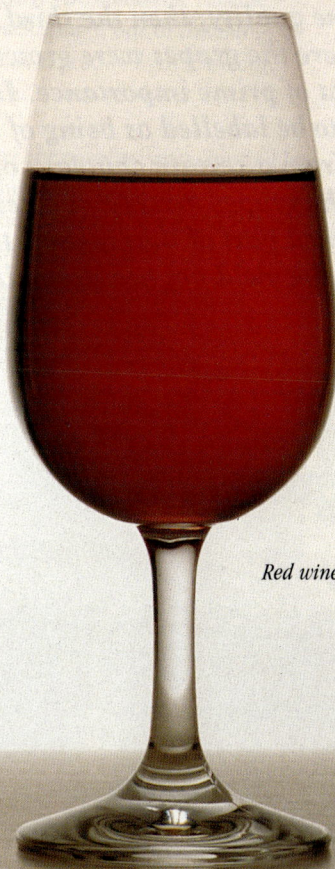

Red wine and rosé

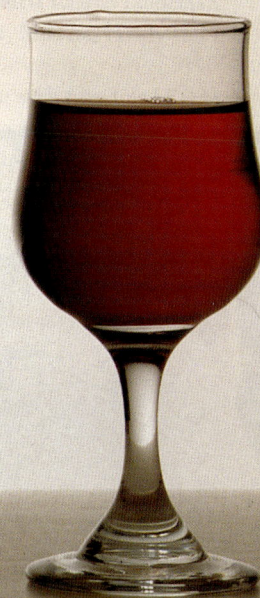

Fortified wines, ports

SOME OTHER USEFUL WINE ACCESSORIES

One I find useful is the champagne bottle sealer. It has a rubber sealer ring at the bottom and two short arms to clasp the thing over the neck opening. Using this, a partly consumed bottle of champagne will last for days or a week in the fridge without losing its bubbles. Another is a simple novelty gadget with a hidden, carved blade, by which you can simply remove the top of the lead or foil neck capsule by rotating it around the top, and so easily get the corkscrew tip to the top of the cork.

One useful device is the Vucu-Vin, a small pump which removes much of the air from a partly-empty bottle through a special rubber cork. Wine so treated can be kept for quite a long time, certainly a week, especially if it is also refrigerated.

Another useful device, available in several forms, wraps around a wine bottle and gives you an instant read-out on the wine's temperature. Handy, but holding the bottle will tell you much the same thing once you've got to know what consumption temperature suits you best for different wines and various seasons.

You can buy many others, such as gadgets to stop bottles dripping. But why bother? Many of these gizmos just get between you and enjoying the wine and, as I've often said, enjoyment is what it's all about.

RECOMMENDED READING: I mentioned winery newsletters earlier, but many of the better wine/liquor retailers put out good to excellent newsletters, and sell wine gadgetry, too. Ask a good 'un near you, and if there isn't one nearby, write or ring one in the major capitals to get on their list — such as Camperdown Cellars, Roseville Cellars and Sheargolds in Sydney; Murphy's and Nicks in Melbourne; Primo Caon's Chesser Cellars in Adelaide; and so on.

RECOMMENDED DRINKING: Try your new champagne cork puller on a bottle of McWilliam's Mount Pleasant Champagne NV Brut, a reasonably priced premium bubbly made from pinot noir and chardonnay in the Hunter Valley. The 'NV' says 'non vintage'.

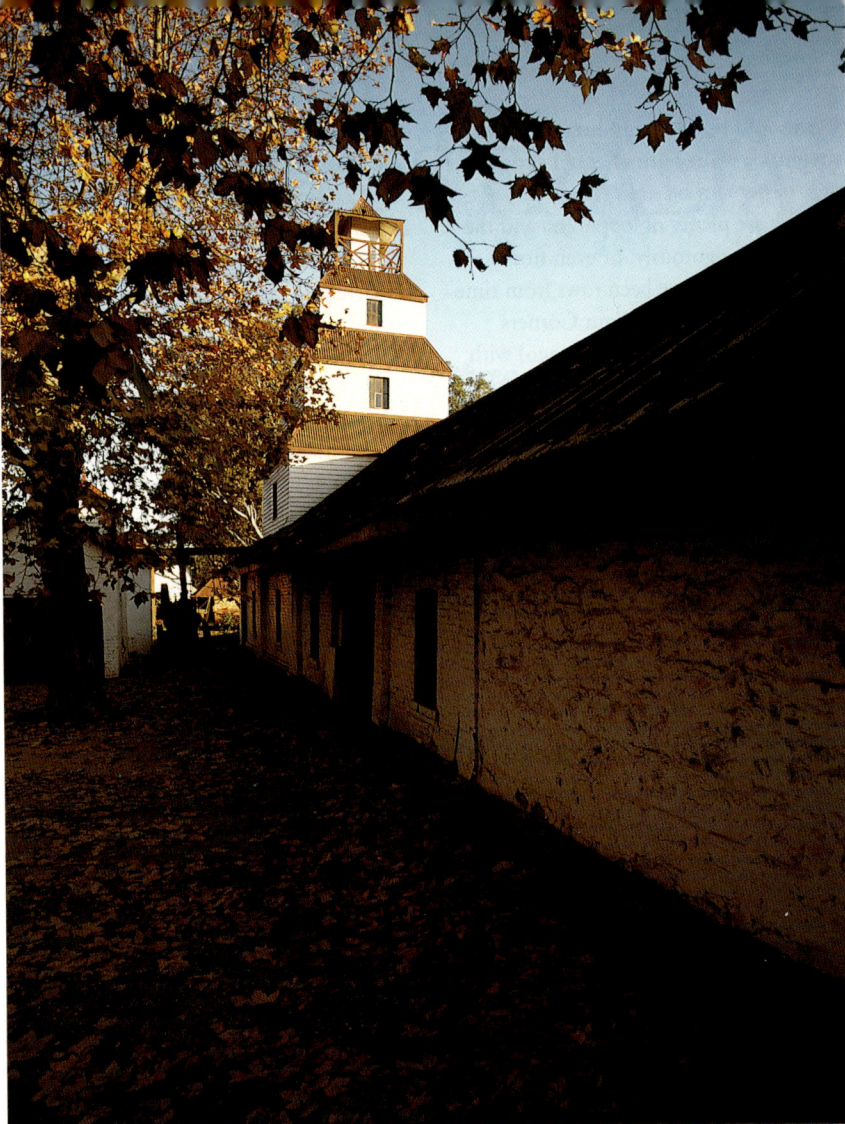

The wooden tower at Chateau Tahbilk in Victoria's lush Goulburn Valley is a local landmark.

on Madeira, thrives in Western Australia.

There's still a tremendous amount of learning to be done, and nature is always teaching us that there is another lesson just around the corner. In Western Australia, for example, millions of silvereye birds feast on the ripe grapes, often destroying the crop. In the Hunter Valley it often pours with rain at harvest time, introducing diseases like Downy Mildew and making access difficult or impossible for the tractors. In Coonawarra and Padthaway, in the run up to the 1988 vintage, devastating frosts descended on the immature fruit hanging on the vines, burning much of it off; not long afterwards, fierce storms swept through the Barossa and Riverland areas. I can remember talking to wine-maker David Watson of Woodlands Wines in the Margaret River area of Western Australia, while researching The Pocket Australian Wine Companion, who said that the kangaroos kept eating his ripe cabernet franc and merlot grapes! Grape-growing wasn't meant to be easy.

THE REGIONS

Why does it matter where the grapes for a particular wine come from? Well, in some cases, it doesn't matter at all, as I've said. Many of the big brand names don't specify where they source (get) the grapes.

Orlando would like us to believe, though they don't outrightly say so, they get all of the grapes for Jacob's Creek Claret from the Jacob's Creek Vineyard (signposted "Home of Jacob's Creek" alongside the main road through the Barossa Valley). But of course the brand is far too big for that and a lot of the grapes come from the generous S.A. Riverland — and elsewhere. Ditto to Wolf Blass Yellow Label, his biggest selling red wine. Hardy's Siegersdorf Rhine Riesling is no longer produced at their Siegersdorf Winery in the Barossa, where the brand first emerged. And Tyrrell's Long Flat Red presumably has some fruit from the Long Flat vineyard — but the Flat is certainly not

long enough to provide 100 per cent of this popular red. And no one would believe that Wynn's Seaview Cabernet Sauvignon still comes from the old Seaview winery at McLaren Vale ...

But none of this really matters, because in all the instances mentioned above, the wines are of excellent commercial quality and you know what you're going to get when you order a bottle at a restaurant. Consistency and drinkability are the names of this game — not places of origin.

If, however, you take the next step and get interested enough in drinking or collecting wine, the vineyard and the source of the wine almost certainly will interest you. In some cases it can even be a virtual guarantee that you'll get a great wine. Several examples spring easily to mind: Orlando's wonderful rieslings from their Steingarten Vineyard, high above the Barossa; Cape Mentelle's super cabernets from David Hohnen's Margaret River vineyards, and the excellent chardonnays emerging from James Halliday's

Coldstream Hills vineyard in the Yarra Valley near Melbourne ... And there are plenty of others, people who obey the letter and the spirit of the laws and conventions of wine.

There are now around 40 distinct wine-growing regions of Australia, some of them sub-regions of others. As I said, just a little knowledge of them will greatly enhance your enjoyment because climate, soil and local factors profoundly affect the taste of the end product.

Let's take a walk, then, through some of the better-known regions and some of their wines. If you're planning a visit to any of them, a copy of The Pocket Australian Wine Companion (Reed Books) will provide full details of cellar door times, phone numbers, credit card acceptance and a host of other facts about them, their owners, makers, services and products. That small book lists all of the wine areas and all wineries; what follows is a thumbnail sketch of some of the key areas around Australia.

VICTORIA

Victoria was to be "John Bull's Vineyard" and indeed its soils and climate generally seem to resemble many of those of Europe. That was the latter half of the 19th century, when wineries flourished in many regions of Victoria. Then the vine disease phylloxera struck, doubtless imported from Europe in soil clinging to the roots of the many vine cuttings.

This microscopic root louse swept through Victoria's vineyards like the plague, and no remedy — not flooding, smoking or poisoning — would stop it. Many vineyards and wineries disappeared, not to re-emerge until the 1970s and 1980s, as interest in wine, especially quality wine, rekindled. A number of wineries carried on through the intervening years — notably Great Western, Chateau Tahbilk and some in the Milawa/Rutherglen areas, such as Brown Brothers, Morris and Campbells.

Today Victoria is emerging strongly as a most vibrant wine State. In researching The Pocket Australian Wine Companion, we counted 126 wineries in the State, second only to South Australia (155), but Victoria is still growing fast and turning out some exceptional red, white, sparkling and traditional fortified wines. They come from makers including Mitchelton, Seppelt, Balgownie, Brown Brothers, Chateau Tahbilk, Campbells, St Huberts and Mildara, plus a host of smaller makers such as Virgin Hills, Taltarni, Hanging Rock and Coldstream Hills.

Murray Valley

The Pocket Companion divides Victoria into these areas : Central and Southern (centred on Bendigo); East Gippsland; Geelong; Goulburn Valley; Great Western; Macedon; Mornington Peninsula; Murray Valley; North-East (Rutherglen and Milawa etc); Pyrenees; Yarra Valley. Like many such divisions, they are rather arbitrary. For instance, the Murray Valley is an enormous area, including wineries as diverse as Bests family wineries and as huge as the juice factories of Lindeman's Karadoc and Stanley's (owned by BRL Hardy) Buronga plants, which depend on the irrigated Sunraysia district for the fruit for their big selling bottled wines and casks.

Among the wines from this area worth a look are those of the Big Three: Lindeman's at Karadoc, Mildara at Merbein and the more anonymous presence across the river and the border of the Stanley Wine Company.

The North East

Heading way upriver to North East Victoria, here is a diverse and very fascinating wine area of Australia. I include Milawa in this general area, even though it is about an hour's drive away, and this brings the extremely diverse wines of Brown Brothers into the area. The area is generally a hot one, hence ideal for the production of some of the world's great fortified wines, but the Browns, among others, encourage vineyard development in some of the higher areas, and along some of the nearby valleys (King and Ovens), which produce excellent fruit.

Of all of the Victorian areas, the North East offers the best and most diverse area for visitors — and for absentee tasters! Unlike many of the Victorian areas, which have only a handful of wineries, often scattered widely, here there are plenty of wineries and lots of different wines and makers to try, all within a reasonable radius within the general Rutherglen-Glenrowan-Milawa triangle. The scenery, too, is outstanding.

In the Rutherglen area you can taste a very wide diversity of products from the superb dessert muscats and tokays of Morris (and Chambers, Campbells, All Saints, Baileys and Bullers) through to

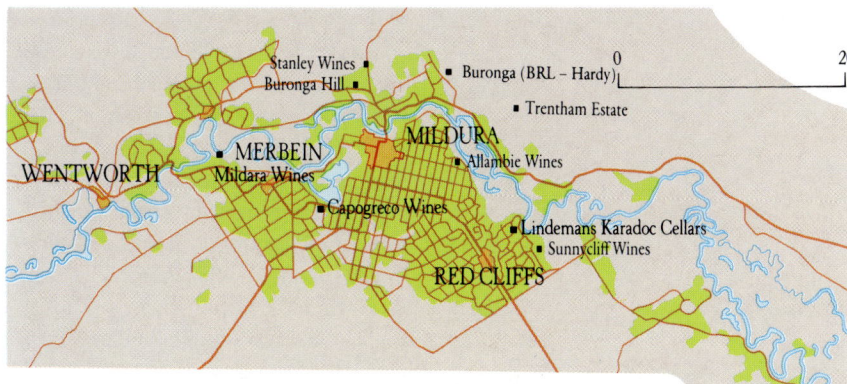

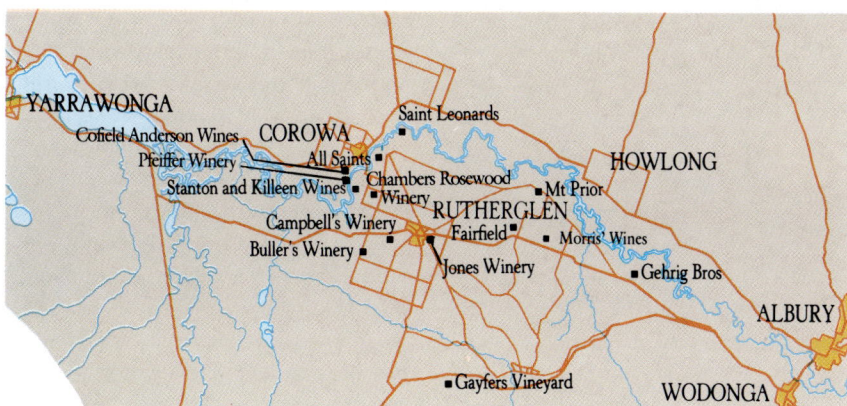

GOULBURN VALLEY

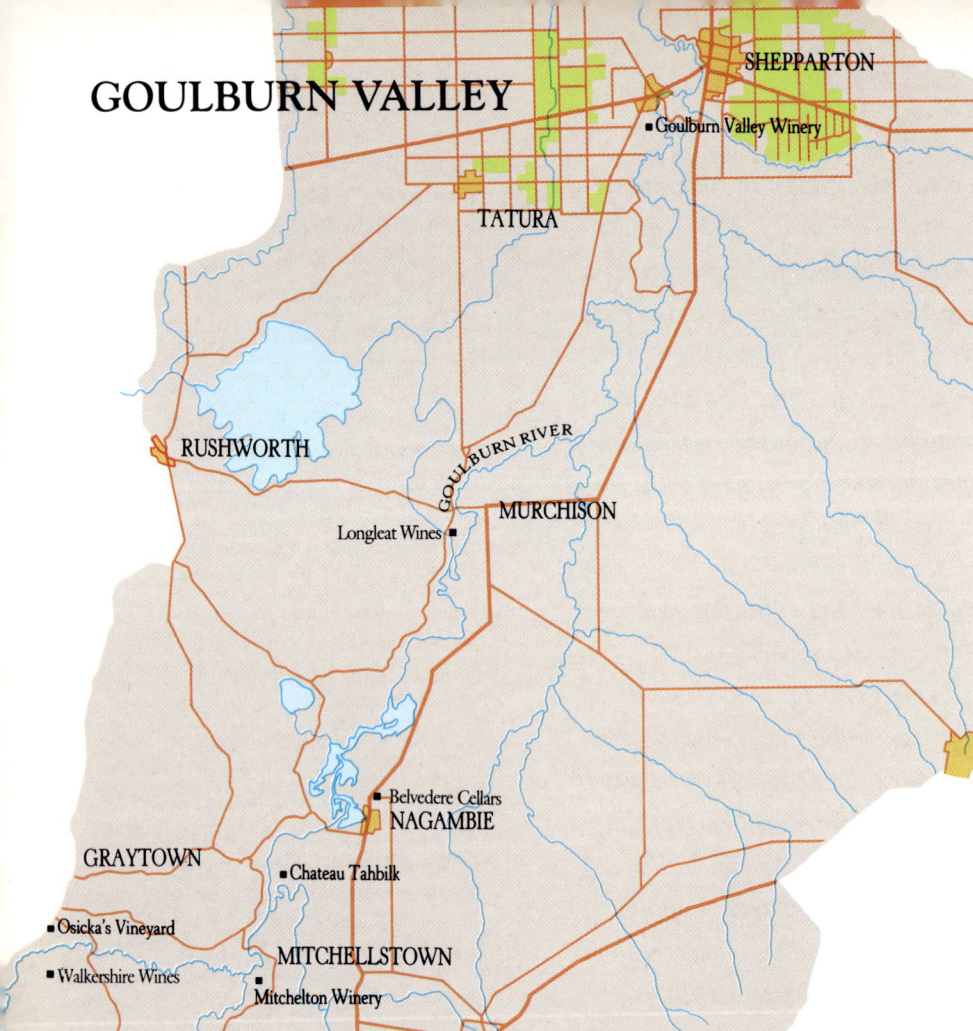

SHEPPARTON

■ Goulburn Valley Winery

TATURA

GOULBURN RIVER

RUSHWORTH

Longleat Wines ■

MURCHISON

GRAYTOWN

Belvedere Cellars ■
NAGAMBIE

■ Chateau Tahbilk

■ Osicka's Vineyard

MITCHELLSTOWN

■ Walkershire Wines

■ Mitchelton Winery

STAWELL

Donaview Wines ■

HALLS GAP

GREAT
WESTERN

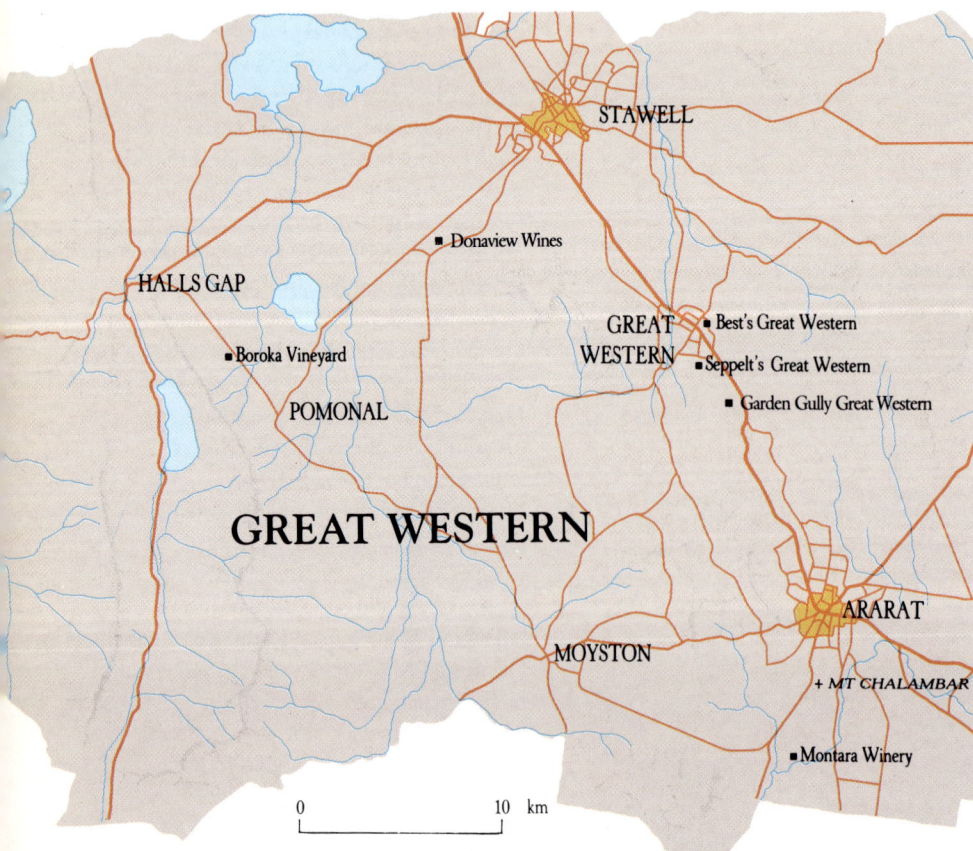

■ Best's Great Western

Boroka Vineyard ■

■ Seppelt's Great Western

POMONAL

■ Garden Gully Great Western

GREAT WESTERN

ARARAT

MOYSTON

+ MT CHALAMBAR

■ Montara Winery

0   10 km

some good chardonnays (Morris, St Leonards, Pfeiffer) and reds (Chambers, HJT, Pfeiffer). The climate leans the reds towards the bigger style, and if you want to see what I mean, try Morris Durif, and some of the local cabernet and shiraz wines.

Goulburn Valley

To the south towards Melbourne lies the Goulburn Valley, scenic and with its historic vineyards. The two most recognisable vineyards, Chateau Tahbilk and Mitchelton, both have symbolic towers though they are poles apart in wine styles and physical appearance. Tahbilk dates from 1860 and Mitchelton from 1969. Cabernet and shiraz appear to do well along this river valley, and it is on traditional and unusually long-lived reds that Chateau Tahbilk has made its name. Mitchelton, with its trademark modern tower, has made some lighter-style reds and some very good whites which have done well in wine shows. Both makers produce Marsanne whites, which I have mentioned elsewhere, and both are worth a visit or if you can't get there, their wines are worth trying.

Great Western

South and west a few hours' drive are two other regions, one traditional and one newer but fast gaining appreciation. Great Western is famous, of course, for the sparkling wine of that name made here by Seppelt. The name comes from a small town of that name, just a few hours' drive from Melbourne. What is less recognised is that from the surrounding vineyards, Seppelt (based in Adelaide and now owned not by the Seppelt family but by SA Brewing Holdings Limited) also make some very good table wines, reds and whites, from fruit from this Central Victorian district. They are wines worth seeking out, as are some of the wines from the other major local maker in the Great Western District, Bests.

To those new to wine enjoyment, Seppelt also make a range, or family, of Great Western sparkling wines, running through various price and quality levels. As the grape varieties chardonnay and pinot noir become more common in our vine-

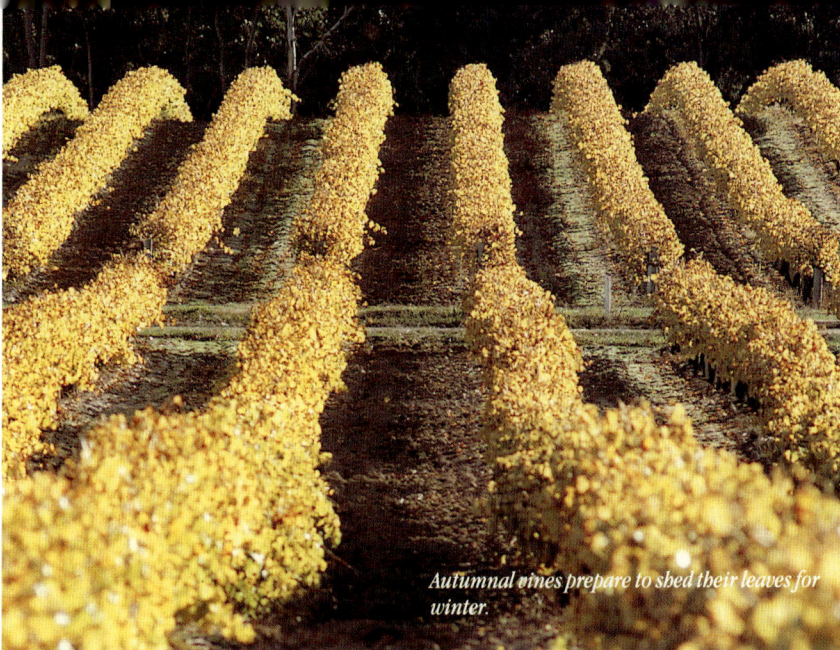

Autumnal vines prepare to shed their leaves for winter.

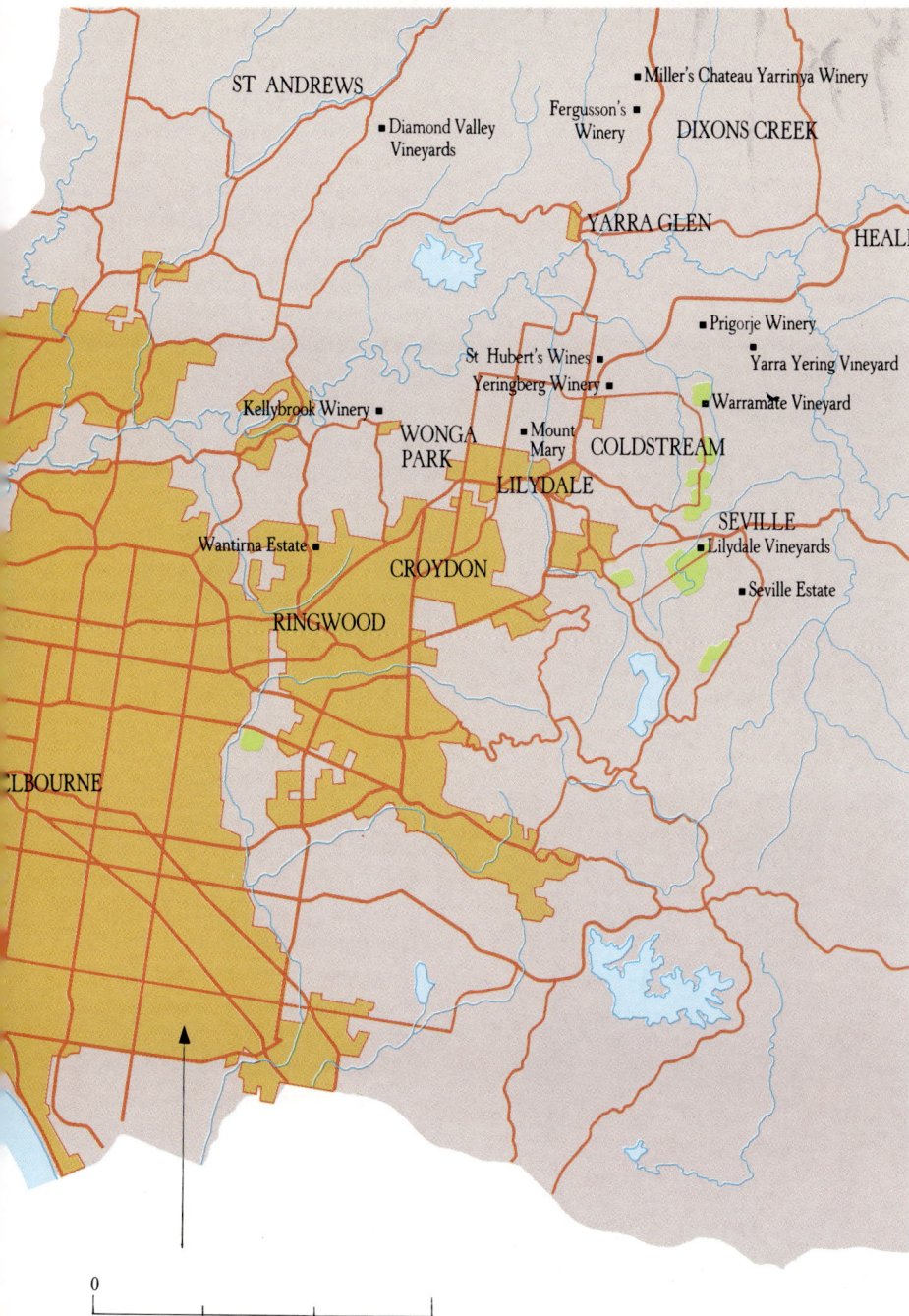

ST ANDREWS

■ Diamond Valley Vineyards

Fergusson's ■ Winery

■ Miller's Chateau Yarrinya Winery

DIXONS CREEK

YARRA GLEN

HEAL

Kellybrook Winery ■

St Hubert's Wines ■
Yeringberg Winery ■

■ Prigorje Winery

Yarra Yering Vineyard

■ Warramate Vineyard

WONGA PARK

■ Mount Mary

COLDSTREAM

LILYDALE

SEVILLE

Wantirna Estate ■

CROYDON

■ Lilydale Vineyards

■ Seville Estate

RINGWOOD

LBOURNE

0

yards, so the sparkling wines of Australia get better. One of the best improvers in this handicap race (with champagne itself as the finishing post) has been Seppelt. Among their Great Western products are some of the best sparkling wines made in this country, and they are worth seeking out, either for interest or for special occasions. Or maybe just for pleasure.

Central Victoria

The area of Central Victoria, centred on an axis between Ballarat and Bendigo and extending westwards to Moonambel and eastwards to Heathcote, has scattered through its rugged region some small wineries (and some not-so-small), making some marvellous wines. Taltarni, Warrenmang, Passing Clouds, Chateau Le Amon, Balgownie, Knights and Yellowglen have all produced some excellent wines, mainly reds but some whites and sparkling wines. I have a feeling it is from this greater region that we will see some of the best Victorian wines emerge, though it may take several decades to happen.

Yarra Valley

Much closer to Melbourne — in fact almost in its outer north-eastern suburbs — is the Yarra Valley, scene of some wine triumphs in the middle of the 19th century and now coming back to form as a premium wine-growing area. The cool climate and the soils seem eminently suited to producing high-quality dry reds and whites such as cabernet, pinot noir and chardonnay and, while these wines are necessarily expensive, they are, for the most part, exciting wines. Makers who stand out — all of them fairly small — are St Hubert, Coldstream Hills, Yarra Yering, Yeringberg and Seville Estate.

Other Areas

Several other areas surround Melbourne at various distances, and most of their wines are hard to find outside Melbourne itself. Geelong, the Mornington Peninsula and Macedon all seem suited to producing good to very good table wines, though again the economies of scale make the final products sit at the expensive end of the scale.

New South Wales

One cannot take a viticultural tour of Australia without looking to the Hunter Valley. Because it was settled so early (the 1830s) and because of its proximity to Sydney (160 km for the Lower Hunter district), it has assumed a place in the Australian wine scene far out of proportion to the percentage of Australian wine grown annually (around 2 per cent).

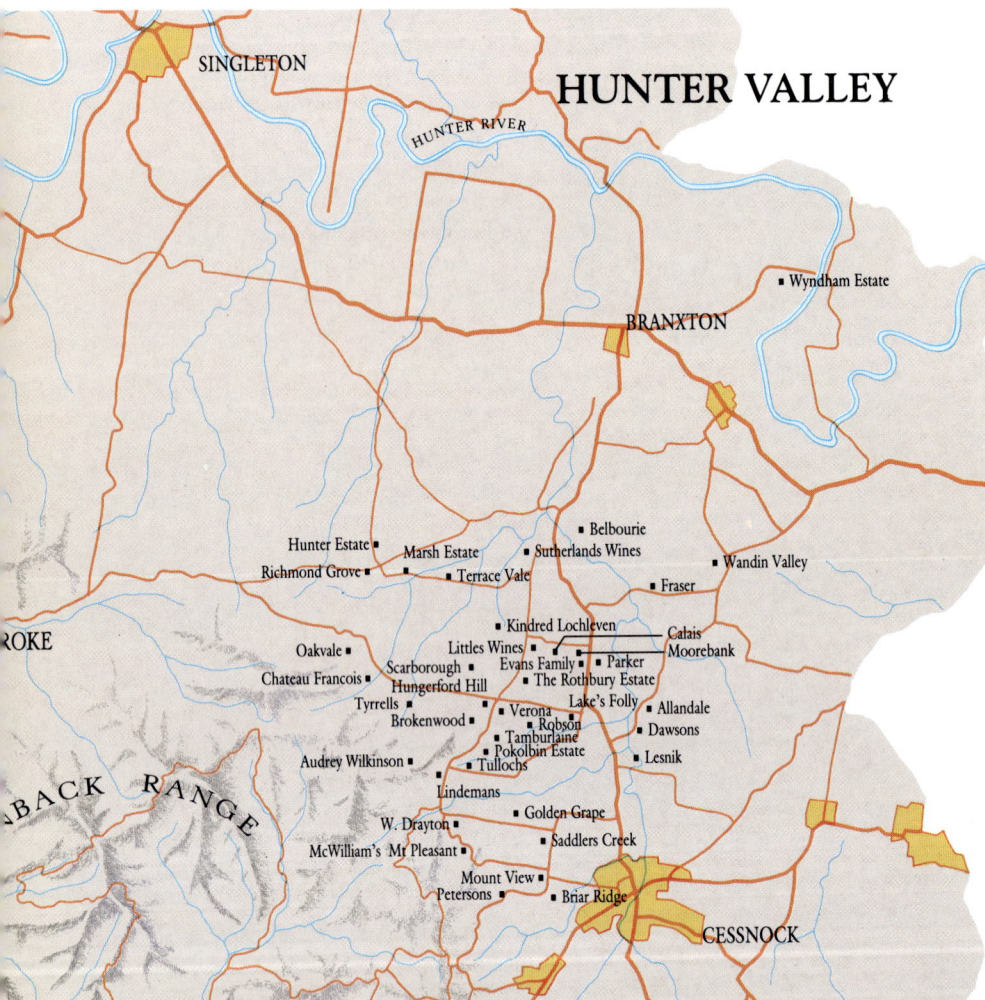

HUNTER VALLEY

Historic reminders for winemakers of harder times gone by.

The Hunter Valley

The paradox of the Lower Hunter is that the wines it makes most excellently are not really the wines that most Australian drinkers enjoy today. As I've said, riesling (or similarly aromatic wines) is the flavour most "ordinary" Australians tend to like, and the Hunter is not good at growing riesling (though the Upper Hunter has made some very good ones).

The Pokolbin region has historically grown two grape varieties well, and may now be adding several others to its quiver. The classic two are semillon, originally inaccurately known as 'Hunter River Riesling', and shiraz (hermitage). More recently, chardonnay has performed creditably here, with evidence that cabernet sauvignon can do quite well, too.

The problem is that most Hunter semillons are not at their best when young, and need at least three, and preferably more, years to age into the great white wines for which this district is rightly famed. With age, these wines gracefully acquire golden colour and delicious, honeyed flavours. Sometimes you'd swear that they are wood-matured, when often they are not. Few people these days have the patience, the capital or the cellar to keep Hunter semillons for five years or more to see them reach their peak drinkability, which is a great, but understandable, pity.

The better makers of Hunter semillons (and indeed most of the better Hunter whites and reds) are Lindeman's (whose wines are quite outstanding), Tyrrell's, The Rothbury Estate, Tulloch, Brokenwood and McWilliam's. The largest maker in the Hunter Valley is the Wyndham Group, which controls the Wyndham Estate winery, on the banks of the Hunter, near Branxton; the Hermitage Winery, Saxonvale, Richmond Grove; and the Mudgee wineries Montrose, Amberton and Craigmoor. The Orlando group, based in Adelaide, owns Wyndham and Montrose.

Because of soil and climate, the Hunter reds (generally hermitage, but in recent years pinot noir and cabernet have improved) tend to be big-bodied wines. Among the greatest and biggest-bodied are some made by Lindeman's from dry years — for example 1965, some of which are

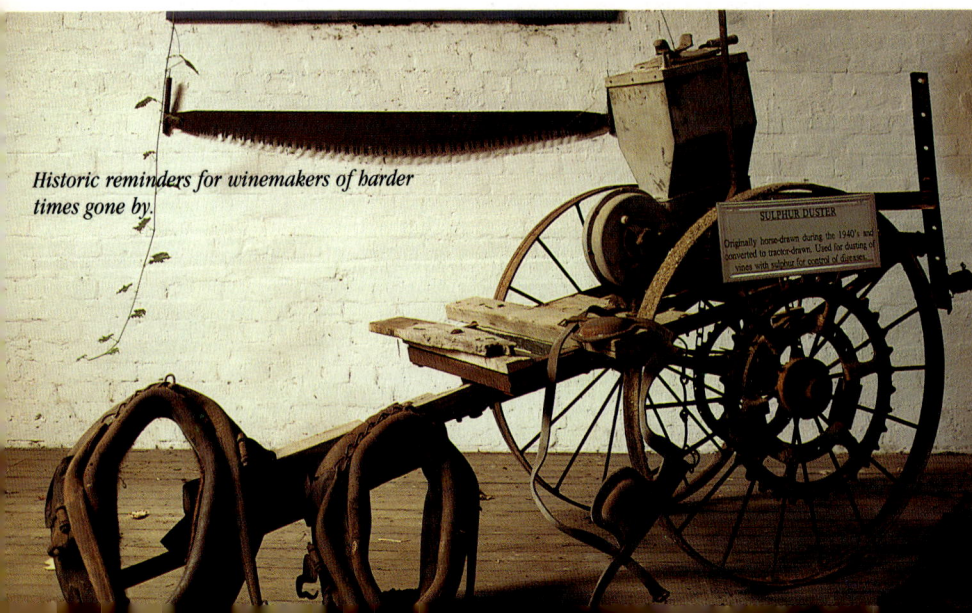

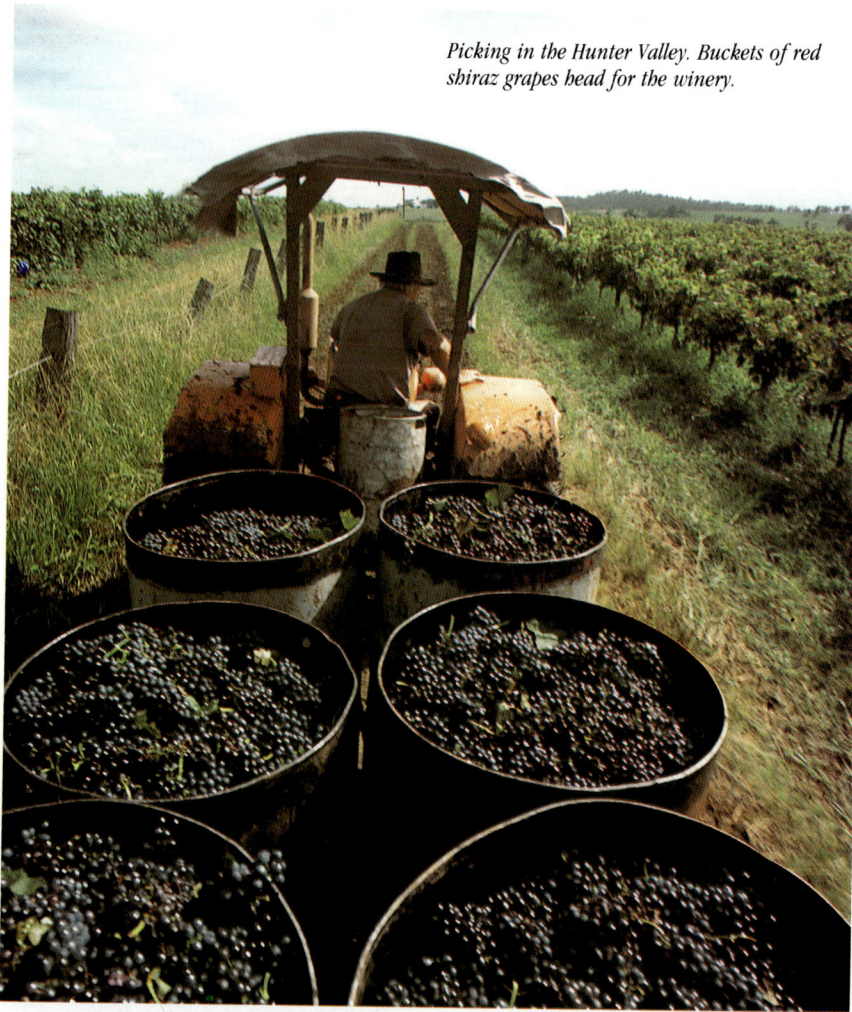

Picking in the Hunter Valley. Buckets of red shiraz grapes head for the winery.

is a rather more up-market destination, but if you are seriously interested in wine, then it's a must stopover, as this winery makes some great Hunter (and other) wines, and they will help you learn about them (and many other world wines) through some of their superb dinners and other events in the magnificent Rothbury Estate Great Hall. Joining the Rothbury Estate Society is as simple as buying a few cases of their wine annually, and it really is worth getting involved.

Of course, there are many other, smaller wineries around the lower Hunter district. Some make some very good wines indeed (for example, Chateau Francois), and are worth exploring. The Hunter now has some excellent accommodation, and restaurants, and the roads from Sydney are now good, for the most part, and the drive is just over two hours. The Hunter is a fun place to while away a couple of days or stay for a week.

Upper Hunter Valley

The Upper Hunter Valley is, as the name suggests, further up the winding reaches of the Hunter River. It is a much newer wine region, and has extensive vineyards, though the wineries are not as well known as those of the lower Hunter (or Pokolbin) region.

The best known winery is Rosemount Estate, producing one of Australia's better-known chardonnays. Rosemount's Roxburgh Chardonnay, in particular, is worth seeking out — a rich, buttery wine of tremendous depth of flavour which has wowed the wine critics overseas, particularly in the United States and the United Kingdom. Arrowfield, at the entrance to the region, is another large maker. There are some good smaller makers, but distance is a problem, and they are far-flung. I suspect that in a few decades we will be hearing a lot more about this district, but it will take one or more large makers (or investors) to move in again to put the Upper Hunter on the map in big type.

Riesling seems to grow here far better than in the Lower Hunter, an hour or two away by car, and so does chardonnay. As is often the way, where white wine varieties thrive, reds seem to falter, and I cannot

still around, at premium prices, of course.

While the Hunter specialises in making good dry reds and dry whites, you can certainly buy and taste many other wines there, sometimes wines from other districts. For example, Rothbury makes a very good chardonnay from vineyards in the Cowra district of central New South Wales; Hungerford Hill some excellent Coonawarra wines; Tyrrell's (among others) have access to large volumes of Upper Hunter fruit; and most major makers here sell a wide range of fortified and even pop wines to cater for all tastes. McWilliams is another large winery, on the slopes of Mt Pleasant, offering a wide range of good wines at fair prices.

I am not convinced, as some suggest, that chardonnay has found another 'natural home' in the Hunter. Tyrrell's Vat 47 Chardonnay is the exception that perhaps proves the rule. Hunter chardonnays from Lindeman's have been a rare disappointment from this magnificent maker, and the chardonnays of Dr Max Lake and oth-

ers have left me cold. Perhaps I need re-education, but I don't think so, and I suspect that's why many major Hunter makers are buying in chardonnay fruit from elsewhere.

Like the Barossa Valley in South Australia, also a highly visible wine/tourism destination, the Hunter has changed considerably in the past decade. But so has the Australian wine industry as a whole. Hunter makers have realised that they must give drinkers what they want — rather than what wine-makers think that the public wants, or what is convenient to produce. The survivors in an area which is a difficult wine-growing district (as are many of the other great wine-growing districts of the world) manage to do this, and the ones who stand out as good and consistent performers who know what wine drinkers like are the Wyndham Estate, Tyrrells and Hungerford Hill (now owned by Brian McGuigan's company).

The Rothbury Estate, with Len Evans as its resident and entertaining Chairman,

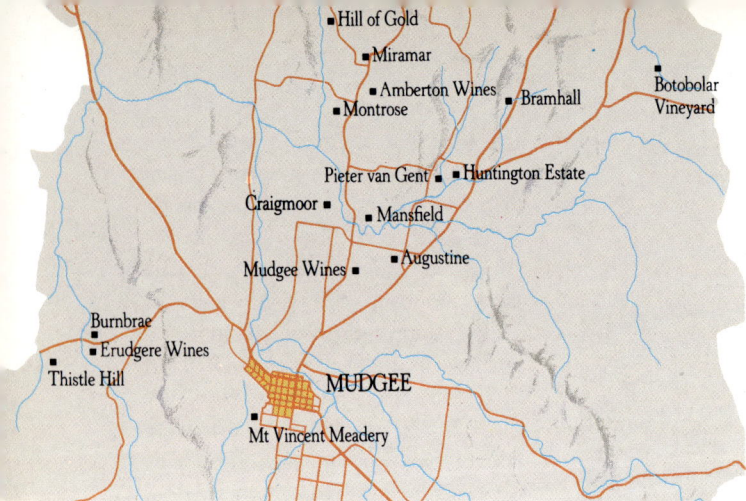

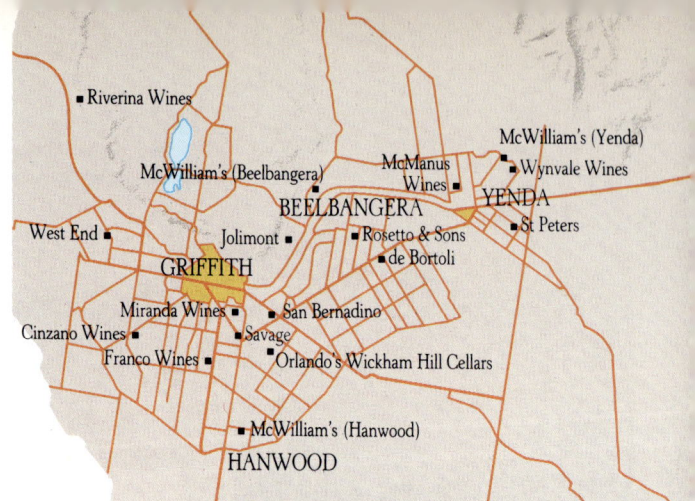

recall really enjoying many Upper Hunter reds. Perhaps that is why Rosemount has invested heavily in Coonawarra, in far-away South Australia, and they make some good Coonawarra reds.

The Upper Hunter, centred on the large town of Muswellbrook, is a district worth visiting if you have time up your sleeve, as the scenery is splendid, the picnic spots abound, the driving is enjoyable and the blue hills roll off into the distance. You can go through to Mudgee from here on the way from the Lower Hunter region, if you really want to do a winery crawl! You can also find some very good wines and some fun times at some of the smaller wineries.

which make impressive wines. Reds seem to be better than whites, though I have tried some exceptional semillons from Huntington Estate.

Botobolar, run by former journalist Gil Wahlquist and his wife Vincie, is an intriguing winery, operated on organic principles. It epitomises the pleasure, involvement and information you can get by taking time and trouble to meet the wine-maker on his/her home ground, to hear what they do and why they do it. And then taste the products.

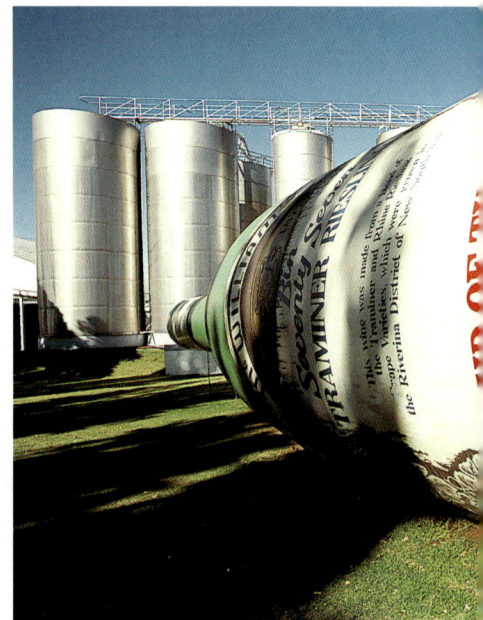

Mudgee

This 'bowl in the hills', further inland from the Hunter Valley, is also a smaller district, but some good and improving wines have emerged from the Mudgee area recently and now, with the interest of at least one major maker — the Wyndham Estate — focused on it, the leap into greater national wine promi-nence may be imminent.

The Wyndham Estate bought the Montrose Group in mid-1988. But even before the takeover, some very good wines were emerging from the winery. This is the largest winery in the area, with the Montrose winery itself, historic Craigmoor and smaller Amberton as part of the group, which is now in the Orlando Wyndham operation.

Scattered around the delightful town of Mudgee are a number of other, smaller wineries. They include Botobolar, Huntington Estate and Miramar, all of

Tending the vines and keeping the weeds and insects under control is a year-round series of chores for the viticulturist.

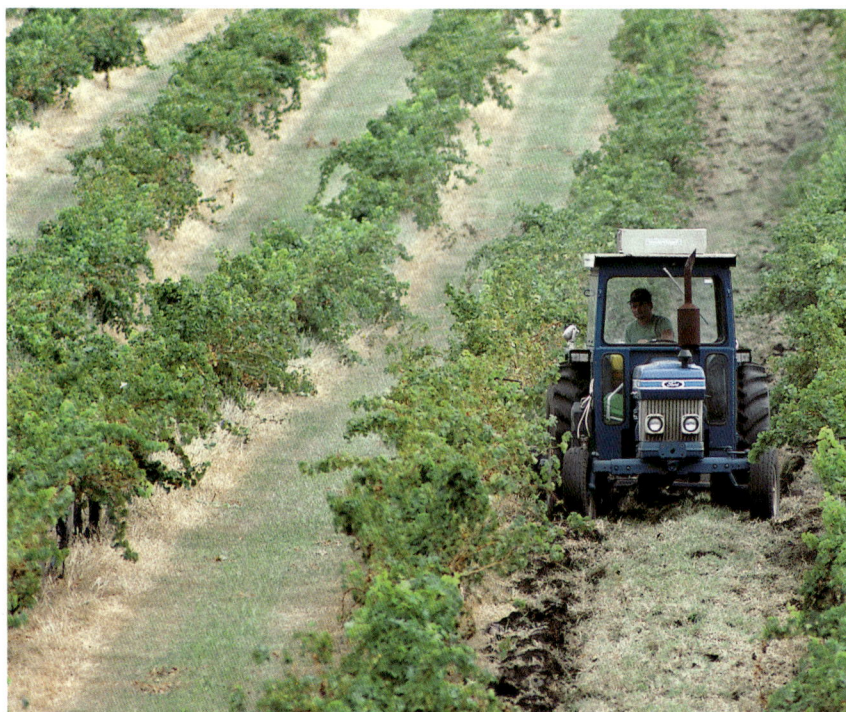

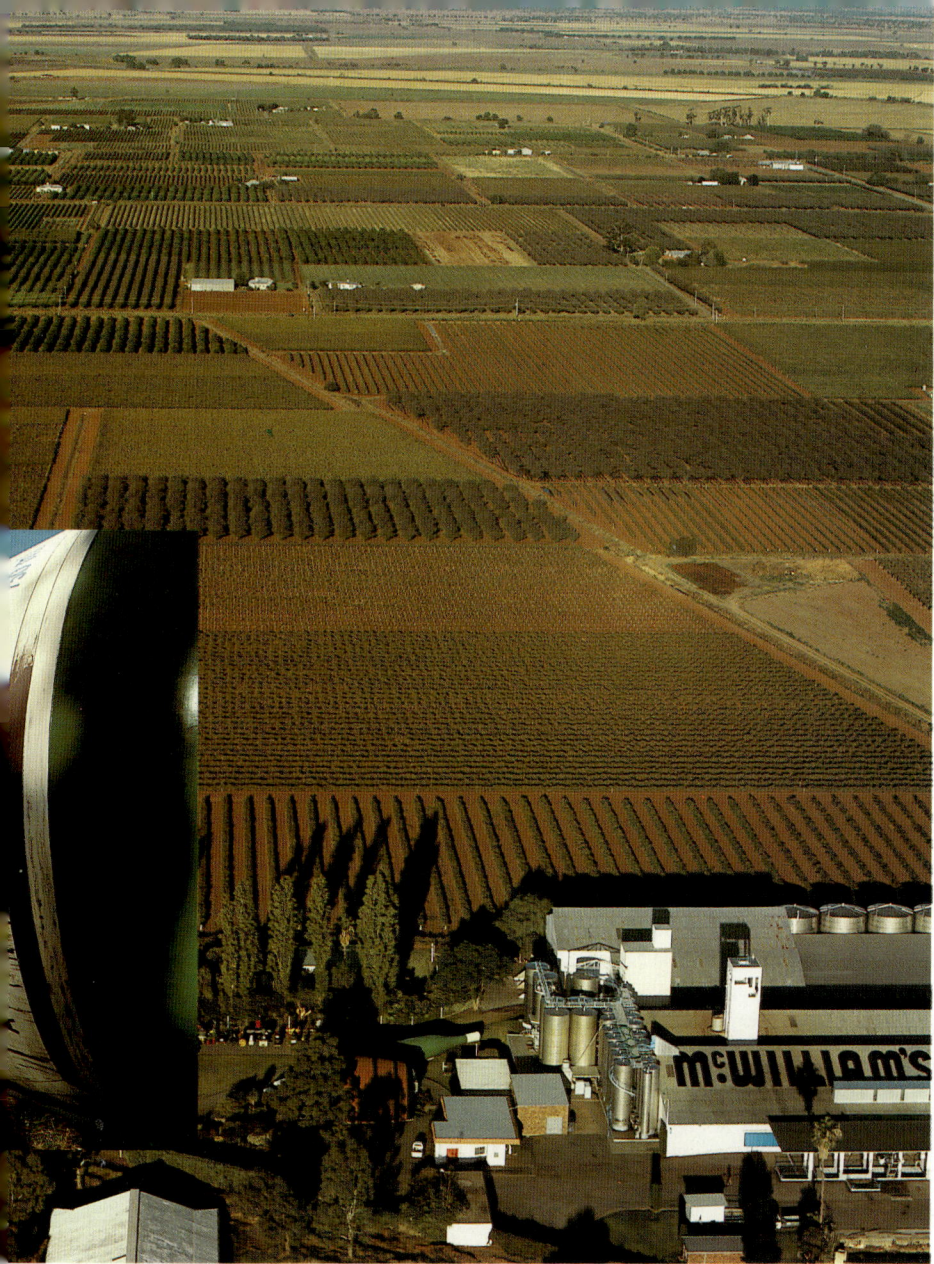

Murrumbidgee Irrigation Area/ Griffith

The M.I.A. produces the best-value-for-money wines in Australia, and has been doing so for a very long time. The area is centred on the large town of Griffith and often, flying over on my way to or from my home in Adelaide, I have looked down from the jet onto this island of green in a sea of Australian red/brown/grey semi-desert.

The M.I.A. is one of the most clearly delineated regions in Australia, as you can see very well from an aircraft. The green is grapes and citrus trees, and indeed the M.I.A. produces around a fifth of Australia's total wine production. The largest maker is family company McWilliam's, with three big wineries in the district (plus the Mt Pleasant winery in the Hunter), making some terrific wines for exceptionally reasonable prices. So, too, do de Bortoli's, and one or two others.

Because Griffith is off the normal tourists' beaten track, disappointingly few wine fanciers spend a few days browsing around to taste what's on offer, in and around the M.I.A. It has been for quite some time, and remains, one of the best wine areas of Australia in which to stock up your cellar with good, and economic, wines that you'll enjoy drinking.

In terms of wine quality, both reds and whites are good. They tend to be 'drink soon' wines, as many have observed. But so what? Most of us drink wines rather than keeping them these days. Rieslings, chardonnays, sauvignon blancs, some excellent sweet whites (notably de Bortoli's), thoroughly enjoyable young cabernets and many good shiraz wines, plus some great fortified wines, emerge from many of the two dozen wineries scattered around Griffith and nearby Leeton.

McWilliam's Hanwood Winery, with its 'Big Barrel', de Bortoli's, Fiumara's Lillypilly Estate and San Bernadino are, among others, worth visiting if you are in the district or passing through. All except Lillypilly have very large ranges of wines available.

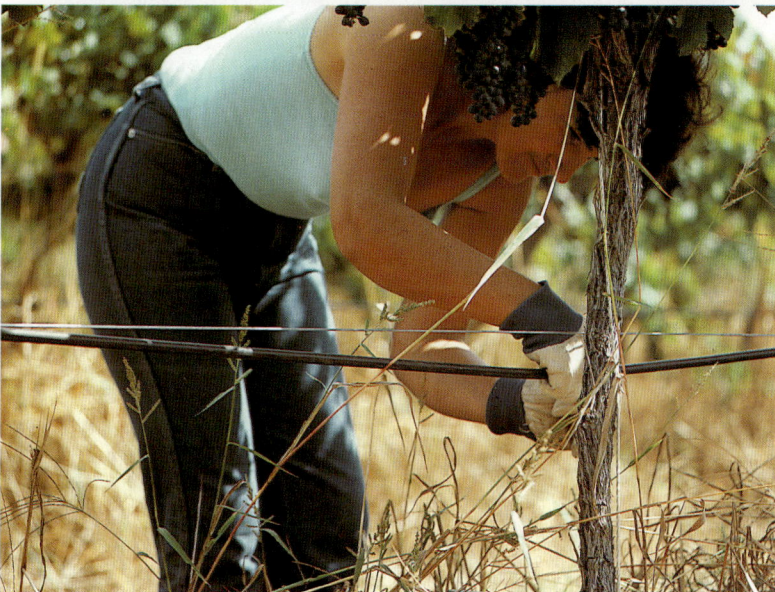

Repairing a drip irrigation system is another ongoing vineyard chore, especially when the fruit-laden vine has to cope with the demands of hot summers.

SOUTH AUSTRALIA

Welcome to the Wine State. The Mediterranean climate has grapevines growing lustily alongside olive trees (often self-sown and lining the roads beside the vineyards), oceans of citrus and almond trees — even avocado and pear orchards! But it's the fruit of the grapevines, of course, that makes just about any wine- drinking Australian murmur approvingly :
'Barossa Valley'.

Anyone interested in wine (or food, for that matter, provided you also enjoy lovely scenery) should, when visiting Adelaide, try to visit the three major key areas scattered within striking distance of Adelaide, that is the Clare Valley, McLaren Vale and the Barossa.

Barossa Valley

The Barossa Valley, an hour or so's easy drive to the north-east of Adelaide, is one of Australia's most important wine-growing and producing areas, arguably the most important, if not the largest grape-growing district. It is certainly home to some of the largest makers, including Penfolds. And it is one of our most historic wine areas, dating back to the 1840s.

Some of the greatest Australian wines have come from this shallow valley and from the vineyards which, like lusty infants leaving the family home, have crept away from it. They've gone to places like the Eden Valley, the Adelaide Hills, Watervale and the Clare Valley, and eventually out along the Murray River stretches to the north and east.

Perhaps one of the greatest legacies the Barossa Valley has given us is our adoption of, and liking for, the marvellous German riesling white grape. The Silesian and German settlers of the Barossa endowed us with this legacy, and Australia (and still the Barossa, with its German settlers and their Barossa-deutsch) make a unique and still little-appreciated dry white wine style from this marvellous grapevine.

Like many Australian wine-growing areas, the Barossa (from Ba-Rosa, or Hill of Roses) is essentially a warm to hot area in which to grow grapes. Hence the increasingly popular moves over the past few decades by some wine-makers to go to higher, cooler areas to grow or find their grapes, mainly in the Barossa Ranges rising to the Valley's east and south. The success of many of these vineyards, and the high quality of much of the fruit now being grown here (by, notably, Yalumba, Petaluma and Mountadam) has encouraged others to plant vineyards in the Mount Lofty Ranges to the south. There will be many more hectares of varieties, such as cabernet sauvignon, pinot noir, riesling, chardonnay and sauvignon blanc, planted in these charming hills and valleys (the 'Adelaide Hills' to the population of Adelaide), which are so cool, green — and atypically South Australian!

The Hills have vineyards scattered throughout but, other than in the northern end (that is, to the east and south-east of the Barossa Valley), there are few wineries yet. Petaluma, with its nearby champagne cellars, entertainment centre and restaurant at the outstanding Bridgewater Mill, is one of the few exceptions. The wines that are coming from these areas are very good, though.

The major makers sited in the Barossa Valley itself are headed by the very large Penfold's Group, with a giant winery in the heart of the Valley near the town of Nuriootpa. As they absorb their company takeovers (Kaiser Stuhl, Wynns, Tulloch, Tollana/T.S.T., Loxton Co-operative and likely others to come), thereby drawing fruit from all over, the overall quality of Penfold Group wines is improving quite markedly.

Orlando and Yalumba are two other major makers based in or near the Barossa whose quality I have praised before and who stand out in this region. Again, like any sensible, pragmatic and flexible wine-making company, both draw fruit from other regions, but they have their roots in the vineyards of the Barossa Valley. Orlando, with the benefits of a multi-national parent (Pernod Ricard), stands out in the quality stakes. But it's hard to get a bad or even mediocre wine from either — and easy to get excellent wines from both labels. Orlando and Yalumba both have very appealing cellar door operations in their respective wineries, too, though I find Yalumba's rustic retreat outside Angaston a little more inviting. Peter Lehmann wines also has an outstanding cellar door operation which is worth a visit.

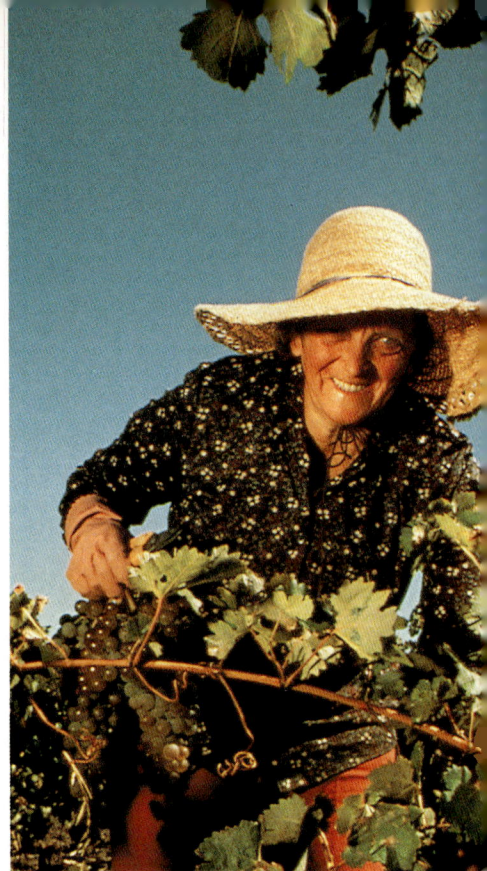

The Barossa Valley largely stands for big wine business now. Seppelt's major wineries in S.A. are here, too, and the comments above apply equally to them. If I had to focus on individual Barossa products I would look to Barossa cabernet sauvignons, shiraz, rieslings (particularly) and some chardonnays for the wines to drink from your table and store in your cellar. For after dinner, the Barossa's ports, both vintage and tawny, are generally exceptional, with superb examples of both styles from Seppelt (the best), Penfold, Yalumba and Saltram.

Seppeltsfield is one of the places you

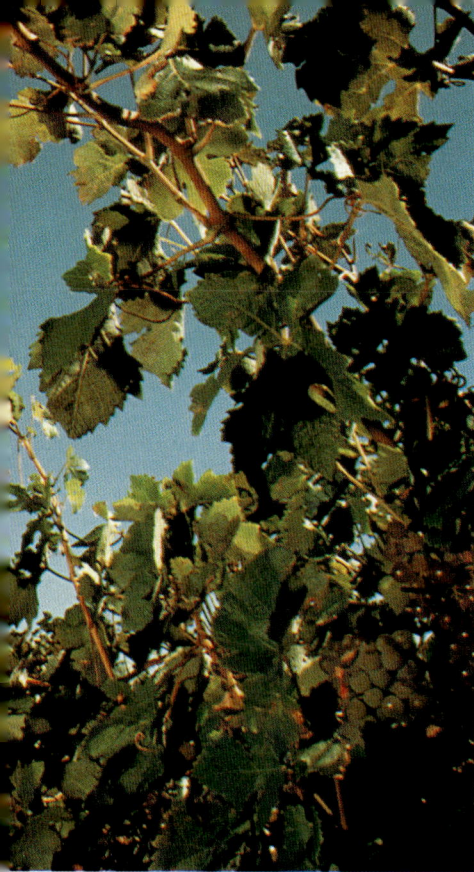

The 'canopy cover' and levels of sunlight allowed through are vitally important, as this Barossa Valley picker demonstrates.

KOONUNGA

STOCKWELL

■ Bilyara Wines
(Wolf Blass)

GREENOCK CREEK

GREENOCK

VALLEY

NURIOOTPA

■ Gnadenfrei
Penfolds ■
■ Tolley, Scott & Tolley
■ Woodley
■ Kaiser Stuhl

■ Seppeltsfield Winery
Douglas A. Tolley
(Pedare) ■
■ Vintners

Masterson ■
■ Saltram

Hoffmanns ■
■ Hardy's Siegersdorf

Bern Kastel ■
Leo Buring Chateau Leonay ■

Veritas ■
■ Basedows

ANGASTON

■ Yalumba

TANUNDA

■ Chateau Tanunda

■ Chateau Rosevale
■ Bethany Wines

BAROSSA

■ High Wycombe

NORTH PARA RIVER

■ St Hallet

BAROSSA RANGE

■ Krondorf

MOOROOROO

Chateau Yaldara ■
■ Chattertons
Wine Cellars
■ Gramps Orlando

■ Karlsburg
ROWLAND FLAT

y Cellars ■
■ Wilsford Wines
Leibichs Rovalley

JACOB CREEK

■ Das Alte Weinhaus

■ Barossa Settlers

LYNDOCH

■ Karrawirra

■ Mountadam

■ Wynns High Eden Estate

WILLIAMSTOWN

SOUTH MOUNT LOFTY RANGES

S

H

shouldn't miss in the Barossa. Not only is it a great, sprawling and fascinating winery. Their wines are tops, and they have the occasional additional attraction of the great hot-air balloon races, which are an unforgettable sight in the still morning air of the Valley.

Saltram, and their wines, tend to be overlooked amongst the Barossa wine-maker. They are discreetly located between the bottom of the Valley and the top. They're just outside Angaston, and are easy to miss if you're driving by. They have consistently made good, sometimes excellent, wines and the company, owned by Seagrams, is an integral part of the Valley and its history. Saltrams also offer some older wines at their cellar door, itself a charming spot.

Among the small- to medium-sized makers, Henschke, Basedow's and parent Peter Lehmann, Douglas A.Tolley's Pedare and (if you believe he's still small!) Wolf Blass all stand out. All of the white and red wines from these and a number of other Barossa makers are good to very good, with some charming characters, wineries and atmosphere behind them.

The Barossa Valley *is* a great place to visit, with some superb wines, great places to stay, plenty of pubs and restaurants, and some lovely scenery. And, whether it's getting a bit touristy or not, it remains today the spiritual and physical home of the Australian wine industry.

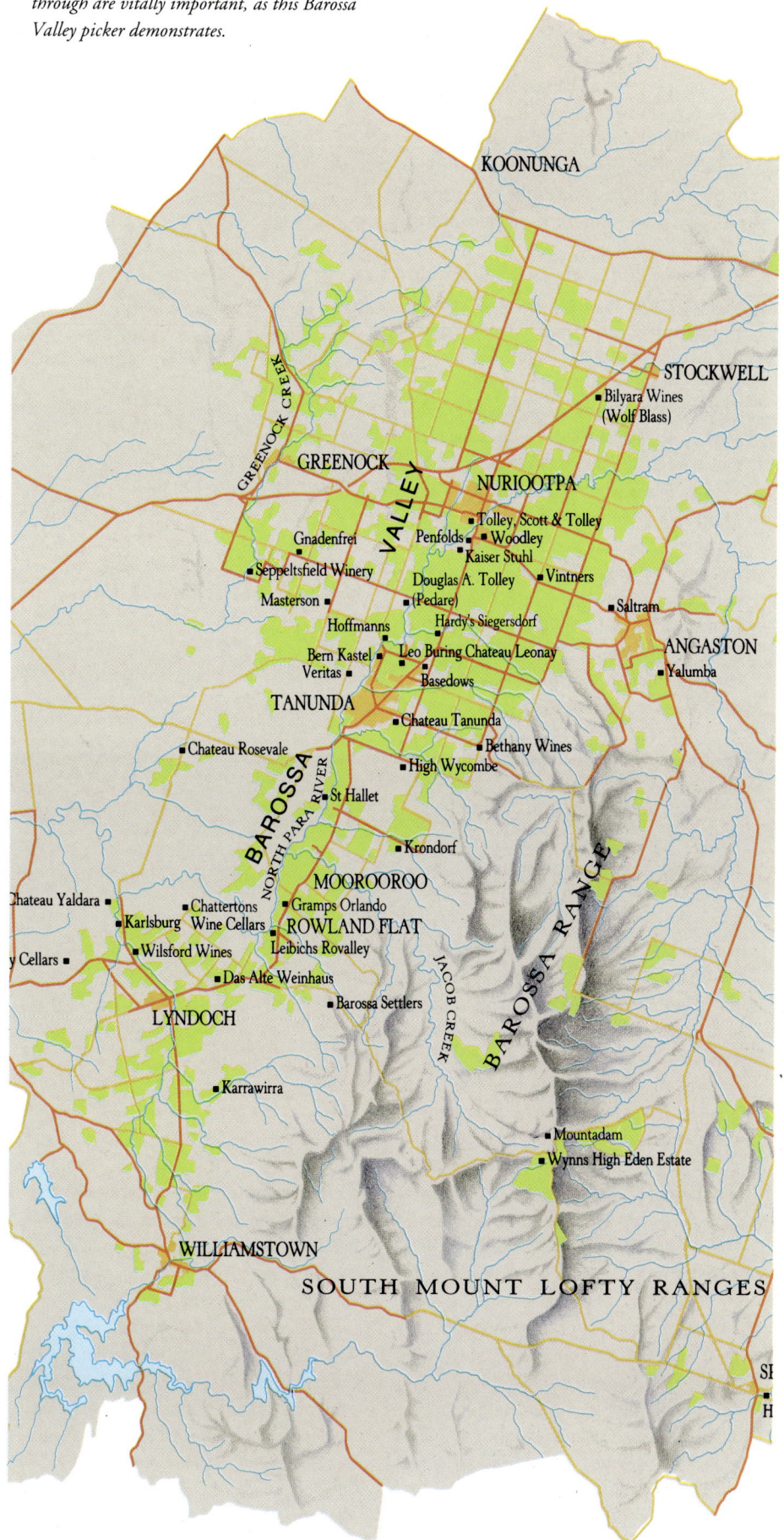

Clare Valley

Not far away from the Barossa Valley, to the north and east a way, is another wine valley, sloping gently but perceptibly uphill from the township of Watervale through the vineyards to the larger town of Clare. The drive from Adelaide is just a couple of scenic hours.

It's a delightful valley, the Clare, with woods, vineyards, creeks and old houses. Halfway up is sleepy Sevenhill and just off the main road is the Sevenhill Winery, run by a Jesuit order with the charming Brother John May as the wine-maker. His wines are worth seeking out, as is the historic church, crypt and old winery.

The major wineries are Quelltaler and Tim Knappstein, bought several years ago by Wolf Blass, though Tim's recently re-emerged to form a partnership with Petaluma; Taylor's and The Stanley Wine Company. Of these, only Taylors remains in its original hands; the others have all changed hands at least once. Among smaller makers are Jim Barry, Dr John Wilson, Wendouree and Jane Mitchell, all making some very good wines, many of quite different styles.

The one enduring truism in the Clare Valley is that it produces Rhine riesling fruit that makes some superlative wines, and most of the makers from here make such wines. I've enjoyed Tim Knappstein's sauvignon blancs (called fumé blanc) and a few chardonnays, but it is certainly riesling that seems naturally at home on the slopes and ridges of the Clare Valley. Other varieties seem to be less attractive, though some admirable reds have come from Stanley (Bin 56 Cabernet/Malbec, among them), the Barrys, Wendouree (huge in power and endurance!) and to some extent reds from Taylors (whose reds in the past have to me had a rather 'furniture polish' character about them, but which have changed in recent years for the better).

The Clare Valley wine-makers have been running a very up-market wine and food weekend, after vintage (in May) for some years. It's been excellent in past years, featuring superb food with some of Adelaide's best restaurants linked to individual wineries, who also feature the new season's juice or young finished wines.

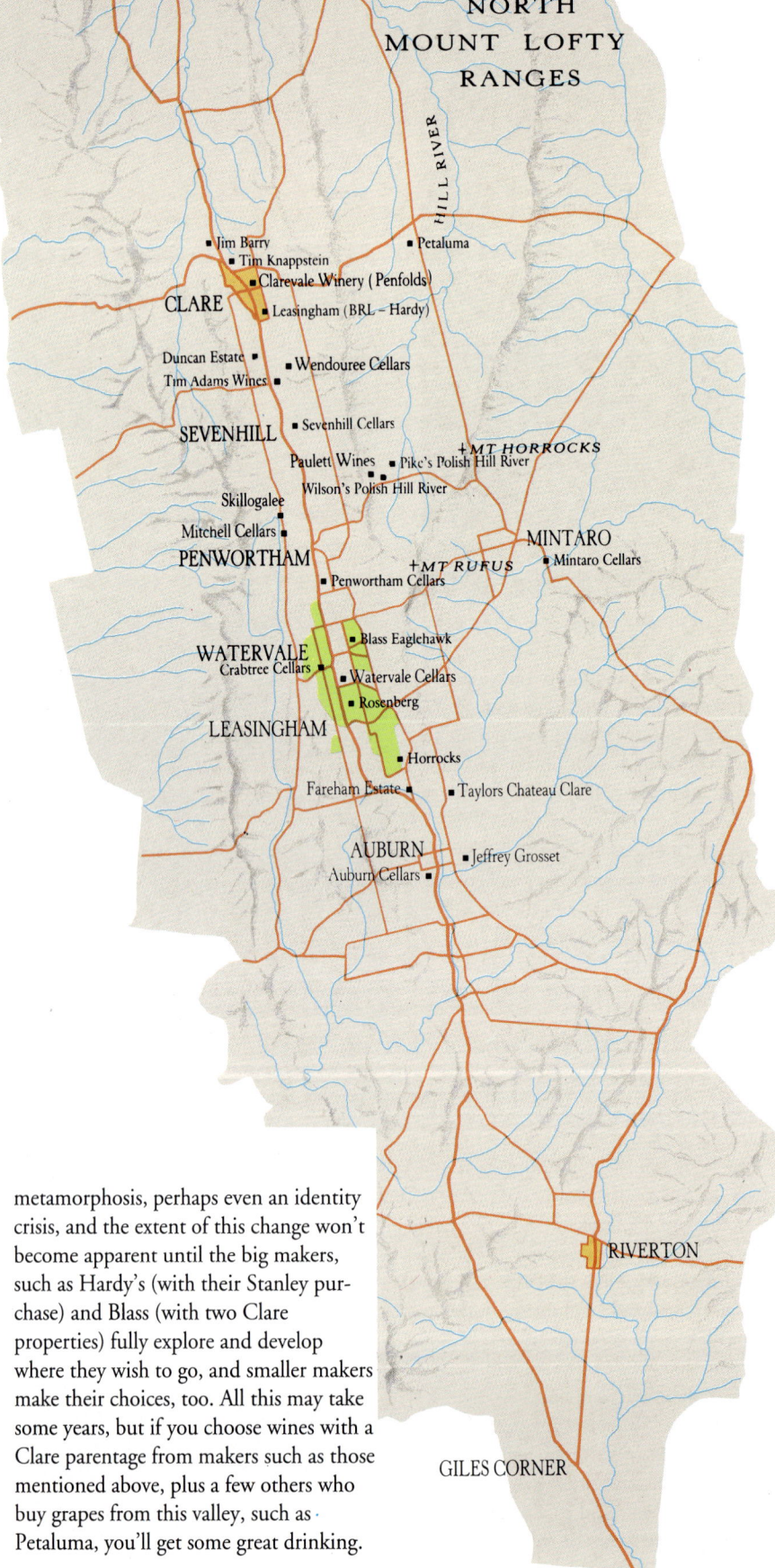

The Clare Valley is going through a metamorphosis, perhaps even an identity crisis, and the extent of this change won't become apparent until the big makers, such as Hardy's (with their Stanley purchase) and Blass (with two Clare properties) fully explore and develop where they wish to go, and smaller makers make their choices, too. All this may take some years, but if you choose wines with a Clare parentage from makers such as those mentioned above, plus a few others who buy grapes from this valley, such as Petaluma, you'll get some great drinking.

CLARE VALLEY

NORTH MOUNT LOFTY RANGES

HILL RIVER

Jim Barry
Tim Knappstein
Petaluma
Clarevale Winery (Penfolds)
CLARE
Leasingham (BRL – Hardy)
Duncan Estate
Wendouree Cellars
Tim Adams Wines
SEVENHILL
Sevenhill Cellars
+MT HORROCKS
Paulett Wines
Pike's Polish Hill River
Wilson's Polish Hill River
Skillogalee
MINTARO
Mitchell Cellars
Mintaro Cellars
PENWORTHAM
+MT RUFUS
Penwortham Cellars
WATERVALE
Blass Eaglehawk
Crabtree Cellars
Watervale Cellars
Rosenberg
LEASINGHAM
Horrocks
Fareham Estate
Taylors Chateau Clare
AUBURN
Jeffrey Grosset
Auburn Cellars
RIVERTON
GILES CORNER

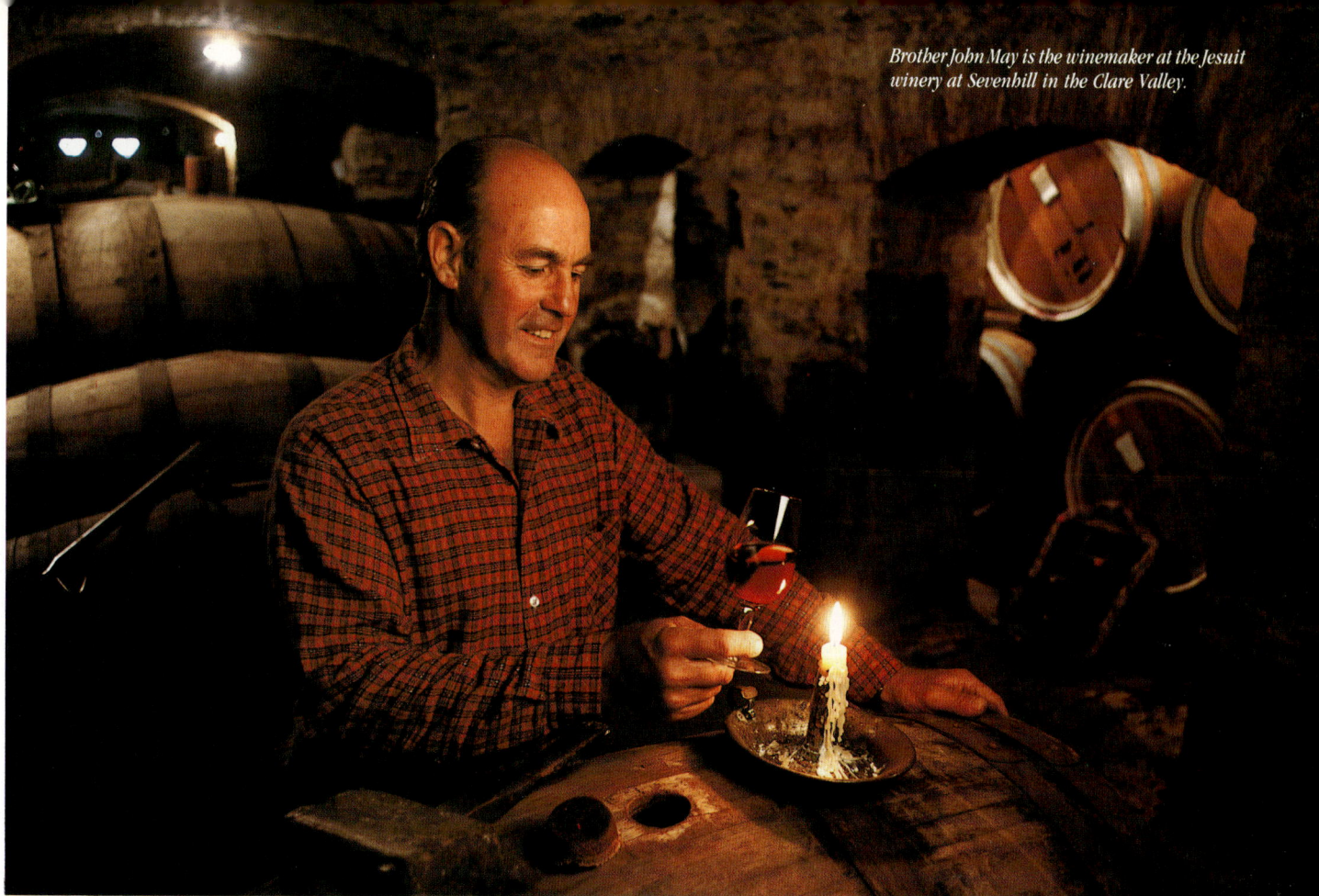

Brother John May is the winemaker at the Jesuit winery at Sevenhill in the Clare Valley.

McLaren Vale

Here, 45 kilometres south of Adelaide, is a true Vale — a shallow valley running from near the coast at the Gulf of St Vincent, gently uphill, through McLaren Vale, McLaren Flat and Blewett Springs to meet the Onkaparinga River at Clarendon. Along the way, and south to Willunga and the escarpment of the Southern Mount Lofty Ranges are extensive vineyards and a host — more than 40 —-small- to middle-sized wineries.

There are also some top restaurants and tourist attractions down south, between Adelaide, Victor Harbour and Clarendon. It is an historic area, with buildings dating from the 1830s and a wine history beginning not much later (the beautiful Chateau Reynella dates from 1838).

Typically, the McLaren Vale area (or Southern Vales to some; they try to change the area's name every now and then because they cannot decide what to call themselves) makes excellent and beautifully flavoured reds, strongly flavoured whites and excellent ports. But the makers in the greater Southern Vales area successfully produce just about every kind of table, sparkling and fortified wine, and do it all pretty well.

The largest maker is BRL Hardy, based at Reynella, 20 kilometres north towards Adelaide and with another large winery in the centre of McLaren Vale itself. Hardy, though now not owned by the Hardy family after being merged with Berri Renmano Limited (hence the BRL) and floated in 1992, is now the second biggest maker in the country, with outposts in the Barossa, Clare, Western Australia and elsewhere, with big vineyards at Padthaway in the south-east of South Australia. Their range of wines is enormous and of high quality. Their Chateau Reynella division makes excellent reds and fortifieds, and the Hardy's white wines are exceptional. Both wineries are thoroughly worth visiting if in Adelaide or down south. The ports of both companies are absolutely outstanding.

Although Wynn's (Penfold's) have two outposts in the Vales, only one is open for cellar door sales and that is the Seaview winery at McLaren Vale. The other is the Glenloth winery at Reynella. Some very good wines are available at Seaview, a once-large winery with an important part in the area's history.

Among the larger district wineries are Pirramimma and the tourist outpost of the vigorous Andrew Garrett company, with winery, restaurant, motel and convention centre at the attractive McLaren's on the Lake operation just outside McLaren Vale.

For the most part the other makers are small, yet produce very good wines. Andrew Garrett himself made the point to me once, accurately, that McLaren Vale produces perhaps the best variety of across-the-board wines of any wine district in Australia, everything from riesling through chardonay and most of the red varieties.

Yet only about 25 per cent of the grapes grown in this area appear as McLaren Vale-labelled products — the rest goes into juice to other wineries or disappears into other people's blends, for example it is a favourite source for Wolf Blass products.

Small makers in this district whose quality stands out are Woodstock (with excellent reds and very good whites), Wirra Wirra (right across the board), d'Arenberg, Middlebrook, Ryecroft and Mount Hurtle at Reynella, operated by the lively and talented Geoff Merrill.

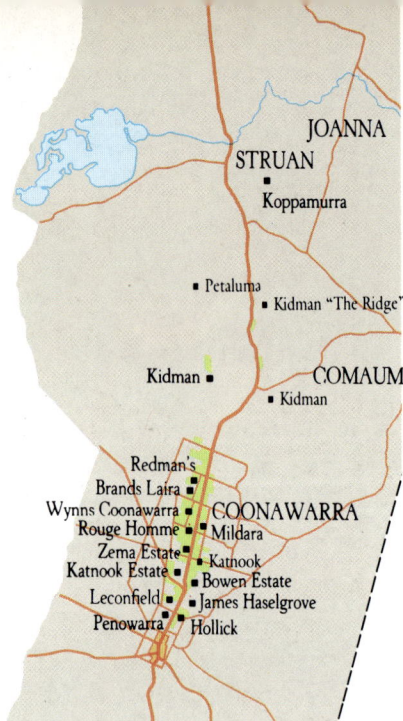

(Map labels, left map:)
JOANNA
STRUAN
• Koppamurra

• Petaluma
• Kidman "The Ridge"

Kidman •   COMAUM
• Kidman

Redman's •
Brands Laira •
Wynns Coonawarra •   COONAWARRA
Rouge Homme •   • Mildara
Zema Estate •   • Katnook
Katnook Estate •   • Bowen Estate
Leconfield •   • James Haselgrove
Penowarra •   • Hollick

(Map labels, right map:)
Lindeman •
PADTHAWAY
• Wynn
• Seppelt
• Hardy

• Brown

KEPPOCH

Coonawarra

Some 400 kilometres south-east of Adelaide is Coonawarra, the area generally recognised as the best red wine-growing district of Australia. The name Coonawarra, by the way, is an Aboriginal one, meaning "place of wild honeysuckle".

A rich, red and cigar-shaped patch of terra rosa soil, plus the climate of the area (cooler than most of the rest of the State) yields grape-growing conditions for fruit, such as cabernet sauvignon, that seem close to ideal. It is not an area that many people visit unless they happen to be passing through this way from Melbourne to Adelaide, though there are some worthwhile cellar door tasting stops to be made, notably at Rouge Homme/Lindeman's, Wynn's, Brands, Laira, Hollick, Leconfield, Mildara and Redman.

The reds of most of these makers, particularly Coonawarra cabernet sauvignon, shiraz and blends of the two (and increasingly a few others in blends, such as cabernet franc and merlot), have made Coonawarra famous, and will continue to do so. Whites seem to present more of a problem, though some makers (Wynn's with their Coonawarra Estate Chardonnay, for example, and Leconfield with riesling) seem to defy these odds.

The coveted Jimmy Watson Trophy, awarded at the Melbourne Wine Show for best one-year-old red wine, seems to enjoy this area, as it returns here with monotonous regularity after the Show each year!

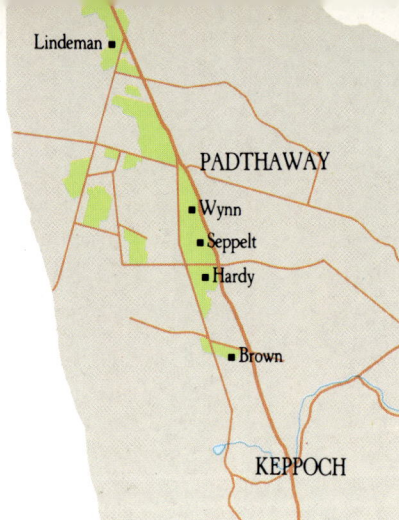

Some of the best reds from this district include Lindeman's St George, Limestone Ridge and Pyrus labels, Orlando's Jacaranda Ridge red, Penfolds stunning Bin 707, Petaluma and the Hardy Collection Coonawarra cabernet sauvignon.

Padthaway

Padthaway is another relatively remote and cool South Australian premium grape-growing region, this time some 70 kilometres closer to Adelaide than Coonawarra, but still far away enough from anywhere to make you put a picnic lunch in a fast car, and be away all day.

Although it's not far from Coonawarra, this area (formerly called Keppoch), was developed in the late 1960s and early 1970s by Seppelt, Hardy and Lindeman's because vineyard land was getting too expensive down the road, and it seemed to have many of the same attributes as Coonawarra possessed. It has produced some of Australia's best dry whites of recent years, most commendably some superb chardonnays. If you want to see what I mean taste the chardonnays under the Lindeman's, Seppelt Gold Label and Hardy Collection labels.

The district is marked by lots of vines and no wineries, but the word "Padthaway" on a major maker's wine label is generally an accurate pointer to high white wine quality.

Other areas

There are, of course, other areas to South Australia's wine atlas. Some of them are vital components of the Australian wine industry, even though one may not see them as often or as prominently as names like Barossa, Hunter or Clare.

Langhorne Creek, towards the mouth of the River Murray, grows some stunning cabernet and shiraz red grapes which go into blends elsewhere and improve them enormously. The individual wines of this area are harder to find, as there are few makers based here.

The **Riverland District** produces huge volumes of bulk and quality wines — and some great value wines — but few large makers are based here. Angoves, owned by the Angove family, is one high-quality maker, selling very good wines, usually at competitive prices. If you are at all interested in wines, Angoves and the local outlets of BRL Hardy are really worth a visit, to seek out wines, all the way from some great fortifieds to some top varietal table wines. Let them know you're interested when you go through the door and you will have an opportunity to taste some excellent products. Finding their better wines elsewhere is often, sadly, a battle. But there is usually plenty to praise in their quaffing wines. They are, after all, exceptional value for your money. These and some other Riverland makers represent some of the largest volumes in the country, in 4-, 5- and 6-litre casks.

There are several good makers on the **Adelaide Plains,** north of the city of Adelaide, especially Primo Estate; and the **Adelaide Hills** I have touched on elsewhere. Sadly, the outer suburban areas of the city of Adelaide, once home to thousands of hectares of vineyards, have largely gone, replaced by houses. Penfold's Magill Vineyard remains, much diminished; Reynella has shed some of its buffer of vines; Hamilton's vines have gone from here; and so it all has gone, and will go ... Grapes cannot economically be grown in the suburbs.

And while areas such as the Adelaide Hills and some other larger areas produce some distinctive wines, they are not areas whose labels, presence or taste variations justify a great deal of further explanation here. Some are, quite simply, efficient makers of what are for the most part very enjoyable wines; look for them and Enjoy! (as they say in the South Australian tourism ads).

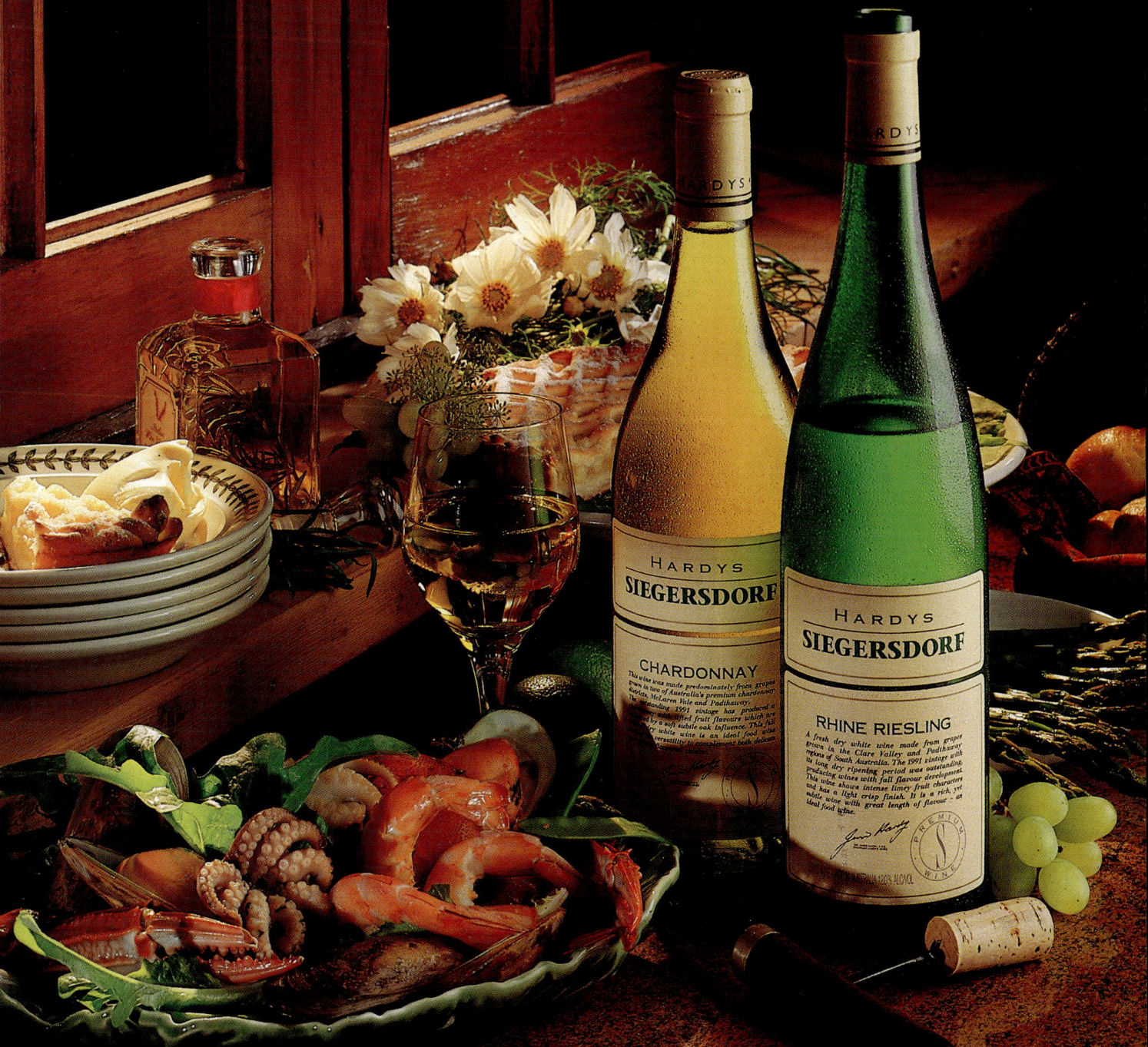

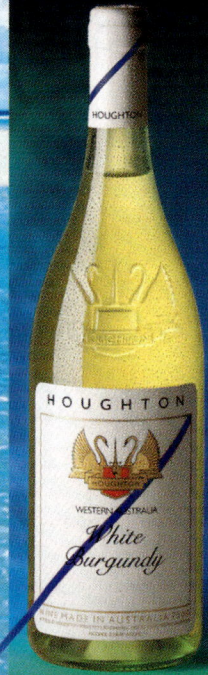

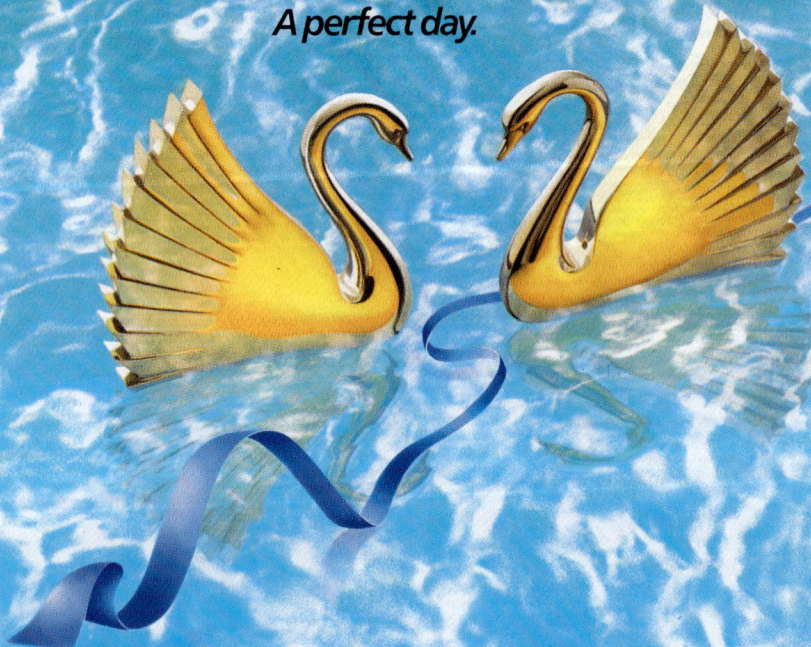

Western Australia

I have to admit I find Western Australia both exciting and disappointing as a wine-making State. Unquestionably, some superb wines have headed East, and many have also been consumed within the ample borders of W.A. There are only a few makers whose products are quite widely available outside Perth. They include the big two, Houghton and Sandalford, plus a few others such as Evans and Tate, the Leeuwin Estate, Mosswood, Plantagenet, Cape Mentelle and one or two others. The areas start with the Swan Valley, just a hop, skip and sip east of Perth along the Swan River. It's a hot part of the wine-growing world, and wines such as Houghton White Burgundy, together with some of its cousins from nearby maker Sandalford, are all the more remarkable tributes to technology for this. Houghton White Burgundy, with its distinctive blue stripe is, I hardly need say, the flagbearer of W.A. wines and is successful because of its distinctive area and grape flavours, which gives it a real difference in taste in dry white wines, and the marketing skills of its makers.

SWAN VALLEY

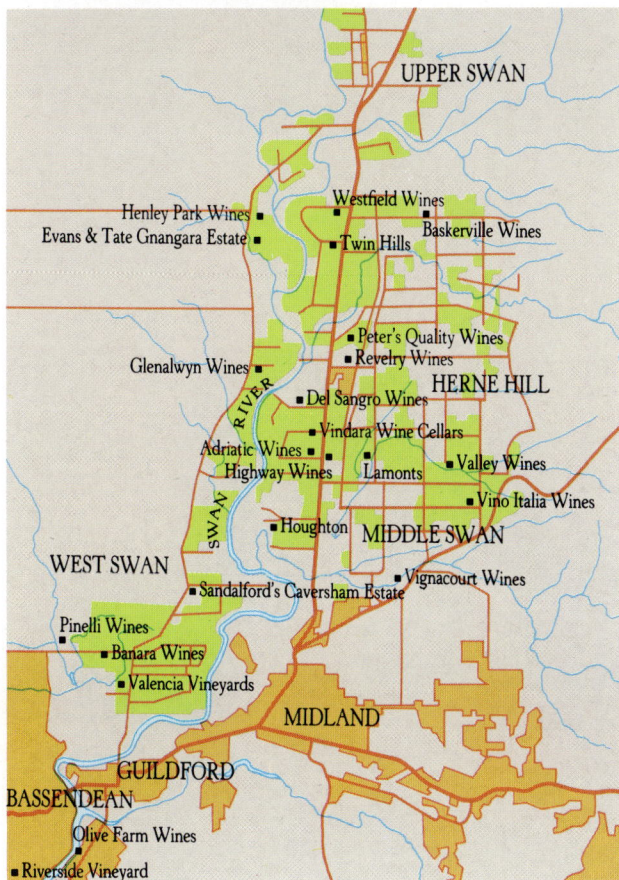
Leeuwin Estate

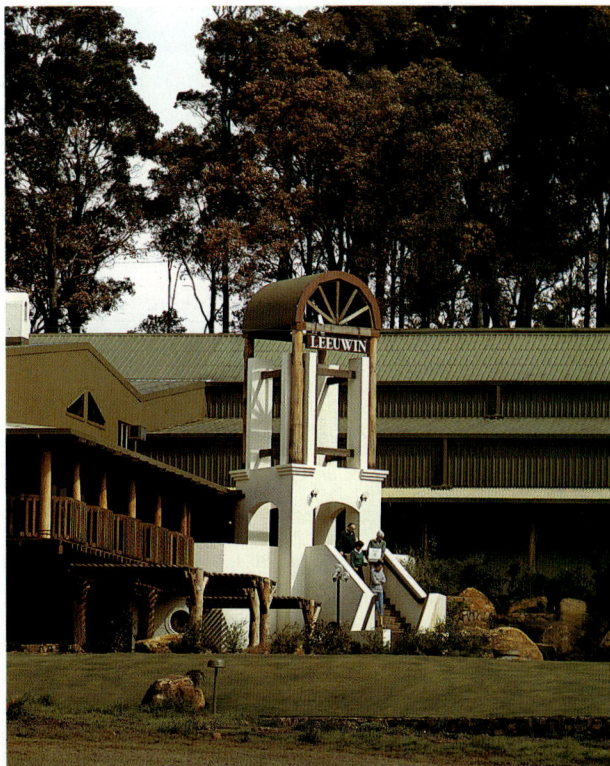

If you want to taste the distinctive wines of the West, it is with these two makers, Houghton and Sandalford, that you should begin.

North of Perth is Moondah Brook Estate, yielding some very enjoyable whites — verdelho, chardonnay and chenin blanc and a large source of the fruit for Houghton. To the east is the Darling Ranges area. South are far-flung and generally small vineyards heading down to the Margaret River region — a long way from Perth. Here are some of the best quality wines of the West from wineries and vineyards including Redbrook (Gnangara), Vasse Felix, Cape Mentelle (reds and whites), Mosswood and Pierro; these last three make table wines, particularly red wines, of exceptional quality, as a rule. Look out for them, but they will be quite expensive.

The Leeuwin Estate makes very fine wines, but the prices reflect the cost of building one of the most astonishing winery monuments in Australia. The modern structure, the inspiration of Perth millionaire Denis Horgan, is certainly worth visiting if you're in this splendid and isolated part of Western Australia.

I'm afraid, however, that I cannot see comparative value in young white and red table wines, however good, priced at $25 to $40 or more a bottle.

There are several other small areas, including the Frankland River and Mount Barker areas. They are isolated, comparatively new and trying very hard, and some exciting wines are surfacing. The winery which stands out is Plantagenet, near Mount Barker. Western Australia has a wine history dating back to the 1830s, but its isolation and the hot climate of the Swan Valley seem to have relegated it to a bit part, and to making some fantastic fortified wines, until the late 1960s. Then it was realised that good table wines could be grown elsewhere in the State, and a Medibank-led wine boom got under way. Now doctors are making wine all over W.A. — or so it seems to me every time I go there.

So things are changing, and like most places wine is made, it takes a long, long time to work out ... well, what works. So, many better things are on the way from the West. Today, only a couple of per cent of Australia's wine comes from W.A. and the State "imports" more than it "exports".

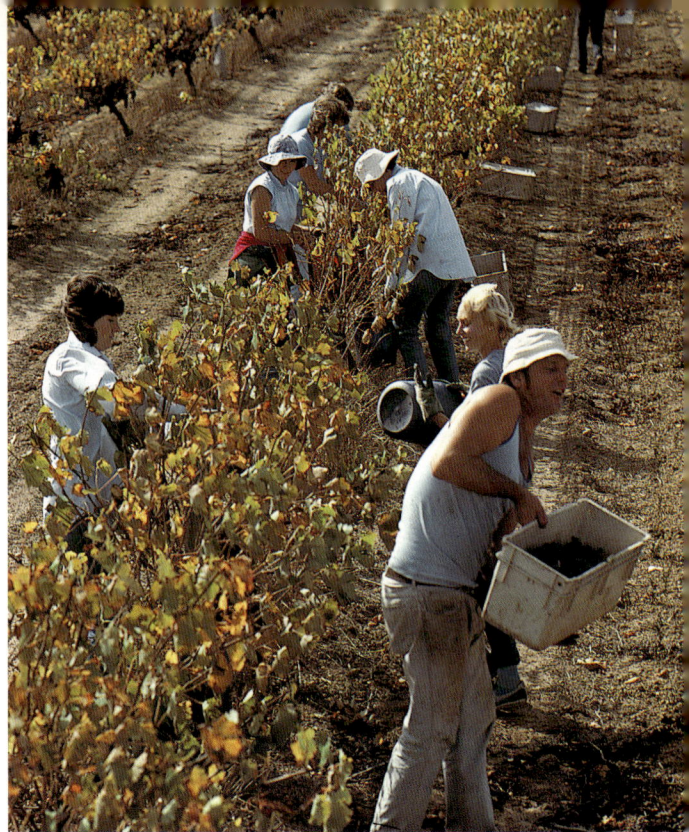

Above: *Hand picking is back-breaking work but preserves fruit quality.*
Below: *Eucalypts dominate the skyline behind the vineyards near picturesque Margaret River, Western Australia.*

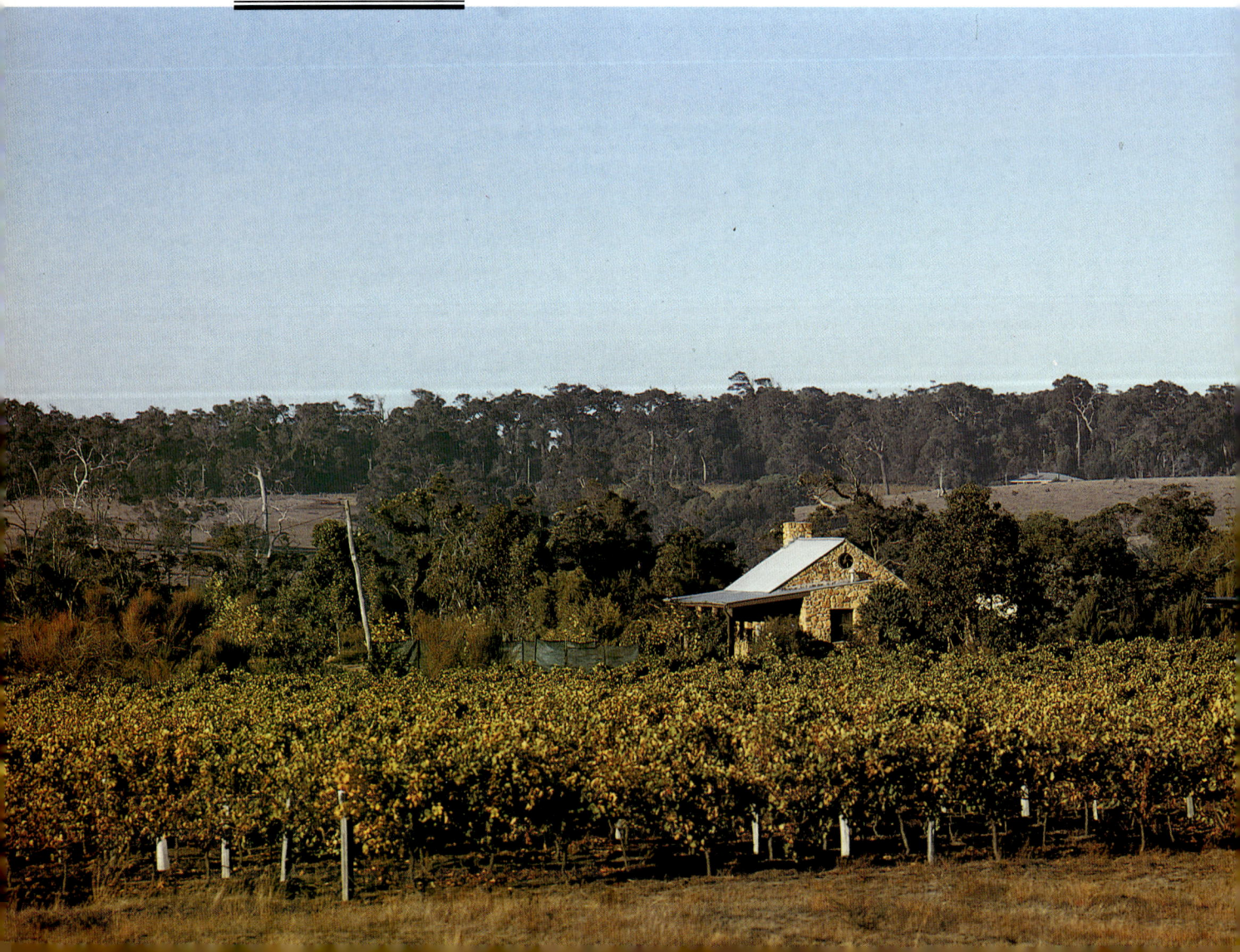

Tasmania

Very, very small quantities of wine are being made in Tasmania. The State can grow good grapes and make good wines, but the climate is cool to cold, which is good for quality but, like making love in the shower, it takes practice.

You won't see much of Tasmanian wine on retail shelves outside Tassie, and what there is tends to be expensive. But it's generally good, and recent enthusiasm shown by French Champagne interests (Roederer, among others) suggests that they recognise climatic similarities between the Champagne District (50° North latitude) and Tasmania (between 41° to 43° South latitude)

In the meantime, if you feel the overwhelming urge to try a Tasmanian wine, try a riesling, chardonnay or cabernet sauvignon from Piper's Brook or Heemskerk, both wineries being sited in the Tamar Valley just north-east of Launceston. I suspect that pinot noir is going to be good from Tasmania, too. Several good smaller wineries, such as Moorilla Estate, operate in the Derwent Valley area, closer to Hobart in the south of the island. Generally, Tasmanian wine quality is high.

Queensland

Again, miniscule production. There are wineries at Roma (outstanding fortified wines), the Atherton Tablelands, and one or two experimental ones elsewhere. But the Granite Belt area around Stanthorpe, south-west of Brisbane in the Darling Downs region, is making some very palatable wines. It is, after all, quite cool there, and a number of other fruits, such as apples, perform well. Also, wineries such as the Robinson Family, Rumbalara, Sundown Valley, Mount Magnus and Old Caves are making some good table wines, including chardonnay.

Elsewhere

There are wines made in the Northern Territory (at Chateau Hornsby, outside Alice Springs) and in the Australian Capital Territory (or nearby). But away from cellar door they are difficult, if not impossible, to buy or taste. And quality from many of these developing areas, and from small makers, is of necessity very variable. See *The Pocket Australian Wine Companion* if you're interested in more details of all of these wineries, and

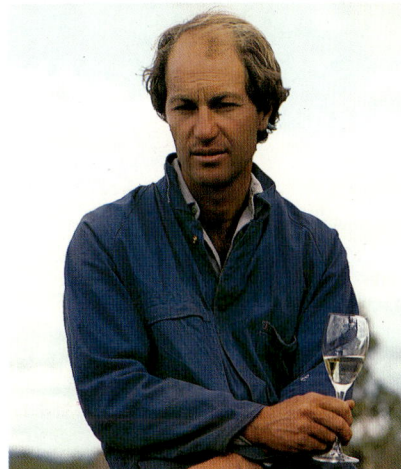

Dr Andrew Pirie is one of Tasmania's most progressive winemakers.

others not mentioned above under areas, as there has not been space to provide a complete listing. Lord knows, I have enough trouble tasting them all!

RECOMMENDED REFERENCE : An attractive plasticised wall map of *The Wine Producing Areas of Australia* available from Lane Printer Group in Adelaide, telephone (08) 376 1188, showing all Australia's wineries and wine areas, about $9.95 plus postage .

RECOMMENDED DRINKING : Something from a different part of Australia — Houghton White Burgundy if you live outside WA, or Tyrrell's Long Flat White if you live in WA.

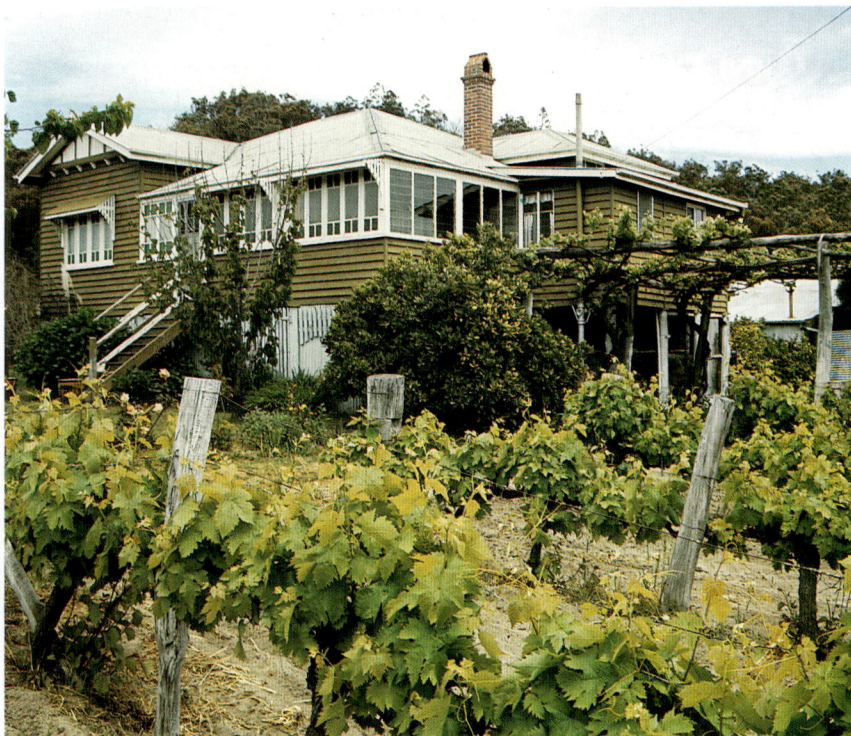

Characteristically Queensland architecture dominates a vineyard at Rumbalara in Queensland's Granite Belt.

VISITING WINERIES

Wine's special qualities are seldom more appreciated than at the place where the wine is made (or at least close by). It's known as the 'cellar door', and visiting and tasting and buying wine there can be either a great pleasure or a tender trap. Cellar door sales areas exist at most of the five hundred and fifty wineries around Australia, and the majority of them have acknowledged that to properly appreciate and assess a wine, a visitor has to taste the stuff – and therefore you can taste it free of charge.

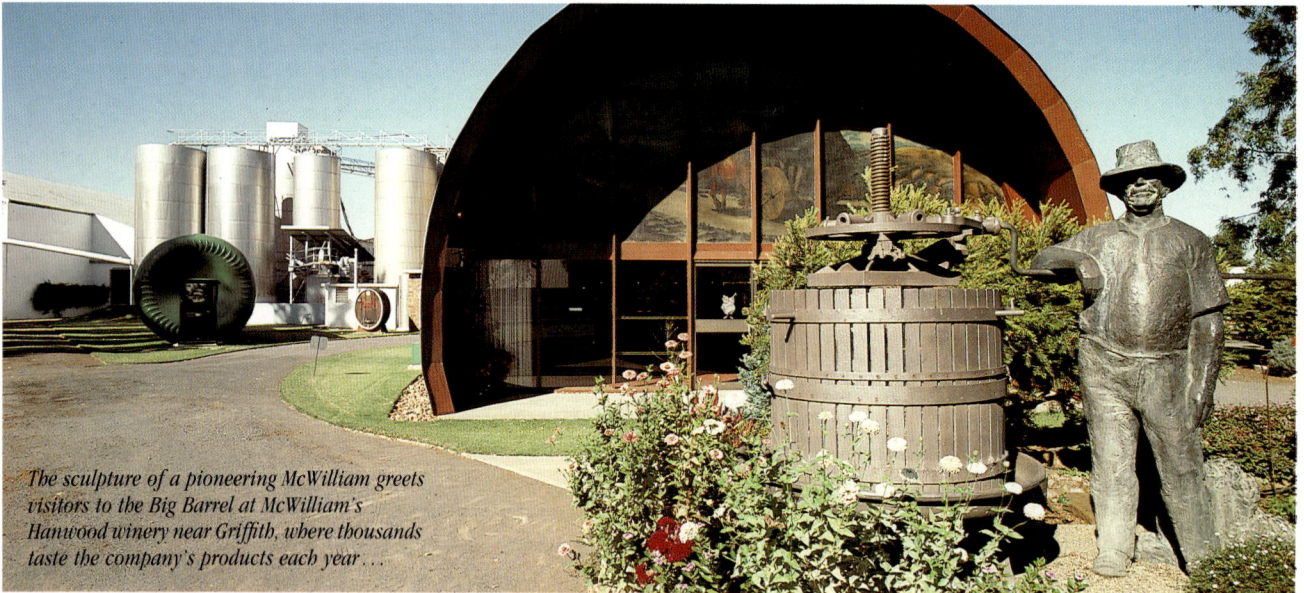

The sculpture of a pioneering McWilliam greets visitors to the Big Barrel at McWilliam's Hanwood winery near Griffith, where thousands taste the company's products each year . . .

That happy state of affairs, though, is slowly coming to an end, as many wineries give away a few per cent of their production in this way and, when you understand that this can make the difference between a profit or a loss for the wine-maker, you can appreciate why an increasing number of wineries are now charging for tastings. The fee charged, if any, is small, just a dollar or two, but the happy days of free tastings, while still with us, seem limited.

Visiting a winery without tasting the product is like, well, having a barbecue without tomato sauce. It's obligatory, and it's an enjoyable and hopefully educational process.

Visiting wineries and tasting wines will help you learn a lot about wines, especially about the vast differences between them. And it will give you an increased appreciation of the essentially rural connections of wine, and the generally delightful nature of many of the people who toil in vineyard and winery to make the product.

But visiting and tasting at cellar door also imposes a few obligations on visitors, gentle though those obligations may be. This brief chapter may help you enjoy winery visits more.

WHICH WINERIES TO VISIT?

If you live in or near Adelaide, Perth or Melbourne, or one of the major provincial centres near a wine area (such as Newcastle, Albury-Wodonga or some of the other larger Victorian cities), you can get to a wine area and back in just a few pleasant hours. Many other Australians and visitors have to drive a little further.

However far you have to go, pre-planning the trip is worth a quarter of an hour or 20 minutes of your time. There are plenty of wine books to consult, plus tourist brochures, newspaper articles and of course your own wine preferences and the recommendations of friends. If you like a wine or know of a good wine-maker, make that cellar door one of your stopping points.

Eating along the way is usually pleasant, so selecting a restaurant (and an increasing number of wineries have them on site), or a picnic or barbecue spot adds an appealing break to the day out.

HOW MANY WINERIES TO VISIT?

This depends on your stamina, but most people seem to find it hard to cope with more than three in the morning and two in the afternoon. Five wineries, or even four, is plenty for a day out, so try to make them as diverse as you can. Perhaps, if you are going to a larger area such as the Hunter, Barossa, Swan Valley or McLaren Vale, you can take in one or two bigger wineries and then make the rest small wineries.

The charm of small wineries is that you will quite likely get a chance to meet the wine-maker or one of his family at the counter, and hear a close-up view of what it's like to grow the grapes and make the

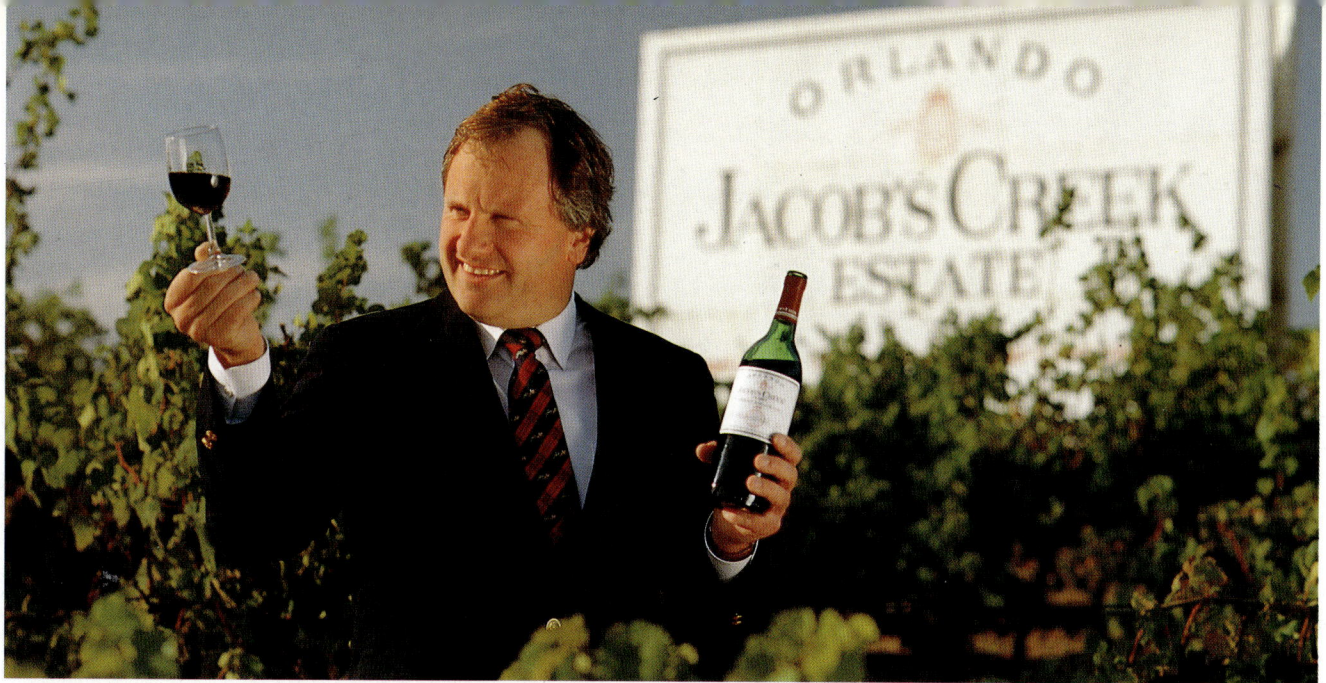

Blending is one of the skills used by big wine-makers to attain large volumes of high quality wine. Robin Day, Orlando's Chief Wine-maker, shows how it's done with Jacobs Creek red.

wine, from whoa to go.

Bear in mind also that most wine areas have attractions other than wineries, and you'll very likely want to see the scenery, the monuments, the wildlife or flowers, the towns themselves, the beaches, the arts and/or crafts shops and so on.

HOW MANY WINES CAN I TRY?

No real limit, within reason. Parties of itinerant boozers from footy clubs tend to get rather short shrift at cellar doors as they are often simply out to have a "good time", beginning at a pub. But if you have any reasonable interest in wine, your interest (at any level from beginner to buff) will be taken seriously by whoever is organising the tasting. They'll try to show you wines you enjoy.

As a rule of thumb, tasting four or five whites, three or four reds and one or two fortified wines is no problem from the winery's point of view.

IN WHAT ORDER SHOULD I TASTE THE WINES?

Sparkling wines first, then whites from fruity through to dry, followed by reds, and then fortifieds and/or sweet whites. Dry biscuits and cheese will help you cleanse your palate, but nibble on them, and try to select biscuits and a cheese which isn't too spicy or too sharp.

CAN I SPIT THE WINES OUT OR DO I HAVE TO SWALLOW?

Of course you can spit them out! But you don't have to. Sipping and spitting is a recognised part of wine tasting, and judging. Almost all wineries either provide buckets or sinks for spitting out tasting wines. (No, they do not recycle these wines!) If you cannot see such a bucket, don't hesitate to ask if you can spit.

You *can* swallow, but be careful. A mouthful or so of each of five wines at five wineries adds up to 25 mouthfuls, which could well be a full bottle of wine. In some circumstances, that could well put you over the legal blood/alcohol limit.

DO I HAVE TO BUY WINES?

No. If you've tried a few wines and you genuinely haven't tasted anything you liked, say so. Explain why, too, if possible. Any reasonable wine-maker knows that their wines will not appeal to everybody. That's the beauty of wine — there's always something else down the road. But the wine-maker quite fairly expects a reasonable level of interest from you. In other words, you shouldn't be coming through the door and drinking his wines if you were not prepared to buy some (however little), if you do enjoy the wine.

HOW SHOULD I PAY FOR ANY WINE?

Most of the usual facilities are available at wineries — all reasonable credit cards, and cheques will be accepted at most with presentation of reasonable identification. Even cash! Freight and insurance will normally have to be paid for together with the wine itself, if you want it sent home.

HOW MUCH WINE TO BUY

Here's one of the traps for young players. The best answer is (unless you really know what you're all about): not too much.

There are several reasons for this advice. First of all is the feeling I hinted at above. Tasting with a wine-maker who is understandably enthusiastic about his or her wines can be heady stuff. They love their "children" and will pour their hearts and souls into praising the wines' extraordinary virtues (and maybe — just maybe — they have such virtues!).

Joining in with the enthusiasm is easy, especially if it is the first winery you've visited that day. The wine is likely to make a very different impression on you when you face a few dozen in your home a few months later.

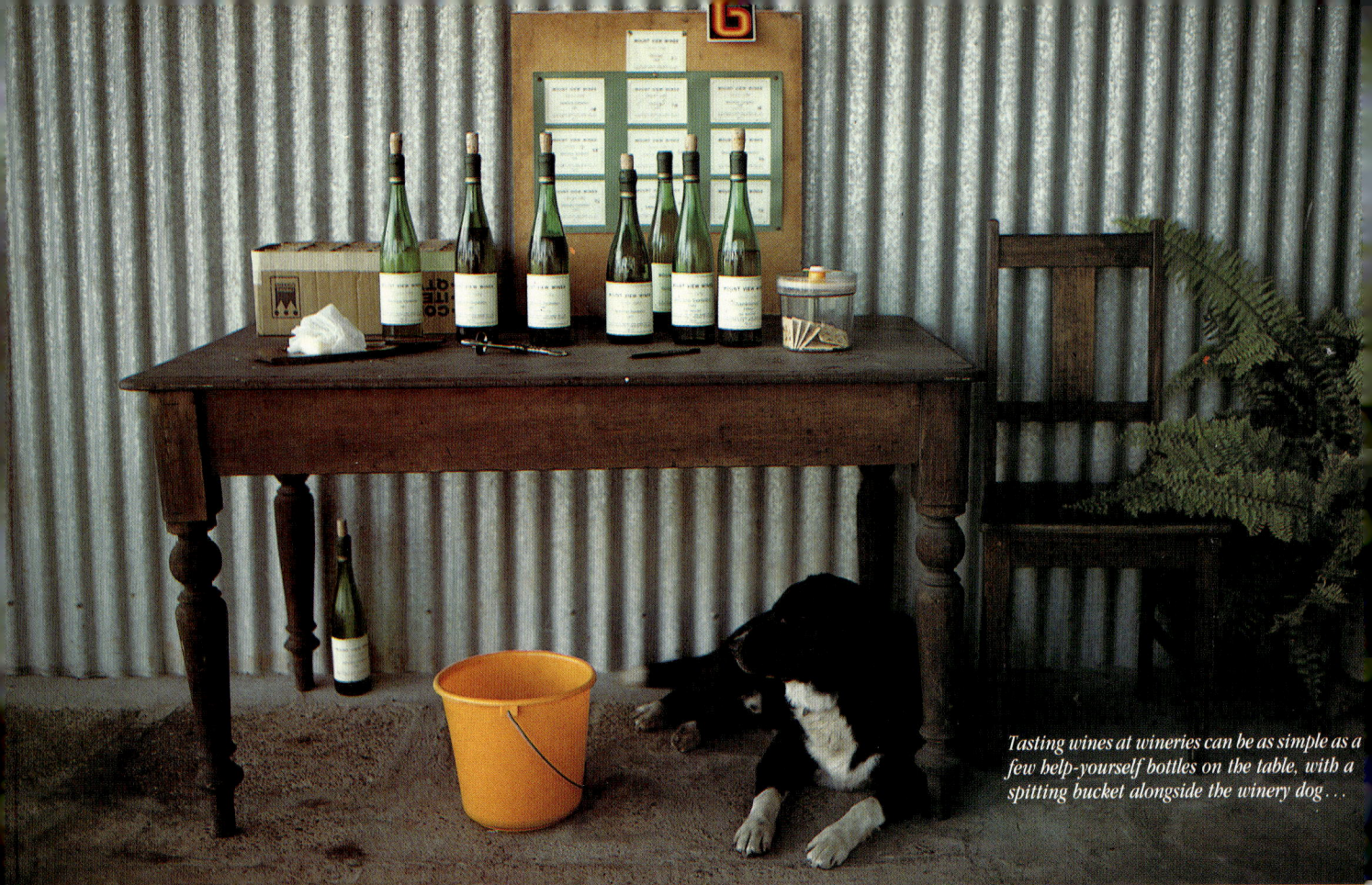

Tasting wines at wineries can be as simple as a few help-yourself bottles on the table, with a spitting bucket alongside the winery dog . . .

Proceed with caution. No bargain is so great that you can't repeat it at some stage down the line a little. Making mistakes in selecting wines is but human, and everyone who has ever had a love affair (even a flirtation) with wine has fallen into this trap. But don't fall too deeply and get stuck with a lot of wine from a few makers. Not at first, anyway. Buy by the several (or even half dozen) bottles at first.

EATING AT THE WINERY

Because wine and food go together so naturally, many people want to eat as they go around wineries. Wine-makers won't thank you for munching away at your packed lunch as other people taste, but many now provide picnic areas — one of the best, by the way, is at Brown Brothers at Milawa, but plenty of others have similar areas, even barbecue spots.

A civilised addition to the winery calendar in recent years has been "Gourmet Weekends" where each winery in an area invites a restaurant or hotel to serve manageable portions of high-quality foods. Two of the best are held in the Clare Valley and McLaren Vale's "Continuous Picnic" each year.

Taking a picnic and enjoying a glass of wine is a great way of touring the wine areas of Australia.

HOW TO TAKE WINES HOME

With care, naturally. Car boots are likely to be a problem (they get very hot in summer); aeroplanes tend to break a few bottles in every case. Buses ditto, and you can also lose your wine by theft. Some form of separate road freight, recommended by the winery, is often a good idea. But insure your wine as part of the purchase deal; any reputable cellar door sales operation will be able to arrange both road freight at fair prices, and insurance.

Individual or loose bottles are a problem, too. If you aren't buying wine in whole cases (normally a dozen 750 ml bottles to a case) ask a friendly cellar door person if you can take the three or so bottles you buy there in an empty carton; you can fill the carton up as you visit other wineries. Try to get a complete dozen, or dozens, as they travel more securely encased in lots of 12 bottles inside the carton. If taking just a few bottles, try to get

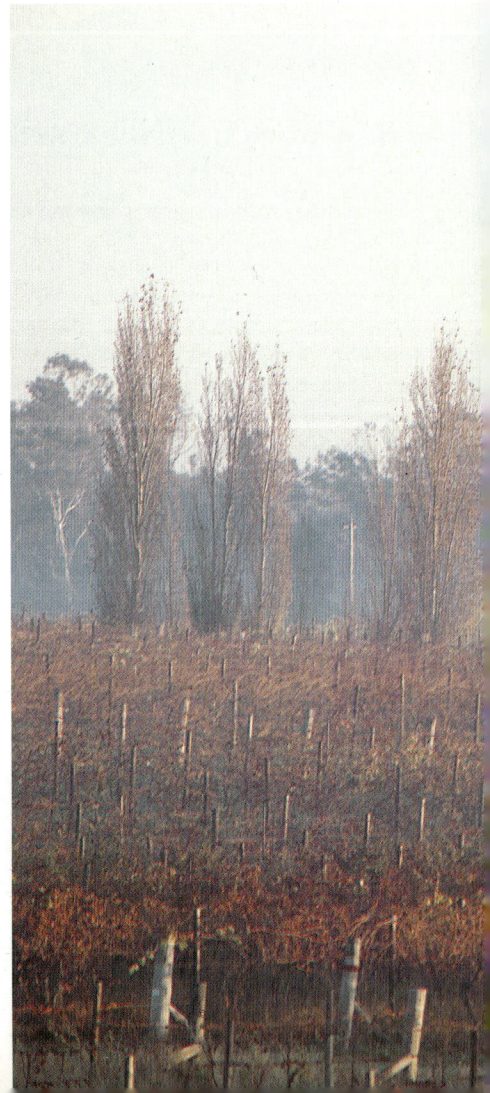

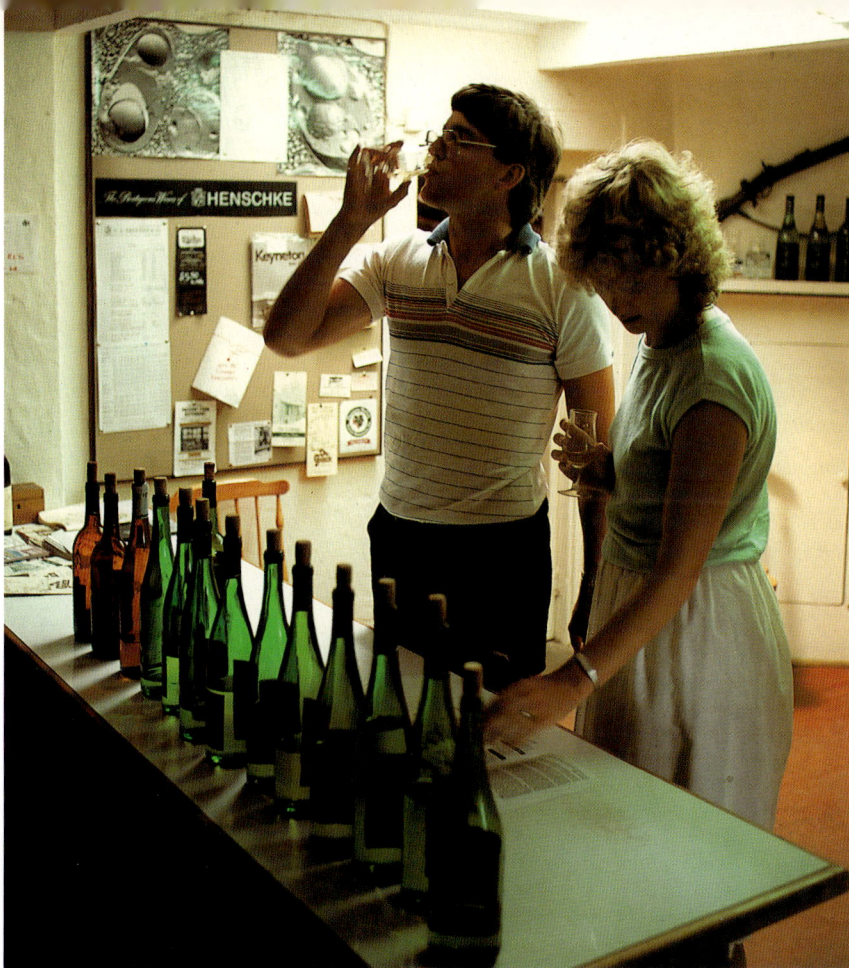

one of the "carry-packs" available in many wineries in capacities of two, three or four bottles each. Maybe also pack them with newspaper or cloth to help the wines survive the journey home.

WILL I SAVE MONEY BY BUYING AT THE WINERY?

The cautious answer to that is: you may, but probably not much. This has been canvassed elsewhere, but wineries are forced by many of their trade customers to keep their prices up so as not to unfairly (as the trade sees it) compete with licensed liquor outlets, which are their largest clients. Occasionally bin-end bargains are to be found at cellar doors, too. But you *will* have a lot of fun, and learn some fascinating things about wines if you plan your winery visits a little, and behave as if you are the wine-maker's honoured guest — which you are.

BE A LITTLE SENSITIVE ...

Wine-makers are there, like most of the rest of us, to earn a living. They are enthusiastic about their products and their premises, normally. Rampaging kids, noisy parties of story-tellers, yahoos in racing cars, Know-All wine buffs who've always tried something better elsewhere, and people who steal tasting glasses and anything else that's not nailed down usually get a hostile reception (and maybe a warning phone call to the next place down the road!).

Wine tasting remains a civilised privilege to be enjoyed, not abused. And if you take a curious yet relaxed attitude about going to the cellar doors of Australia's wineries, you'll have a great time, and you'll most likely Meet your 'Maker there!

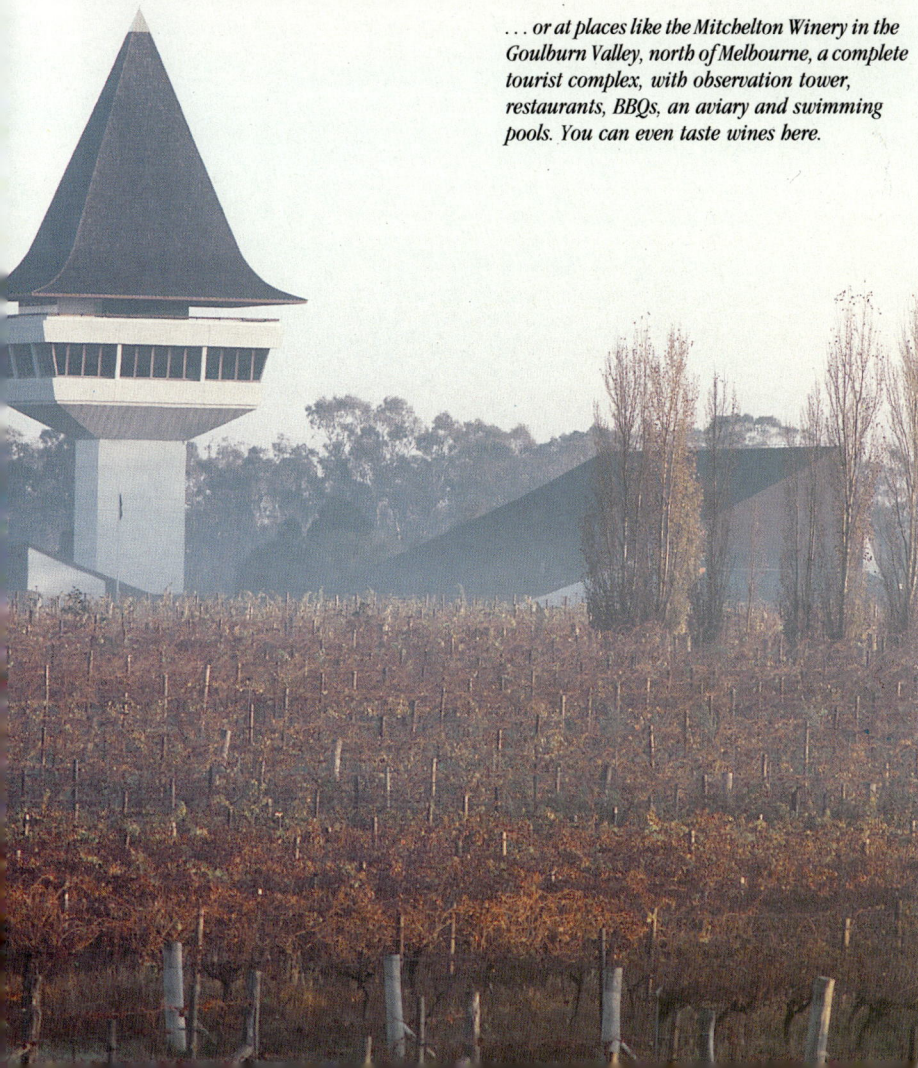

. . . or at places like the Mitchelton Winery in the Goulburn Valley, north of Melbourne, a complete tourist complex, with observation tower, restaurants, BBQs, an aviary and swimming pools. You can even taste wines here.

RECOMMENDED READING: A good winery tourist map. Most wine areas produce their own, often in conjunction with local (or State) tourism bodies and tourist centres.

RECOMMENDED DRINKING: A half bottle (375 ml) of Hardy's Siegersdorf Rhine Riesling. Then you'll be able to drive safely.

COLLECTING WINES

You don't need a stone cellar. A few traps to avoid in storing wine.

You can collect wines at varying levels of interest. Many people who know little about wine keep a few bottles here or there — sometimes for the right reasons, sometimes for the wrong reasons. I kept a few bottles of quite old Grange Hermitage for years because they'd belonged to my Dad. Sentimental but silly, as by the time I came to drink them they'd had it, because Dad had not stored them properly. (He kept them under the bar in his family room, where the kerosene heater was...)

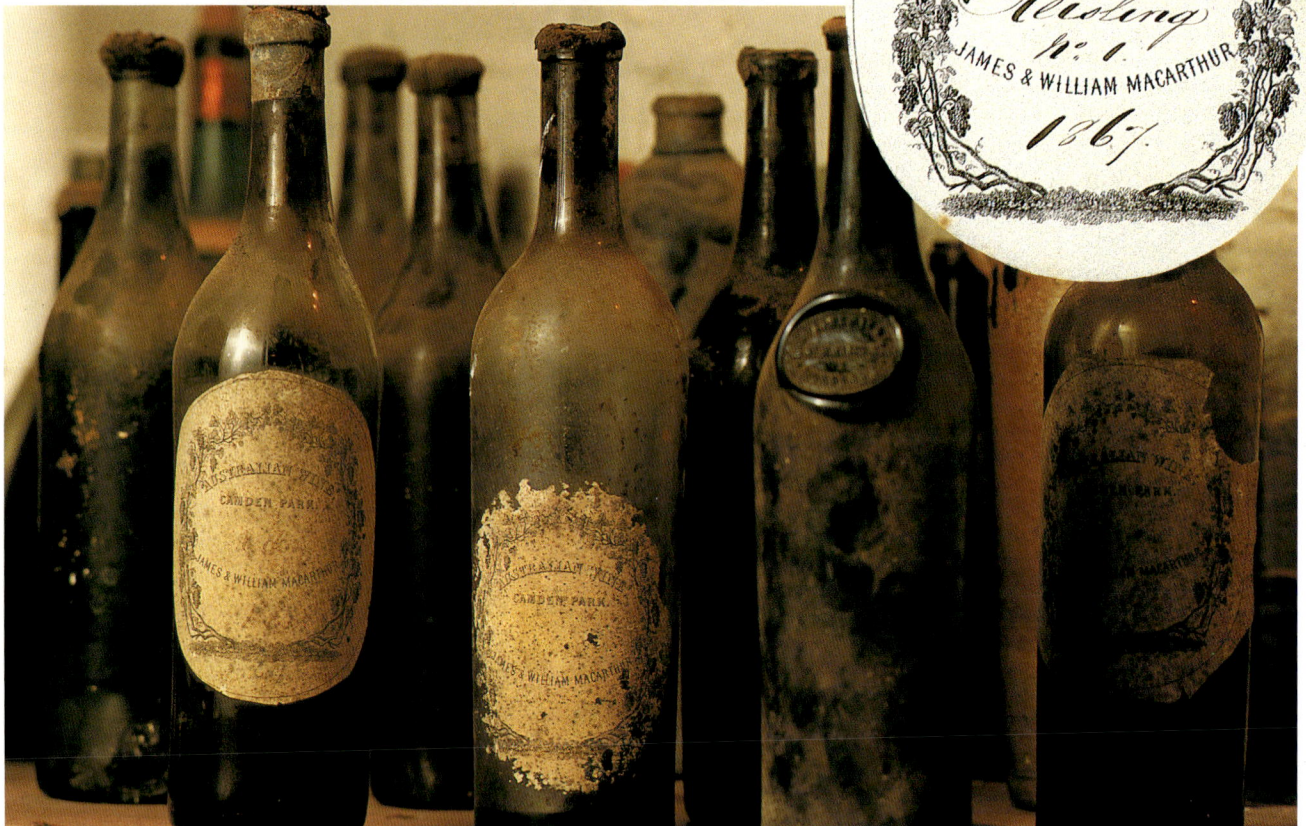

I should say up front here that not many people collect wine. The wine trade knows that 95 per cent of wines bought in liquor stores or pubs are consumed within 24 hours. Who'd want to make wines that last?

Nevertheless most commercial wines will improve with some bottle age. But why collect wines at all?

Well, first, we have ready access to a reasonable range of wines.

Secondly, wines, or some of them, improve in quality (or drinkability).

Thirdly, maybe to make a monetary gain, or alternatively to save yourself money because you bought cheaply and can continue to drink economically, compared with inflating wine prices. (In fact wine prices have in reality fallen over recent years in real terms, largely because of the continuing high level of competition between Australian wine-makers.)

The fourth reason may well be because you enjoy collecting things, possibly to celebrate an anniversary.

A final reason may be the sort of sentimental reason I cited above — as a reminder of good times, good company, a winery visit or travels elsewhere.

Collecting wine is not difficult, no matter where you live or work, for in some cases, if you are lucky, you may be able to store wine at a work place or somewhere other than home.

You've already heard about the importance of temperature in successfully storing wine. It is important, though wine does have a reasonable tolerance. As temperature rises, the ageing process accelerates, though there is a band where the change will not be as rapid as it might seem. That "tolerance band" lies roughly between 5°

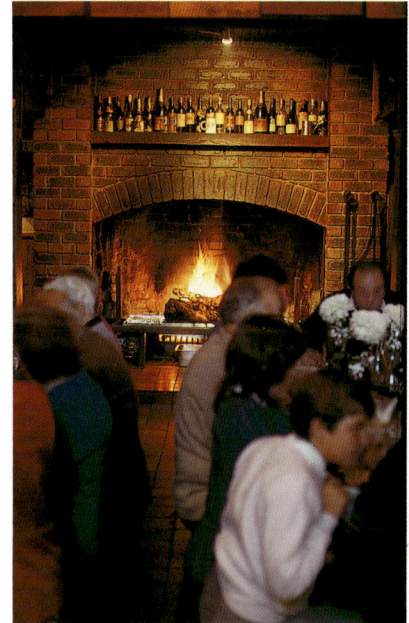

and 20°C. Below 5° the wine will age quite slowly; above 20°, quite fast through to deterioration. Inside this band, change is reasonably stable even though you are storing your wine at an average of 12°C and your neighbour is storing it at 16°, say.

Fluctuation, especially violent fluctuation, is the change which will do damage to your "cellar".

So, if you want to store wine you need a place where the temperature doesn't go much below 5° or much above the low 20's, and preferably changes only slowly throughout the year. Of course, an underground stone cellar is good because temperatures will change less there than most other places, and there are quite a number of houses (in cities like Sydney, Melbourne, Adelaide and elsewhere) built of stone blocks where such a storage arrangement is quite possible. Just watch for damp coursing, which will grow mould on the bottles and corks and may damage

Wine	Cost	Start drinking
12 bottles of Hardy's Siegersdorf Rhine Riesling	*$96*	*After 1 year*
12 bottles of Pike's Clare Rhine Riesling	*$115*	*After 18 months*
12 bottles Gramp's Chardonnay	*$84*	*After 1 year*
6 bottles of McWilliam's Elizabeth Semillon	*$60*	*After 2 years*
12 bottles Penfolds Bin 389 Cabernet/Shiraz	*$90*	*After 2 years*
12 bottles of Yalumba Galway Hermitage	*$70*	*After 1 year*
12 bottles of Seaview Shiraz/Cabernet	*$70*	*After 2 years*
12 bottles of Tyrrell's Long Flat Red (Hermitage/ Cabernet/Malbec)	*$85*	*After 2 years*
6 bottles of Yalumba Family Series Coonawarra Cabernet	*$53*	*After 3 years*
6 bottles of Seppelt's Fleur de Lys Vintage Brut	*$54*	*After 1 year*
6 bottles of Bridgewater Mill Sparkling Rhine Riesling	*$54*	*After 1 year*
6 bottles of Hardy's (young) Vintage Port	*$60*	*After 4/5 years*

Total cost around $891

Here's our Cellar Starters' list, with approximate retail prices per dozen. Now you don't have to buy all of these — maybe pick out the ones you fancy — but it's a reasonably balanced cellar which would cost you less than $900 for 114 bottles of white, red, sparkling and fortified wine. So you'd be paying an average of $7.81 a bottle. Only a smallish cellar, but with some good wines. (Notice the commercial riesling from Hardy's... it could be any good riesling, such as Orlando, Pewsey Vale, Stanley or Peter Lehmann.) All will improve with some bottle age, and all are nationally available at what must these days be considered reasonable prices.

You might consider that with buying in cheaper wines, or drinking flagon or cask wines for everyday occasions, you'll get through a couple of cellared bottles every fortnight. Averaging it out, your wines will therefore last you about a year. Doesn't seem like long, does it? And if you want them to improve, you shouldn't start drinking any of them for a year, at which point the riesling will probably be two years or so old, and the reds three or four years. The semillon and chardonnay can probably do with an extra year or so, to be opened between about two-and-a-half and four years.

You must therefore have a little patience, some discipline (especially at the end of dinner parties!) and must also be prepared to add bottles to your cellar as you subtract.

In fact I think the ideal small cellar is about 12 dozen, which should be added to a little faster than you are drinking them for a couple of years so you can build up to the desired level and then remain at that stock-holding level. You have to plan forward, but your planning will be rewarded. Remember again: keep opening them regularly to see how they're going. This means about every six months.

or remove labels.

But there are plenty of other places where small to medium quantities of wine can be stored with reasonable safety for a reasonable time. Cupboards, nooks and crannies, studies and stairwell crevices are all possibilities. Installing insulation is often possible (using Pink Batts or similar insulation, perhaps left over from other work or expansions) to keep your temperature stable.

Where possible stay away from attics, cupboard tops, high shelving and similar locations. I'm always horrified to see some restaurants storing wine around the tops of rooms, where temperatures are highest — I can see why (because floor-level space is at a premium) but the effect on the wine over a year or more will almost certainly do some damage to its quality.

Remember, too, that you should sit down before starting to collect wine and define your aims. Initially they will probably be something like: "I want to have 12 dozen bottles of medium- to good-quality wine, perhaps biased towards reds, but not necessarily so, which I can regularly rotate, and which will provide me over the next couple of years with moderately aged wines to serve at my lunches or dinners or other special occasions."

This is a realistic and economic way of starting a wine cellar. I went to see Fred Hamood, who runs Dulwich Cellars, an excellent liquor store near me in Adelaide. Together we worked out what you might buy, using "reasonably" priced commercial wines which are nationally available and which will repay one to three, maybe a few more, years of cellaring (the vintage port will need more, if young when bought). You might be able to get some of them cheaper by shopping around, so try.

STORAGE SYSTEMS

There are plenty of commercial storage systems around, most of them expensive. Remember that you can't drink them, and that they don't improve the wine! If your cellar is out of sight, don't bother spending a lot of money on expensive racks. If a rack of 48 bottles retails for $144, then you are effectively adding $3 a bottle to the cost of your wine (at least if you write the cost off in the first three or four years). That's relatively expensive drinking, so you should ask yourself whether you want it to be decorative, or simply practical and out of sight.

There are dangers in decorative systems, as I've said. Putting wine where people can see it means conditions are not likely to be ideal, perhaps even perilous to the wine's "health" because of temperature fluctuations.

So perhaps build a wine storage racking system yourself in a safe and stable place. Get some wooden boxes, use timber offcuts, weld steel strips together, use off-cuts from suitable sized plastic tubing ... use old cardboard wine cartons if you have to (provided they won't get damp). The storage systems advertised in glossy magazines and elsewhere may look good, but storing your wine in the living room, where the temperature goes up and down all the time, isn't the wisest thing to do with your valuable wine.

If you must display wine somewhere, don't display the lot. Use the wine you'll be drinking next and keep the rest in a cooler, more stable environment.

MAKING MONEY

Making money from wine is like making money (or aiming to make money) from anything else. If it was easy we'd all be doing it. You need to spend a lot of time studying what's in demand, which way trends are going, the trends in wine styles and what has historically done well. I've sometimes thought that there must be more wines on the market in Australia than there are horses racing ...

You *can* make money from wine, just as you *can* make money from punting, but it probably isn't worth the time and trou-

ble unless you make a virtual occupation from it. In my view, it's better to get pleasure and enjoyment from ageing wines for your pleasure, and that of your friends and guests. Bear in mind also that buying and selling alcohol without a liquor licence is unlawful in most places.

The other point to be remembered is that simply being old isn't enough to make a wine valuable. It depends on its rarity. There are still a lot of bottles of Seppelt 1944 Para Liqueur Port out there, so it will fetch only about $45-$50 a bottle at auction. Penfold's famous 1955 Grange Hermitage, though, will get you up to $500 a bottle. And the earlier Granges from the 1952, 1953 and similar vintages were not commercially released and are breaking auction records every time bottles find their way out of the hands of well-connected owners! These rare vintages of the 1950s are fetching between $1,000 and $2,500 a bottle, because of their scarcity.

Just out of interest, though, here are a few example of how a small selection of wines have improved in value over the years, selected for me by my good friend, the eminent Adelaide auctioneer and wine authority Colin Gaetjens :

Wynn's (black label) Coonawarra Cabernet Sauvignon 1978 would have retailed for about $5/$6 a bottle when released, is now worth about $15 or more. **Hardy's Eileen Hardy Dry Red 1970** (a great vintage, the first of these wines) sold for about $5 and now fetches about $30 a bottle.
Wolf Blass "Jimmy Watson" Black Label wines of the early 1970s sold on release about $6 and now get about $25 a bottle.
Penfold Grandfather 1945 Port (current releases are non-dated) sold in the early 1970s for around $6 — now about $60-$70 a bottle.
Penfold 1966 and 1971 Grange Hermitage originally cost between $12-$16 a bottle, they're now worth $150 and $225 respectively.

In considering whether you can make capital gains out of wine, then, remember these key points. Most wines in this country are made in commercial (i.e. large) quantities to be consumed not long — a few years, generally — after making. Only the wines with big 'asset backing', such as the French First Growths, Penfold's

Grange and so on, will appreciate in a reliable and rewarding way. The way to take advantage of cellaring is to buy good wines, mature them yourself and drink them yourself so that you do not incur the cost of someone else cellaring them on your behalf.

KEEP A RECORD

A cellar book is a good idea, however simply done. List your wines, and log them in and out. If you have the time, list what you paid for them and comment on how you liked them when you opened them.

These days you can use a computer to do the same thing. Indeed, you can now buy several personal computer programs to help you keep track of your wines.

HOW LONG WILL AUSTRALIAN WINES KEEP?

Generally, not as long as their best French counterparts, a factor partly of cool-climate vs warm-climate wine-making. But almost all Australian commercial bottled wines costing over about $5 a bottle will improve with a few years' bottle age, with good reds eight to 10 years. Wine-makers often give best-estimate recommendations, as do wine magazines. But they are only rules of thumb to be considered in tandem with storage conditions and vintage variations.

SHOULD I RE-CORK?

No, unless you are keeping or dealing in wines over about 12-15 years' of age. Consult an expert if you feel you need to put new corks in older wines.

Penfold run regular 'clinics' for the owners of older Penfold reds such as Grange, St Henri and so on, where they can have their wines inspected, possibly tasted and sometimes recorked by the wine-maker.

RECOMMENDED READING: Robin Bradley puts out his regular *Australian Wine Vintages*, with opinions from the actual wine-makers as to their wines' progress, sponsored by Benson and Hedges.

RECOMMENDED DRINKING: If you're on the learning curve (who isn't?) get a bottle of a great Australian red and taste it when it's young, so you know what to look for ... Penfold's St Henri (Saint On-ree) of a recent vintage.

Buying Cheaper Wine

Everybody wants to buy cheap (or cheaper) wine. Very few of us would admit that we like to pay more than we need to for anything, and with wine a particularly powerful Scrooge instinct seems to come into play! I worked for a large wine company for five years, and the question I was most often asked on social occasions was: 'What's cheap and good?' There was a positive answer. The company, like most others making a wide range of products, had bits and pieces, discarded lines, products with imperfect packaging and lines being quit for various other commercial reasons. This was known internally as the 'Deleted Products' list (that is, deleted from the company's main wholesale and retail lists).

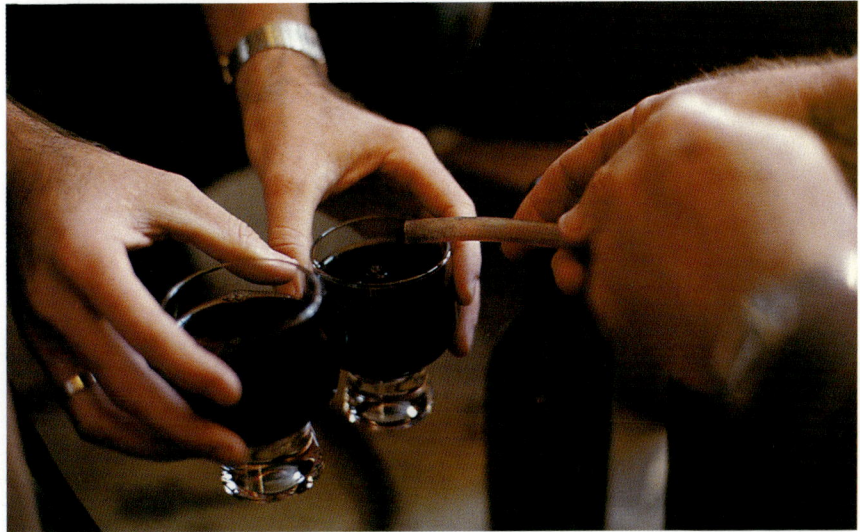

Tasting a red wine from the barrel is a good idea before buying a bulk wine.

On this list, printed out every few weeks by the company's computer department, were some things I wouldn't drink in a fit; some moderately good wines; some interesting curios; some reasonable quaffers (including flagons) and, every now and then, some stunning bargains. On one occasion in 1988 the company had 1,500 cases (that's 18,000 bottles) of an excellent 1985 Rhine riesling that they quit at just $3 a bottle. Why? Because a very small number of the bottles had faulty corks. Some leaked a little and so the fill was a little below the 750 ml contents printed on the labels. So rather than unpack the lot and find the bad 'uns, or hassle with a very few disgruntled buyers, they very reasonably decided to put it all on the Deleted Products list to get rid of the problem quickly, and get some cash at the same time.

I bought quite a lot of this wine, and shared some with friends, and only ever found two bottles that were 'corked' (the air had got in and the wine had gone sour). The overwhelming majority of bottles were absolutely terrific drinking, bearing in mind that I happen to believe that Australian rieslings are among some of the best wines we can make.

As I write this I am drinking a 1987 Watervale Rhine Riesling that another major maker quit at $3 a bottle because they couldn't be bothered selling it to the trade in the quantity they had (a few hundred cases).

You've got to be lucky, or have a friend in the business, to crack bargains like this, though. But there *are* other ways of finding bargains in wines, and here are a few clues to help you spot them.

WATCH THE BARGAIN BINS

If you are looking for a recognised, quality brand in a retail outlet these days you'd expect to pay at least $5.99 to $8.99 and up a bottle, often a lot more.

Nevertheless, liquor store owners often need to clear crowded shelves. They have leftover odds and ends and just can't move quite good wines because they are not brand names, are not advertised, or for some other reasons. There are sometimes some odd bargains around which, while there's no surefire way to spot them, can give you a big saving if you can sniff them out. Example: some companies put brand-ed products (let's say it's Chateau Mayne's Coonawarra Cabernet/Shiraz, normally selling for $7.99) into special label jobs. It might be sold as National Trust Dry Red, Cootamundra Bowling Club Dry Red or Townsville Library Centenary Cabernet/Shiraz. The label may or may not indicate the maker's name, but if it's a large maker, it'll almost certainly be a good commercial wine.

And it may be going really cheaply. If the conditions listed above apply, it's probably worth risking three or four bucks to try it. If it tastes good, run back and buy a case or two!

You'd also be surprised at the number of big branded wines sold under different labels. They seldom sell big quantities under these special labels, so the 'fathers' of these ideas usually have to quit varying quantities at the end of the day. They end up in bins in stores, restaurants, wineries, offices ... Pick them out from the ruck, and you can save quite a lot of money.

Some of the direct buying lures aimed at wine drinkers.

Making friends with your local wine retailer can be an investment in drinking economically. He or she will be flattered by your interest, too.

But, as always, taste critically if you can, to see whether you like it first.

SAVING AT CELLAR DOOR

Cellar doors at wineries sometimes sell wine cheaply. I say *sometimes* because they generally find it difficult to do so because of opposition to low prices from the people who are their main customers — the wholesalers and retailers, who have to mark products up to make a profit themselves. These sorts of wines may well be in the 'bargain bins' as described above.

Every now and then you'll find a bargain, and not just at the big boys' cellar door sales operations. They get rid of discontinued lines which can't be sold elsewhere when they have 50 or 100 or 500 cases left, when vintages have changed, when labels have been re-designed or there has been some other aberration in the making, marketing, selling or distribution systems.

Retailers themselves can offer bargains frequently, and they are often worth grabbing with both hands. Several cases come to mind. When Penfold's bought Wynn's a few years ago they had to honour sales commitments to sell some splendid Wynn's Coonawarra reds very cheaply. Hardy's bought Chateau Reynella, and in early 1983 sold a poultice of wines to Melbourne-based merchant Dan Murphy, who quit large volumes of excellent Chateau Reynella wines at what appeared to be absurb prices — in some cases for $1 a bottle!

Maybe those mad discount days have gone, though I suspect it will happen again from time to time.

ADVERTISING WINE BARGAINS

Watch the display ads in the main newspapers, especially those that run long typeset lists of wines with prices. The ads

that show all of those pictures of products, or bottles, are called 'co-op advertising' in the liquor business; that means the liquor maker or agent is invited, even coerced, into paying the retailer to have his labelled bottle put in the overall advertisement. Many sales deals are done over this 'co-operative' formula, so real bargains are hard to find in this area — notice how all the prices are pitched at those $5.99-$6.99-$7.99-$8.99 (and so on) 'price points'?

While I'm spilling trade secrets, some of the consumer wine publications also sell pictures of bottles to liquor makers. They conduct tastings to assess quality (which

are probably quite fairly done, though we have no guarantees of this) and then they tell some liquor companies that their products have done well, and invite them to have the labels/bottles pictured in the relevant magazine in colour, at $200 or $300 per label.

The consumer/buyer should know these things — as the differences between paid advertising and independent editorial comment is becoming increasingly muddied, as it is in motor cars, food, real estate and many other areas of business.

It is all about *selling* things, of course. But good contacts and a desire to find a bargain can help you seek out the occasional bargain lot. Stay alert!

BUYING BY MAIL

It is possible to buy wine by mail and save money. But you do have to exercise care and think a bit about what you're doing. There is always, obviously, a price of one kind or another for saying Yes to convenience.

There are now many organisations spruiking wine by mail, by brochure, by cassette and through various other sales mediums. American Express and Cellarmasters are two such organisations offering many very good wines, often with the additional attraction of enabling you to try a number of products you normally may not find or get around to tasting, wrapped into one simple deal.

The Australian Wine Club, based in Melbourne and started by Bill Jane (brother of racing and motorsport champ Bob Jane) and his three daughters, is another good commercially operated wine club. Their newsletter is better than most, and they run some keen bargains and good wine recommendations, from all over Australia.

WINE CLUBS AND SOCIETIES

With so much variety around in the wine-making business, it's simpler to let others do the deciding for you. Or is it?

We all know how hard it is to try lots of wines when you're so busy working, running a family or socialising. The Wine Society, based in Sydney is one of the original Australian wine clubs. This is a true co-operative, based on non-profit share-holding and an idea sensibly borrowed from a similar organisation in the U.K.

One of their more attractive schemes, still operating, is to supply members monthly (or less frequently, as requested) with a mixed dozen bottles of wine at a guaranteed price. They can be ordered with a bias towards red wines, white wines or whatever. But this does again enable members to try wines they may never otherwise manage to taste. If liked, these wines can be ordered in larger quantities from the Society. Prices are on the whole very fair, with an occasional scoop bargain purchase.

The Wine Society puts out a bulletin, conducts tastings, sells all sorts of interesting and appealing wines (and other beverages). Compared with the American Express and some similar schemes, it is less 'glamorous' and the wines are somewhat less up-market, but in my view, it is a very good way to buy wine sensibly and eco-

nomically. You can will your Society shares on to your children, too, if you so desire — an interesting wine legacy.

WINE MERCHANTS' HOME ORDERS

Quite a few of the more entrepreneurial wine merchants have started their own mailing list newsletters, and a few are very good. Dan and his son Phillip Murphy in Melbourne are among the very best wine merchants in this country, and perhaps anywhere, in terms of their experience in the wine business, the range of products and buying power. There are others such as Crittendens in Melbourne, Camperdown Cellars and Kemeny's operation in Sydney plus others in Perth, Adelaide, Hobart (Aberfeldy Cellars in Tasmania is quite exceptional, and has a very good newsletter) and Brisbane ... There are always bargains of one level or another to be found in-store, or more particularly through their newsletters.

Many suburban liquor merchants run small wine groups, and they are also a good way to get to know what's currently good in wine.

They all chop and change, as the liquor business is a cut-throat one, and there's plenty of movement, with new operators constantly emerging.

Farmer Brothers in Canberra operate a large wine business which provides an honest-to-goodness, hard-sell newsletter. They sell good wines cheaply, deliver all over Australia and they know their wines.

Mail ordering from these sorts of operations is a smart way to buy wine as cheaply as you can reasonably get good wines in this country. You'll see plenty of their ads in the major metropolitan newspapers.

BOTTLING YOUR OWN

By this I mean you actually bottle wine which has been made by others.

Of course, you *can* make your own, and plenty of people have fun doing so, as many thousands of people enjoy making their own beer. For a start there is no tax on the stuff you make yourself (which is somewhat less attractive with wine than with beer, as taxes are lower on wine).

But wine-making is a complex business, and much can go wrong without ready access to high technology, good yeasts and laboratory skills. There's not much point ending up with alcohol if the beverage which contains it is not drinkable, far less enjoyable!

You can buy bulk wine from many wineries, especially the smaller ones, usually contained in 20 to 50-litre plastic drums. The next step is to put it in bottles yourself, or have a bottling party. Or you can have the bottling party at a winery. Some wineries encourage this — for example, Maglieri's and Tinlin's, both near my home south of Adelaide.

Be cautioned, though. The bottles and plastic hoses *must* be clean. Airborne or other infections which get into dirty containers, or unsterilised hoses or bottles can ruin your wine, as can bad corks or other contaminated equipment.

Home brewers are well aware of the need for careful and thorough hygiene, and taking a leaf from their book is worthwhile, even if wine (especially port, with its much higher alcohol level) is somewhat safer, as the alcohol content should be higher than most beers.

It can be a lot of fun to have a bottling party with a group of like-minded friends. And you can save some money — though I suggest not a lot over the cost of buying good commercial wine, already bottled, from major makers.

A WORD OF CAUTION

Taste before you buy wine you are unsure of or have not tasted previously. Be cautious about small or unknown makers. Be very *wary* of door-to-door liquor salespeople (particularly if they are selling imported wines). Unlabelled wines can be dangerous buys, if you're unsure what they really are or where they come from. And old or damaged stock might be suspect. Stay away from cask bargains (they've probably had it), and be careful of flagon 'bargains'.

Yes, it's nice to drink wine cheaply. But not bad wines! Cheap wines you've got to throw away or you don't like are actually expensive wines, because you paid out money and got nothing in return.

RECOMMENDED READING: *The Good Australian Wine Guide* is a neat little book produced by Penguin, in which Melbourne wine writer Mark Shield and colleague Phillip Meyer taste and review 1,000 wines and rate them for quality and value.

RECOMMENDED DRINKING: The wine that they considered "Best Wine" was Mildara's 1988 Coonawarra Cabernet Sauvignon, and indeed most of this makers' reds are excellent. Also try their Jamieson's Run reds (and whites).

PULLING THE LAST CORK

*This chapter should really be titled 'Pulling the First Cork'
– I hope you aren't about to pull your last! There is so much
pleasure to be had from wine, in all its manifestations,
that your pleasures should have just begun.
This book was started because I thought my first wine book,
UNDERSTANDING AUSTRALIAN WINE, needed revision and
expansion to help people like those who've said to me over the
years, 'I like drinking wine, I don't know much about it, but I
know what I like.' Such a comment, or feeling, is the perfect
recipe for finding out more about wine, enjoying it more,
collecting it (if you wish), and for ordering better wines
wherever you go in Australia or overseas.*

The wine buffs may still frighten a few of us, whether they're wine waiters, pseuds or people who do know plenty about wine, and who should know better than to show off . The trouble is, wine is an infectious enthusiasm and we all, myself included, want to share the flavours and pleasures of wine with others.

Quite often when I go to restaurants I am asked to choose the wine. I'm also a creature of habit, and I must confess that I enjoy it when others choose wines they have enjoyed, and maybe I haven't tasted before. I also enjoy finding a wine that I really enjoy (especially if it's reasonably priced), and I go back and order it again. The wines that *I* enjoy tend to have several things in common: they are strong on fruit flavours (and if wooded, are not overly wood flavoured); they have their various components in balance; and they are reasonably priced.

Is that what you want in a wine? I suspect it might be because, if you're like me, you want to enjoy drinking it, probably with food. Why?

Each year the range of flavours and differences of wine gets renewed with the new vintage. I wish I *could* taste them all, but neither my liver, nor my time, nor my bank balance, are up to it.

I must also confess that I'd like to visit all of the wineries in Australia; I have visited many of them in the course of various jobs — though not all 600 or so. But new wineries and new wine-makers and new ideas are popping up just about as quickly as corks are being popped from bottles.

I like visiting wineries not just because I enjoy tasting and drinking different wines. The beauty of wine areas as diverse as Margaret River, Western Australia, or Clare in South Australia, or the Hunter or Mudgee in New South Wales, or Coonawarra's isolated, almost barren seclusion ... or even around my home at McLaren Vale, South Australia ... continues to delight me with the brown-and-green and then green-and-brown annual cycle of vines renewing themselves. And then there are the things around them, the mountains, bays, rivers, forests, and the inevitable Australian plains, some of which in our ignorance we call valleys.

A few years ago I went to the Napa Valley (which is to California what the Hunter Valley is to Australia) and I was enchanted to find in that Valley some of the same sorts of vineyards, similar vines and wines, equally enthusiastic people — and a burning desire to make great wines. And the Californians (and some others in the U.S.) *are* making great wines, as we undoubtedly are in Australia today.

I suppose it is the constantly changing cycle, the link with the land, the pleasure of the product and the nature of the people who grow and produce it that makes this industry, and this product, a special one in California, in New Zealand, in Australia and even back where it started, in France, Germany, Portugal and Spain and elsewhere in the Old World.

There is an affinity among wine people, whether they belong to the smaller

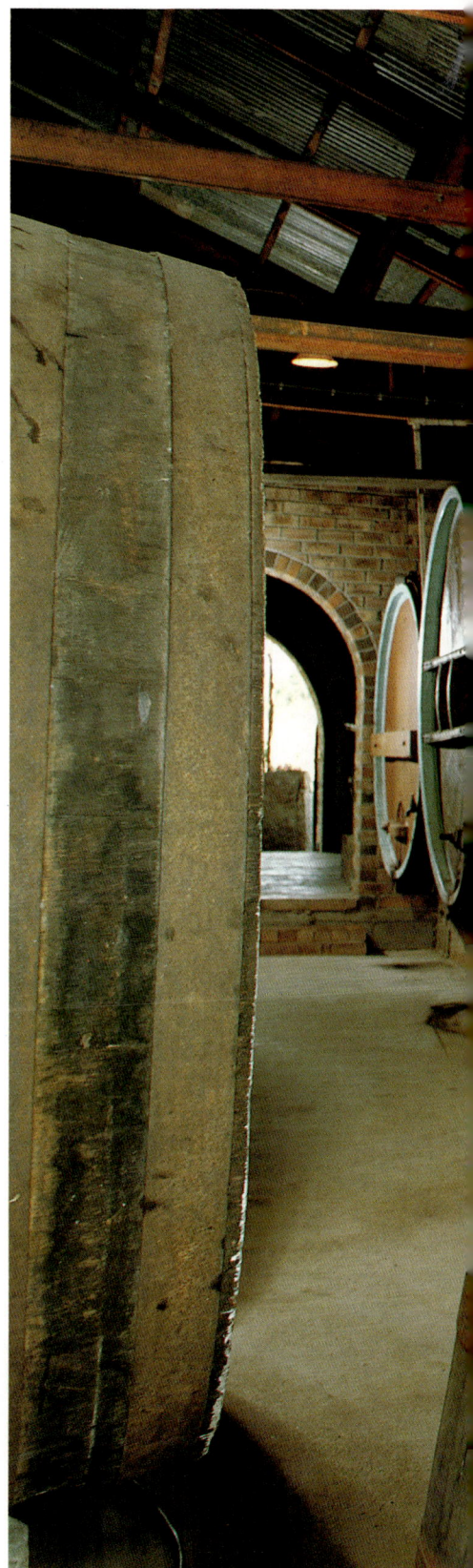

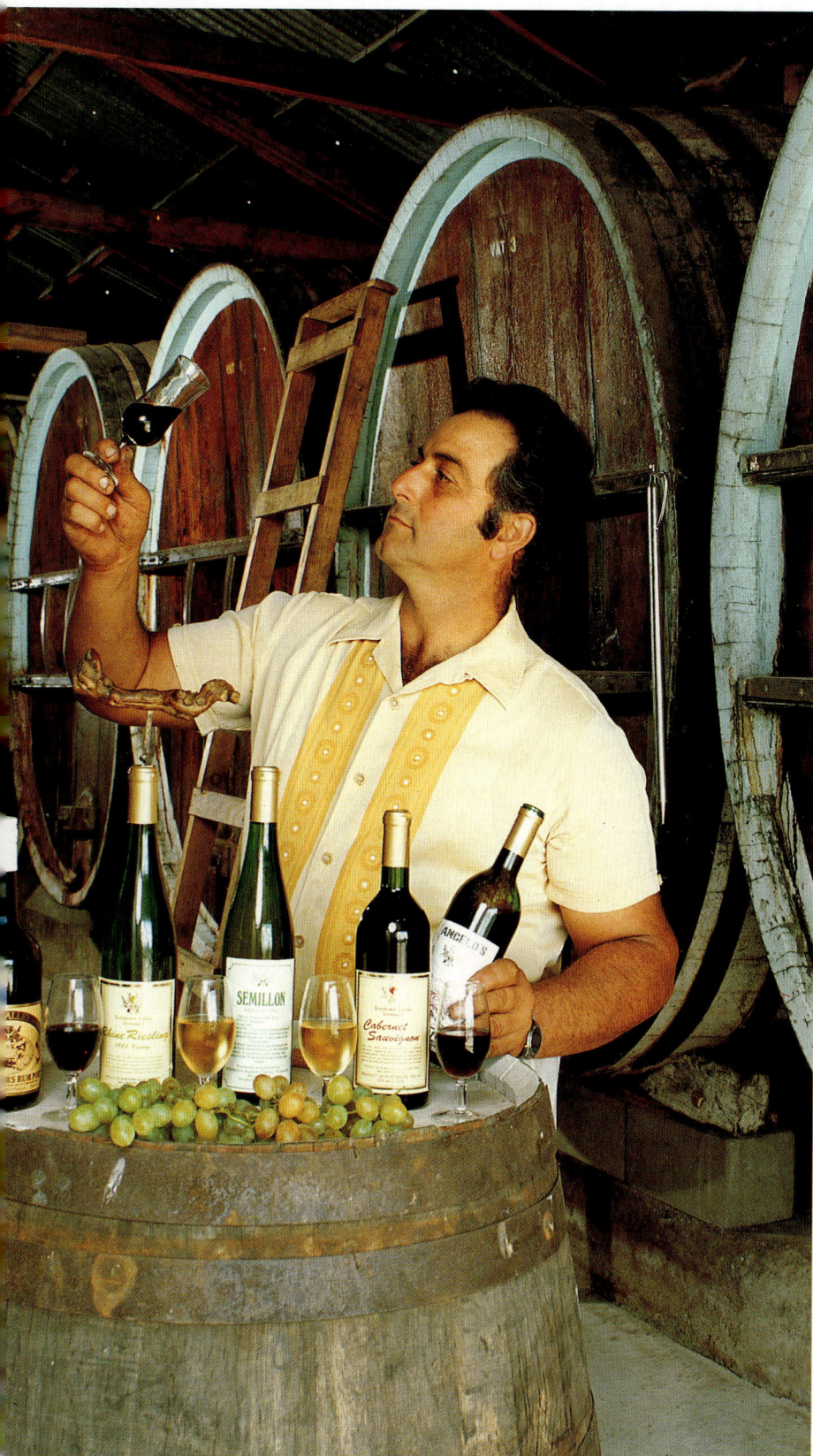

*Not everyone has the opportunity to have a cellar like this. But Australian wines are still remarkably good value for money, and you **can** build up a cellar if you have the enthusiasm and a few spare dollars.*

ranks of wine-makers or the larger ranks of wine drinkers, all over the world. They are civilised people.

And in the countries of the New Wine World, such as the United States and Australia and New Zealand (most obviously), some amazingly good wines are, increasingly, being made today. Indeed, I know that in Australia we are making wines which on average leave the French and the Germans and the Italians for dead.

This outstanding value-for-money component that Australian wines offer has, with a lot of help from the competitive Australian Wine Show circuit, led to a great export boom. I believe it will continue, and that we can carve for Australia a powerful new position in the world of wine over the next few decades. After all, we have the skills, the technology, the climate and, quite importantly, the clean land to grow the right grapes. And we do not necessarily just have to look to traditional wine-drinking (i.e. also wine-growing) countries for our markets, as countries such as Japan will soon offer enormous opportunities.

Our Australian wines are world class — no one in the world of wine can buy for the equivalent of five or six or seven dollars such a range of rieslings, or chardonnays, or cabernets, or even blended cheaper wines as we can pluck from our retailers' shelves in just about any populated part of Australia in the early 1990s.

I said at the beginning that we live in this new, Golden Age of Wine. Many of us can even afford to drink them daily, unlike our predecessors of decades or centuries past. Wine is the drink of the Twentieth Century, and perhaps more so, of the Twenty First Century.

We must learn, if we do not know already, to drink, enjoy and use it sensibly. It is the drink of moderation.

Wine is everlastingly different, more pleasurable, more diverse, more interesting, more personal ... just like food. In that sense, food is addictive! And yet while I need to eat food to stay alive, I cannot say the same thing of wine. Yet my life would be much the less for its absence, as much for social as for physical reasons. My feelings here are, admittedly, rather ambivalent. The drink *is* just a drink; but it is also somehow a very *special* drink. It's not like beer, or whisky, or lemonade or even milk or tea.

I enjoy drinking wine with food and good company. That is the bottom line of all this, I suppose, and I wish nothing more than some of the things said in this book help you to enjoy it too, in all of its wonderful diversity.

A FEW WINE BUZZ WORDS . . .

Wine, like anything else, has its own language. Describing flavours and tastes in words is as difficult with wine as it is with food. But human communication being what it is, we try to put into words what we also put into our mouths – and the following glossary of terms is just such an attempt.

Given that you won't understand what some of these terms mean until you actually taste the physical or chemical sensations involved, this is a quick guide to some of the more common terms used in winemaking and wine drinking. Some of the terms are obvious (acidic, sweet, dry); others are less obvious, even obscure (full-bodied, corked, volatile). You might never use any of these terms if you are, like me, a drinker and enjoyer. But you'll be certain to hear a few of them from time to time over dinner tables, or to see them in magazines or wine-writers' columns.

(Terms in SMALL CAPITALS are more fully explained elsewhere in the glossary; some of them also have pronunciation guides.)

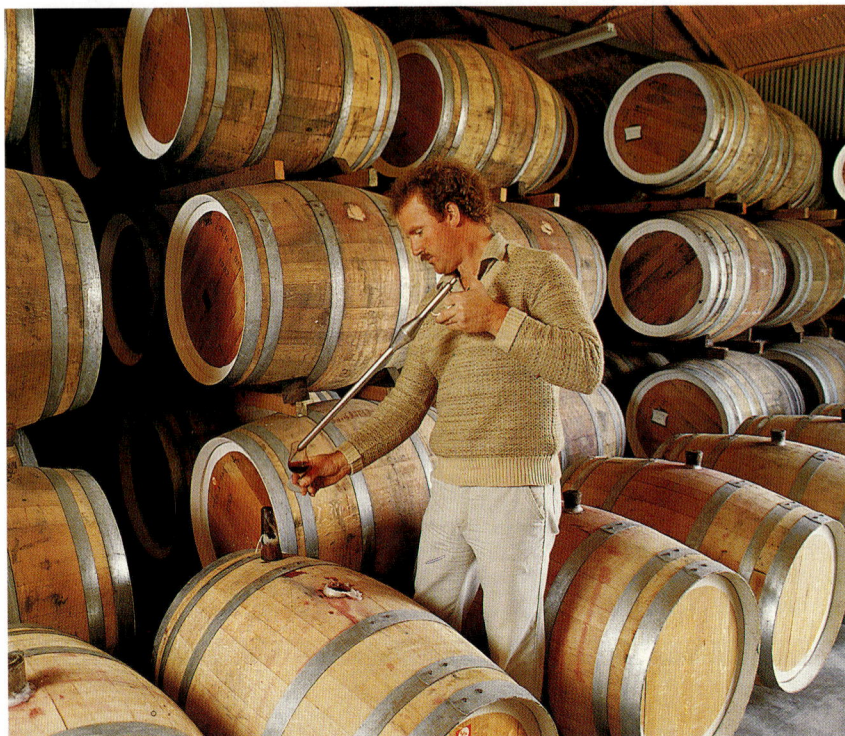

Bill Hardy makes the fortified wines and brandy for his family company, Hardy's Wines, but he also enjoys the simple pleasures of drinking wine socially.

Acetic acid

This acid (CH_3COOH) is the component that turns wine into vinegar, by oxidation (or exposure to air). Obviously, not desirable unless you want to put it on your salad. An excess of it in a wine makes the wine VOLATILE. A faulty cork can cause the problem.

Acid

Acids of various types are present in wine, and are essential to your enjoyment and to the wine's longevity. Too much can spoil the wine, even turn it into vinegar; too little also affects the wine's quality. It needs to be present in BALANCE with other components of the wine.

Aftertaste

The flavour that lingers on in your mouth after tasting or swallowing, and which can be either pleasant or unpleasant — or non-existent, which would indicate a neutral flavoured wine. Harsh or unpleasant aftertaste may indicate the presence of ACETIC ACID in the wine.

Alcohol

The substance which makes the difference between grape juice and wine! Alcohol is produced by FERMENTATION and in this context means ethyl alcohol (C_2H_5OH), produced by the action of yeasts on grape sugars during the fermentation. 'Alcoholic' usually means high in alcohol. Its ability to relax and provide enjoyment, or to intoxicate (make drunk) is fairly well appreciated, but alcohol also has an important bearing on the taste of wine.

Amontillado

A wood-matured fino sherry. A dry fortified wine, usually with a rather 'nutty' type of taste. *Pron. ay-mon-tee-ard-oh.*

Ampelography

The science of classifying different grape varieties. There are thousands, and sometimes the differences are apparently insignificant. One of the ways of telling the differences, when everything looks the same (like chicken sexing, I guess), are the subtle differences in the shapes of grapevine leaves.

Aperitif

French term for an appetiser drink; here, means a pre-dinner (or pre-lunch) glass of wine, sometimes a sherry or perhaps a sparkling wine.

Appellation

A system for guaranteeing the origin (and sometimes the quality) of a wine. From the French Government controlled 'Appellation d'origine'.

Appellation Controleé is the way the French choose to control and promote their area wines from, say, the districts of Burgundy, Champagne or Chablis.

Similar systems are now being used in parts of Australia, and the promise is to provide the consumer with a "warranty". So far it doesn't mean much here, and some Europeans are still grossly overcharging for these wines.

Aroma
The smell of a wine, usually meaning pleasing smells, rather than OFF ODOURS. Young wines often have more obvious odours, normally associated with grape varieties, and wood often comes through the nostrils with reds.

Astringent
Tannins produce astringent tastes in wine. You can detect astringency by the involuntary 'puckering' of your mouth, as the tannins hit your taste buds. Tannins come from grape skins, seeds and wood.

Auslese
A German term meaning the selection of riper-than-normal grapes for wine-making. Its use on Australian labels usually designates a fruity white with rather more sweetness than normal.

Austere
Means different things to different palates, though generally meant to indicate a wine that has recognisably strong flavours with nothing too dominant.

Balance
The assessment that a wine has flavour components in harmony, no one being too dominant.

Baumé
A measurement of the sugar content of grapes. The Baumeé figure roughly translates to the alcohol content in the finished wine (as percentage of alcohol by volume). For example, grapes at 10 Baumé will produce a wine with about 10 per cent alcohol. *Pron. bow-may.*

Beerenauslese
Another German term one level up the sweetness (sugar) scale from AUSLESE. Very ripe grapes help make such sweet wines. *Pron. beer-en-ows-lazer.*

Big
Powerful in flavours or bouquet.

Bilgy
Term evocatively describing unpleasant wine characteristics emanating from slime bacteria caused by waterlogged oak barrels.

Bitterness
Unpleasant characteristic in wine, usually detected on the aftertaste. Not to be confused with acidity.

Blanc
White, as in sauvignon blanc, the white grape variety. 'Blanc noir' is creeping in as a term to describe white wine made from red grapes. *Pron. blonk.*

Bland
Wine-tasting term denoting a wine without character, though not necessarily having any wine faults.

Blend
Mixing of two or more grape varieties to increase quality or maintain consistency. Can also be a 'blend of areas' of origin.

Body
Full-bodied means with fullness of flavour in the mouth; conversely 'light-bodied' means the opposite. Some makers (for example, Huntington Estate at Mudgee) label their reds F.B. or M.B., for full bodied or medium bodied, a useful guide for potential drinkers.

Botrytis cinerea
A parasitic fungus which, if present in a vineyard, can attack ripe grape berries, removing water and concentrating sugar and flavour constituents. Helps make some of the world's greatest sweet white wines (for example, the wines of Sauternes in France). See NOBLE ROT.

Bottle
Usually means a 750-millilitre glass container to hold wine. Various shapes are made by glass makers such as A.C.I., for example champagne, riesling, hock, claret and burgundy bottles. Half bottles (375 ml) of quality wine are becoming popular.

Bottle age
Time spent in the bottle after making and possible wood ageing. "Will improve with bottle age" means the maker suggests the wine should taste better with several years' proper cellaring.

Bottle variation
Difference in the character of a wine from bottle to bottle in the same wine. These otherwise unexpected variances can be due to storage conditions, cork differences, unclean bottles or other factors beyond the wine-maker's control.

Bouquet
The smell of a finished wine. May be affected by time spent in the bottle. *Pron. Bo-kay.*

Brandy
The spirit of wine (although of course there are also fruit brandies). By Australian law anything labelled simply 'brandy' must be made only from fresh grapes, and after distillation must be stored in wood for a minimum of two years. (There are whispers of change to this law).

Breathing
Allowing a wine to come in contact with air before serving. There is little agreement among wine enthusiasts about whether this practice enhances wine enjoyment or not. It may occasionally let an OFF ODOUR (for example sulphur) dissipate, but I have considerable doubt about whether it 'improves' most wines.

Bright
Perfectly clear wine with no suspended particles. Bright colour is an important pointer to wine quality.

Brut
Dry, usually as the term is applied to sparkling wines. Commercial brut styles usually have a small amount of liqueuring added to sweeten the wine somewhat. *Pron. Broot.*

Buff
In this context, a wine enthusiast or devotee. Its use is usually pejorative, as in "Cripes, that stuck-up wine buff!"

Burgundy
Famous wine-producing area in eastern France.

In Australia the term has been rendered almost meaningless as a guide to taste, but can mean a softer style of red wine.

Cabernet franc
Relative of cabernet sauvignon and a red grape used in the blends of some Bordeaux wines. When well done, adds pleasing complexity and fruit flavours.

Cabernet sauvignon
Red (or black) grape variety, widely considered to produce the finest red wines in the world. The classic centrepiece of the Clarets of Bordeaux, France. Widely grown in most areas of Australia and still gaining in popularity. *Pron. Cab-er-nay so-vin-yon.*

Capsule
In wine, usually a reference to the cylinder of plastic or lead that is used to wrap the neck of wine bottles, hence 'neck capsule'.

Carbon dioxide
CO_2. This gas is a by-product of fermentation, and with still wines is dissipated into the atmosphere. However when a secondary fermentation is induced inside a champagne bottle the CO_2 dissolves in the wine, producing the famous bubbles upon opening. Not desirable in still wine.

Carbonated
Sparkling wines made cheaply by the direct injection of CO_2 into the wine. They are both cheaper and coarser on the palate than bottle-fermented wines.

Cassis
A liqueur made from blackcurrants. Sometimes used to add a dash to champagne.

Chablis
Famous wine area of France, producing some excellent dry white wines, mainly using the chardonnay grape variety. Now widely used in Australia to designate a dry white wine of unspecified grape origin. *Pron. Chab-lee.*

Champagne
Another French wine region, this time giving its name to bottle-fermented sparkling wine. In Australia wines so labelled must be fermented in a bottle, not in a tank, and not carbonated. Standard champagne bottles hold 750 ml; magnums 1.3 to 1.5 litres, Jeroboams 3.2 litres, Rheoboams 4.8 litres, and so on. The biggest is the Nebuchadnezzar of 20 litres or 26 bottles. By agreement with the Europoeans, generic terms like Champagne for Australian sparkling wines will be phased out by the turn of the century.

Chaptalisation
Adding sugar (cane, beet or any other) to fermenting grape juice in order to increase alcohol levels in the finished wine. Illegal in Australia (and usually unnecessary), but widely practised in Europe, where sunlight levels can be low, thereby yielding low natural grape sugar levels.

Chardonnay
White grape variety producing some of the world's best white wines, notably in Burgundy and Chablis, also Champagne, in France. Now

widely and increasingly grown in other countries, notably the U.S., Australia, New Zealand and South Africa. Accepts wood maturation gracefully. *Pron. Shar-donn-ay.*

Charmat
Monsieur Eugene Charmat was a Frenchman who developed a method of making sparkling wines in pressure tanks, thereby reducing the cost. Many Charmat-method sparkling wines are produced in Australia, and they are very economical and usually good drinking.

Chenin blanc
White grape variety which makes the wines of the Loire area of France. Here in Australia it tends to make rather neutral flavoured white wines though Houghton in Western Australia make some good ones. Sometimes wood matured.

Cigar box
An aroma akin to the smell it describes though, in a red wine, not as unpleasant as it sounds. Combination of the fruit, wood and other constituents of a red wine, notably some of the great Clarets.

Claret
Originally the English word for the wines of Bordeaux (and probably derived from 'Clairette' or light red). Like Burgundy, it has become somewhat meaningless when applied generically to Australian wines, other than to signify a red wine, perhaps a more full-bodied example.

Climate
The climate (meaning temperature, humidity, rainfall, winds and so on) has a great deal to do with the quality of fruit from grapevines and therefore with the quality of the finished wine. 'Cool climate' is now the vogue word for growing areas of Australia, and elsewhere, which seek to produce higher quality fruit, and this is often associated with altitude. 'Micro-climate' refers to the variations in climate within one general vineyard area — for example between the top and bottom of a sloping vineyard.

Cloudy
A cloudy wine has suspended particles in it, obscuring the colour. An indicator of problems in a wine.

Cognac
Brandy area of western France, the products of which are generally acknowledged to be the best in the world. V.S.O.P. is one style, meaning 'very special old pale'. It is a distilled wine, aged in wood for lengthy periods. *Pron. Conn-yac.*

Colour
In wine an extremely important indicator of quality and condition. Darker colours usually indicate older wines (but may also indicate a more intense wine).

Cooler
Mixture of wine and fruit juice. Fashion fad imported from the U.S. several years ago, though there's really nothing new about it — think of Hock, Lime and Lemon — or Champagne and Orange juice! With 3 to 6 per cent alcohol content and bubbles and sugar to disguise this, it can be a potent drink for the young.

Coonawarra
Australian wine region in the south-east of South Australia, not far from the Victorian border. Cool, produces some of the best red wines in Australia, especially cabernet sauvignon. Top makers include Wynns/Penfolds, Lindeman/Rouge Homme, Hollick, Brand, Mildara, Hardys and Redman.

Cork
The bark of a tree (*Quercus suber*), mainly grown around the Mediterranean end of Europe. Becoming scarcer and therefore more expensive, leading many wine-makers to use 'agglomerated' cork — that is instead of one whole piece of cork to keep the wine away from the outside air, little bits of cork which are glued together to make a cylindrical stopper. Corks can fail, leading to wine which is ...

Corked
A wine whose quality is adversely affected by contamination. Easy to pick–the wine smells earthy. Unusual, but it can happen.

Corkscrew
Device to removed the cork from the bottle's neck. Good ones are a treasure, bad ones frustrating and annoying. The hip pocket 'Waiter's Friend' is good if well designed and soundly made; worth spending a bit more to get a good one.

Crush
The free grape juice from the grape berries. Sometimes used to denote the size of a winery, for example "They have a crush of 10,000 tonnes". The crusher is the area of a winery where the ripe, picked grapes are dumped for the initial extraction of the juice.

Crust
A deposit sometimes found in red wines and ports, particularly vintage ports. Comes from grape solids and, while it may not look terribly inviting, it is harmless and can be removed by straining or decanting. Smaller wineries tend to produce wines with a crust because they may not have the technology to entirely remove these solids before bottling.

Crystals
Tiny tartrates which may sometimes be seen in the bottle or on the bottom of the cork. Again, sometimes found in the wines of smaller makers who don't have the wherewithal to remove them. Harmless.

Cuveé
Most generally a blend. Often used in relation to champagne, as in "This cuvee is an outstanding one." *Pron. Coov-ay.*

Decant
Transfer of wine from the bottle into another container, usually a glass decanter. According to your viewpoint, it achieves one of three purposes: aerates the wine and possibly dissipates any unwanted odours; allows you to leave any crust in the bottle; and looks more attractive than putting a bottle on the table (which few people worry about today, anyway!). Any clean strainer (or a specially designed wine strainer) will do the trick if decanting wine or port.

Demijohn
No, not a partially complete outdoor toilet! A narrow-necked jug, usually wrapped in wickerwork, which holds liquor, often sherry. Used to be quite widely used in Spain and Portugal.

Demi sec
French term meaning semi-dry. In Australia usually means 'half sweet'. Often applied to cheaper sparkling wines.

Dessert wine
Just what it sounds like — wine designed for consumption with sweeter foods. Usually a sweeter, richer style of wine, such as sauternes, port, muscat, tokay.

Distillation
Process by which most spirits (in the case of wine, brandy) are made. Heating up an alcoholic beverage vapourises the alcohol at a lower temperature than water, so the alcohol can be captured and concentrated. There are various types of 'stills' to do this, including pot stills and continuous stills.

Dosage
Also known as liqueur d'expedition, this is a small amount of sugar (usually cane sugar) added to sparkling wines before it is sealed and sold, to give them an extra touch of sweetness. *Pron: Dose-aarj.*

Drunk
1. Person adversely affected by consumption of too much alcohol.
2. Condition of being under the influence of excessive alcohol consumption: a good reason for drinking wine, in moderation and at meal times.

Dry
Absence of res6idual sugar in a wine.

Earthy
Tasting term meaning that the wine has the flavour or odour of the soil. Hunter wines occasionally have this quality, as do some others. It is not necessarily unpleasant.

Estery
Class of organic compounds formed by the reaction of acid with alcohol. This happens in ageing bottles of wine, such as vintage ports and old, dry wines. 'Estery' means strong scents coming from esters derived from bottle maturation.

Ethyl alcohol
See ALCOHOL.

Fermentation
The process of converting sugars (in this case, grape sugars) into alcohol by yeasts.

Filtering
Modern wine-making calls for a good deal of filtering as today's drinkers expect clean, bright wines. Various types of filters (such as

Micropore) and filtering compounds (such as diatomaceous earth) are used to remove solids from wines.

Fining
Way of clarifying wine before it is bottled, for example by the use of egg whites; different from filtering.

Finish
End taste of a wine after it has been swallowed or spat out. High tannin contents might produce a 'firm finish', or lack of flavour might yield a 'poor finish'.

Fino
A very dry style of sherry. See also FLOR.

Firm
Term referring to the taste experience at the back of the palate, caused by TANNINS.

Flabby
Similar to 'fat', meaning the wine has unpleasantly voluptuous flavours on the back palate. High in glycerine in character, soft and broad flavoured.

Flagon
Glass container usually holding two litres, referred to in the U.S. as a 'jug' wine. The name probably derives from a contraction of the words 'half gallon', as this was the original size. Connotes cheaper wines, though some good, sound, Australian reds can still be found in these containers.

Flat
Uninteresting, little flavour. In sparkling wines, of course, little or no bubble left in the wine.

Flavour
The taste of wine.

Flinty
Term usually applied to dry whites, especially of the CHABLIS type. Traces of gun flint on the palate — steely.

Flor
A yeast which grows on the surface of a wine, especially sherry, giving it a 'nutty' character. Usually applied to flor fino sherries.

Flowery
An attractive scent reminiscent of flowers. 'Floral" and 'fragrant' are similar words of approval often applied to pleasing young white wines, especially rieslings.

Fortify
To add grape spirit to a wine. Fortification increases alcohol content and helps preserve the wine. Fortified wines include sherries, ports, muscats, tokays and vermouths.

Foxy
If you've ever smelt a fox or fox skin, you'll understand! In wines, often applied to the native North American vines from the family *Vitis labrusca*, which have it obviously, noticeably on the BOUQUET.

Free run
The juice released from the grape berries when first crushed at the winery — before being pressed further. Usually the highest quality juice because it contains fewer or no extractives from

the skins, stalks or seeds.

Fumé blanc
Dry white wine, usually with wood character. Intended to describe wines from the sauvignon blanc grape variety, though the words on a label are no guarantee that this is the case. *Pron. fume-ay-blonk.*

Gamay
Red grape grown in France, where it helps produce Beaujolais wines. Probably related to pinot noir, it also produces lighter style reds, though of lesser distinction.

Gewurztraminer
See TRAMINER.

Grange
Adelaide suburb and vineyard which gave its name to the famous Penfold's Hermitage red wine which bears this name. The great vintages were 1955, '62 and '65, closely followed by '66, '71, '76 and '86.

Green
A wine not ready for drinking, or made from underripe fruit. One which has malic acid content.

Grenache
Red grape variety widely grown throughout Australia for use in red and fortified wines, now unfashionable. Can still make some good ports and rose wines, occasionally good reds.

Grog
E. Vernon (1684-1757), who ordered the watering of rum. He always wore a grogram cloak, and so was called 'Old Grog'.

Hard
Term which, with 'harsh', refers to bitter and dry tastes associated with tannins on the finish of some wines.

Heat degree days (HDD)
The figure for heat degree days is derived from a viticultural formula which indicates the effect local climate has on the speed of ripening, and hence the quality of the resulting grapes. The lower the HDD number is, usually, the higher the quality of the resulting wines, as cool conditions prolong ripening.

Herbaceous
A taste which can be related to herb flavours. Some reds, notably cabernet sauvignon, and some whites (sauvignon blanc for example) are sometimes described as being herbaceous.

Hermitage
Synonym used frequently for the red grape variety shiraz.

Hock
English name for dry white wine, now little used. Comes from the German town of Hochheim, where Rhine wines are made (using mainly riesling grapes).

Hogshead
Wood barrel for storing and usually imparting oak flavours to wine. Contains about 300 litres.

Honeyed
Relates the flavour of honey to some wines.

Aged Hunter semillons are often said to taste 'honeyed'.

Hot
Refers to slightly burning sensation in the mouth produced by some wines. Usually indicates a high level of alcohol, as with ports.

H_2S
Hydrogen sulphide. Rotten egg smell in wine, caused by wine-making or storage fault, usually very obvious even in minute concentrations. Very bad wine fault.

Jammy
Term usually applied to red wines. Heavily pressed fruit from hot- climate vineyards sometimes produces broad, 'jam-like' flavours in these wines. Less common now that temperature control equipment and night grape-picking can help avoid these often coarse, sometimes unpleasant, tastes.

Jeroboam
See CHAMPAGNE.

Jimmy Watson
Melbourne wine merchant and wine-bar owner, now dead, who donated a Trophy for the best one-year-old red wine at the Melbourne Wine Show. Much sought-after by wine-makers, though there is some dispute about whether such a young wine (the bulk of which is usually still in oak barrels when judged) can be reasonably assessed commercially.

Kerosene
Description sometimes applied to aged Australian rieslings. Presumably caused by the similarities of some compound in these wines to petroleum compounds, which is not as silly as it sounds, as both substances emanate from organic substances.

Lactic
An acid character evident on the palate of some wines, resulting from malolactic fermentation.

Late picked
Grapes picked when riper than average, hence with higher levels of sugar. Can be used in the production of spatlese and auslese wines.

L.B.V.
Late Bottled Vintage — a Portugese port term meaning a young port wine made in the vintage, given some wood treatment and designed for comparatively (i.e, against vintage port) early drinking. Some are made in Australia, though it is an unusual type of wine here.

Lees
Deposits in cask or bottle, notably the residue in champagne bottles from dead yeastcells after the secondary fermentation is complete. 'Lying on lees' is the process which helps lend bottled fermented champagne its yeasty flavour.

Legs
Columns of wine, especially fortified wine, which trickle down the side of a glass. Supposed to indicate high alcohol content in a wine.

Luscious
A full-flavoured, rich, ripe, fruity and sweet-

flavoured wine.

Maderise

Wine characteristic named after fortified old wines of Madeira. Supposed to indicate bottle-developed character resulting from the oxidation of the alcohol content to acetaldehyde, producing an OXIDISED, almond-like flavour in wine and fortified wine. Also gives a brown colour.

Magnum

Large bottle containing the equivalent of two ordinary bottles of wine, or 1.5 litres. Magnums should age more slowly than 750 ml bottles of the same wine, which is another way of saying they should last longer. Some wine-makers (not many, but Redman, Taylors and Leconfield among them) bottle reds in magnums.

Malbec

Red grape variety grown in areas of France. Slowly gaining approval in Australia as a blending partner with other reds, notably cabernet. Used in many good wines, such as Jacob's Creek Claret, to soften and make more enjoyable when young.

Malolactic fermentation

A technical problem for wine-makers which seldom affects drinkers these days. It is (if you really want to know!) the decomposition of malic acid by bacteria to give lactic acid and carbon dioxide — which means that if it happens in the bottle it can blow the cork out. Malic acid is a complex compound $(COOH.CH_2CH[OH].COOH)$. Its arrival is referred to as 'malo' by wine-makers, and they like to see it happen to their wines in the barrel rather than in the bottle.

Marc

Leftover solid material after the pressing of the grapes. The dry residue of grapeskins and seeds.

Marsanne

White grape variety, grown in the Rhone Valley of France but only in a few Australian areas, notably the Goulburn Valley of Victoria, where it makes dry white wines which, with age develop a honeyed character.

Mature

Usually applied to wines with some age. A mellow flavoured and coloured wine. Usually means an attractive older wine.

Medals

Awards from Australian wine shows for well-made wines. The Capital city wine shows are the most reliable indicators of quality. Gold medals are awarded to wines attaining 18.5 points or more out of 20; Silver medals 17.0 to 18.4; and Bronze medals 15.5 to 16.9. Generally any wine of recent vintage that has won any medal at a Capital city wine show should be worth drinking.

Meniscus

The upper part of a liquid column made convex or concave by capilliary action. In our context, the shallow part of a wine against the top edge of a glass, where you can more easily assess the colour of the wine.

Mercaptan

A chemical which can be formed in wine and which lends its host some very unpleasant characteristics. Derived from H_2S or rotten egg gas.

Merlot

Premium red grape variety, usually blended with other reds, such as cabernet sauvignon. Widely grown in France and used as a blend in areas such as Bordeaux. Can lend a pleasingly 'velvety' texture and agreeably fruity flavours to a red wine blend.

Methode champenoise

The authentic French method of making bottle-fermented Champagne. *Pron. Meth-od Champ-en-wahz.*

Mistelle

Grape juice (which is of course sweet as the sugar is still there), used as a sweetening agent. For example, in vermouth.

Mondeuse

Red grape variety not much used in Australia, but used in blends with others, for example, by Brown Brothers with cabernet and shiraz.

Moselle

Australian version of the wines of the River Mosel, in Germany, where riesling is used to make the local wines. Here, it means a light, fruity and pleasantly cheap white wine, though it will probably not have anything to do with the riesling grape variety.

Mousy

A description of a wine with an unpleasant taste and smell. Possibly one with some bacterial disease.

Mulled wine

Heated wine (usually red) with added herbs, spices, sugar — and Lord knows what else! Use the cheapest wine you can (if you have to do it at all), because it will only get worse. Normally only concocted by frustrated skiers when there is no snow around.

Muller Thurgau

White grape variety, a cross between riesling and sylvaner, developed in Switzerland, and tolerant of colder ripening climes. Not much grown in Australia because there is little climatic need to do so, and also because the resulting wines tend to be a little coarse in flavour. New Zealand grows this variety quite well.

Muscadelle

White grape variety linked with the muscat family. Makes some of the great Australian fortified wines. Also grown quite widely in France for inclusion in sweet whites.

Muscat

A name (or a prefix) given to a large family of grapes of colours ranging from very white to very black, and quite a few other colours in between. In general, however the Muscat families share several characteristics: they are good bearers and have rather broad and obvious flavours. Therefore they are ideal for cask and flagon wines, for which they provide much of the base material. From this widespread family of grapes comes, among others, Muscat of Alexandria (occasionally labelled 'Lexia' in Australia), Muscat Blanc a Petits Grains and Muscat de Frontignan.

Must

Grape juice (usually fresh), which includes the skins and the seeds, after the initial crushing process.

Neutral

Little flavour — nothing bad, but not much to commend it, either.

Noble rot

A fungal infection (BOTRYTIS CINEREA) which attacks ripe grape berries and helps make some of the world's greatest sweet wines.

Nose

The smell or bouquet of a wine. To 'nose' a wine is to smell it.

Nutty

Sherries can occasionally smell nutty, as with FLOR sherries.

Oak

Various types of wood are used to store wine in, and usually also to impart extra and more complex flavours to them. French, American and German oak barrels are widely used in Australia. They are getting quite expensive as oak trees get scarcer.

Oenology

The science of wine-making. A wine-maker who goes to wine school is taught by oenologists. *Pron. En-ol-o-gee.*

Off odours

Unpleasant or unexpectedly displeasing smells in a wine.

Oily

Pips and stalks in grapes can inject 'oily' flavours into a wine. Not good.

Olfactory

Relating to your sense of smell.

Oloroso

Sherry-style old and sweet to semi-sweet wine. Can be matured in wood and also be quite luscious.

Overripe

A wine made from grapes which were too ripe when picked. See also JAMMY.

Oxidation

Oxygen presence causes decomposition in wine, turning it eventually to vinegar. Try it. Leave an open bottle of wine in the cupboard for a few days — and it'll taste frightful! Higher temperatures speed the process.

Palomino

Rather neutral white grape variety, used in sherry-making.

Pedro

Pedro Ximinez (or PX) is another grape variety used in sherry- making and in some bland white wines.

Peppery
A not entirely unpleasant spicy characteristic sometimes found in young red wines (especially shiraz wines) and ports. Rather raw, biting and with a characteristic reminiscent of black pepper.

Perfumed
Similar to some perfume smells — usually a result of a fermentation by-product.

Petillant
French word meaning lightly carbonated (sparkling) wine.

pH
Wine-making term relating the measure of the acidity or alkalinity of a solution, in this case, a wine.

Phylloxera
Phylloxera vasatrix is a resilient vine louse, a parasitic plague of which swept through Europe's vineyards late last century and almost ruined them, then moved to Australia. The only known 'cure' is to replant the grapevines whose roots it attacks with vines planted on American rootstocks, which are resistant to the louse — maybe explaining its origins.

Pinot noir
The red grape of Burgundy and one of the varieties which also helps make Champagne in France. Generally produces lighter styles of red wines though they can, when well made, have intense and deep flavours. We're still playing around with it in Australia, but getting better by the year. *Pron. peen-oh-n'war.*

Port
A fortified red wine, the name coming from Oporto, on the River Douro in Portugal. An after-dinner drink (in Australia generally, at least) of quite high alcohol content (17-20 per cent). There is considerable confusion about port wines which can be simply summed up TAWNY PORTS are blended wines which have usually been kept in wood barrels by the maker for some years in order to mature them for drinking when sold. VINTAGE PORTS (which bear a year of origin on the bottle) are usually sold early by the makers and you, the consumer, are expected to do the cellaring until the wine is ready for drinking. Australia makes excellent examples of both styles, though the market is shrinking. See also RUBY PORT.

Pot still
Traditional method of BRANDY distillation.

Pressings
What you get when you use a bit of mechanical muscle to squeeze extra juice, more highly flavoured (and with more tannins), from the skins, seeds and pulp of the grapes.

Pricked
A wine which smells of ethyl acetate which can be said to be becoming VOLATILE.

Puncheon
Larger oak barrel, holding about 500 litres of wine.

Pungent
Strong and aromatic, maybe too much so.

Punt
Concave base of a bottle, usually a champagne bottle as it helps retain strength— though lots of other table wine bottles seem to be adopting this (expensive) pretension.

Px
Pedro ximinez, a white grape variety sometimes used in sherries.

Racking
Transferring wine from one cask (barrel) to another for a variety of reasons.

Rancio
Oxidised character evident in older sweet wines and some sherries. In this context, not necessarily a fault. A bit like the affectionate comment : "He's a terrific bastard!"

Residual sugar
The natural grape sugar left behind (usually by design) after the fermentation has finished. Characteristic of many modern white wines, usually pleasant though sometimes cloying if overdone — or done in the wrong type of wine.

Rhine riesling
Literally, the riesling grape derived from the Rhine areas of Germany. One of the world's classic grapes, and one which does a different, and magnificent job, in many of the better Australian white wines. A grossly under-estimated and misunderstood variety, which still and probably always will make some of the finest Australian white wines.

Rosé
Again, a much misunderstood wine style. *Should* be the classic summer red of Australia. Light, fresh and fruity wine made from red grapes, either sweet, medium or dry — but best as a dry, yet flavoursome, young wine. *Pron. rose-ay.*

Ruby Port
A lighter style of vintage port, without the tannins or the acid, which is nevertheless bottled early to be enjoyed for its rich fruit and complex spirit characters — while still relatively young. There are minor differences in the definition of this port style, depending on whether you want the Portugese rubies, which tend to spend more time in wood, or Australian, which are fresher.

Sauvignon blanc
White variety of grape from Bordeaux and the Loire areas of France, where it makes superb sweet *and* dry wines. Its grassy/steely and sometimes asparagus-like characters attract (like oysters, with which it is often well matched) either love or loathing. Do try a good one or two, though, as it is *different*. *Pron. So-vin-yon-blonk.* Sometimes blended with ...

Semillon
Another great French (especially Bordeaux) white grape variety, which makes quite different wines in Australia in different regions. Usually makes dry, sometimes wood-matured, full-bodied whites in Australia, notably in the Hunter Valley.

Sharp
Acid taste on the palate. Worth thinking about, not necessarily unpleasant.

Sherry
Delightful aperitif drink, originally from southern Spain (*Jerez*) and widely made in Australia, though slowly losing its marketplace popularity. A FORTIFIED wine which can be sweet, medium or dry. Also see FINO and AMONTILLADO etc.

Shiraz
Excellent and very versatile Australian red grape variety, also widely referred to (especially on wine labels) as HERMITAGE. Makes some excellent and often reasonably priced red wines from most areas, and is best noted for its parentage of Penfold's GRANGE Hermitage brand.

Soft
Wine-tasting term. No harsh sensation on the palate and after-palate.

Solera
Method of producing some fortified wines (sherries and some ports) by rotating wine through casks to blend very old with new wine to attain consistency.

Sour
Bitter, unpleasant.

Spatlese
Late-picked style of fruity and/or sweet white wine. *Pron. Sh-spayt-lay-za.*

Spicy
Some TRAMINER wines, among others, can have this character.

Spritzig
A small amount of CO_2 in a wine, such as a rose. Leaves a slight fizzing sensation on tongue. *Pron. SPRITZ-ZIG.*

Spumante
Italian sparkling wine. Here it usually means sweet, sparkling and cheap. *Pron. Spew-man-tay.*

Stalky
Tasting of grape stalks — rather like OILY.

Sulphur Dioxide
SO_2. Chemical used as an anti-oxidant in winemaking, also for sterilisation. The smell of sulphur can be present in a newly opened bottle of wine, but it should dissipate. With today's truth-in-labelling laws, referred to on food and wine labels as 'Preservative (220) added'.

Sultana
White, heavy-bearing and large-berried grape. One of the most grown in Australia, it has a dual purpose — that is, it can also be used for dried fruit and as a table grape. It makes rather coarse white wines, and a lot of it goes into cask and flagon brands.

Supple
Favourite word of wine writers, meaning they like it but can't find the right words to describe its pleasant taste.

Sweet
More than fruity — pertaining to sugar.

Sylvaner

White grape variety making so-so aromatic whites.

Syrah

Best red grape variety of the Rhone Valley of France. Simila,r if not the same, variety as SHIRAZ. Also spelt 'sirah', but it is not the same variety known as petite sirah in the United States (which is probably the variety properly labelled 'durif').

Tannin

A vital ingredient (and preservative) in wines, especially red wines. It comes from the stalks, skins and pips on grapes. The taste of tannins on the palate when the wine is young give that bitter, puckering taste on the palate. A complex and important constituent of wine.

Tart

Taste of acidity, of malic acid, in a noticeable way.

Tartaric acid

The main acid in wine. (COOH.[CH.OH]$_2$COOH).

Tawny

Blended PORT.

Tirage liqueur

Sugar solution which is added to a base wine to turn it into champagne. The secondary fermentation converts this into a small amount of extra alcohol and CO$_2$, which is dissolved in the wine.

Traminer

White grape variety, widely grown in various parts of the world, producing wines with abundant fruit flavours, though not necessarily sweet, and often with spicy overtones. "Gewurztraminer" is often used to designate this spiciness. *Pron. Tram-een-ah.*

Trebbiano

White grape variety from Italy (also known as ugni blanc). Added in some parts of Australia for fairly ordinary medium to dry whites, sometimes blended with others.

Ugni Blanc

Synonym for TREBBIANO white grape.

Ullage

The air space between the top of the wine in a bottle and the bottom of the cork. If excessive, the wine is "ullaged", and may not last as long as it should.

Varietal

Wine made from a particular grape variety (for example, Rhine riesling). Opposite to generic wines (for example, chablis). *Pron . Var-rye-et-al.*

Verdelho

White grape variety used on the island of Madeira. Mainly grown in Western Australia for dry whites, but also used there for excellent fortified wines; used in the Hunter Valley for some dry white wines.

Vermouth

Wine fortified and to which many flavour components are added, for example, herbs, flowers, roots. *Pron. Ver-muth.*

Vigneron

Grape-grower.

Vigorous

In wine, a lively taste or feel. In a grapevine, very fast growing, sometimes a bad thing.

Vin

Wine (French). As in *vin ordinaire* : ordinary wine. To vinify is to make grapes into wine. *Pron. Vann.*

Vinegar

Wine spoilt by the vinegar bacteria — deliberately or otherwise. Not pleasant to drink, either way, and a major wine-making fault, easily detected.

Viticulture

The agricultural skill of growing grapevines.

Vinosity

Wine-tasting term pertaining to alcoholic strength of a wine and the grape character of the wine.

Vintage

The period of picking the grapes each year, as in "the vintage". Also the year a wine was made ('vintaged').

Vintage Port

See PORT.

Vintner

Wine-maker.

Viscous

Thick appearance in wine; showing the presence of glycerol.

Vitis

Vine. *Vinis vinifera* — the grape-bearing vine responsible for most of the world's quality wines. *Vitis labrusca* North American native vine (see FOXY).

Volatile

A wine spoilt by the presence of ACETIC ACID is said to be volatile, or have volatile acidity (v.a.).

Wine

The fermented juice of grapes.

Wine Shows

The Royal Agricultural Societies in the various capital cities organise wine judging on a circuit which usually begins in Sydney (the judging is done before the Royal Easter Show) and runs Brisbane-Melbourne-Perth-Adelaide-Hobart-Canberra. The Canberra Show is open to entries which have won medals in the other shows. The experts seem to agree that the wine shows to watch (because standards are highest) are Sydney, Adelaide and Canberra.

Woody

Strong bouquet of wood (oak) in wine, not necessarily offensive, but possibly very obvious.

Youthful

Wine showing pleasantly young characteristics — fresh perhaps.

Yeast

Single-cell organisms responsible for conversion of grape sugar into ethyl alcohol in fermentation.

Zinfandel

Red grape variety widely grown in California. Little grown in Australia, though some is planted in Western Australia, especially in the Margaret River region. Does quite well in California, where it roughly equates in importance to SHIRAZ in Australia. Wines made from 'Zin' tend to be BIG and high in alcohol.